Hypertension
Community control of high blood pressure

Julian Tudor Hart MB BChir DCH FRCP FRCGP

Formerly Lecturer, St Mary's Hospital Medical School
Medical Research Council Epidemiology and Medical Care Unit,
St Bartholomew's Hospital Medical School
General practitioner, Glyncorrwg Health Centre,
West Glamorgan, 1961-87

Foreword by Peter Sleight, Field-Marshal Alexander Professor of
Cardiovascular Medicine, University of Oxford

THIRD EDITION

RADCLIFFE MEDICAL PRESS   OXFORD

British Library Cataloguing in Publication Data
A catalogue record for this book is available from the British Library

Typeset by Intype, London
Printed and bound in Great Britain
T.J. Press (Padstow) Ltd, Padstow, Cornwall.

Contents

To Mary, Robin, Rachel, Ben and all the people of Glyncorrwg

The inquisitor: They say it is their mathematical tables and not the spirit of denial and doubt. But it is not their tables. A horrid unrest has come into the world. It is the unrest in their own brains which these men impose on the motionless earth. They cry, 'the figures compel us!', but whence come these figures? They come from doubt, as everyone knows. These men doubt everything. Are we to establish human society on doubt, and no longer on belief?

Bertolt Brecht – *Leben des Galilei*

Foreword to the First Edition

By any definition – and there are many of doubtful validity – hypertension is a common malady. It is also much in the public eye. In fact it is widely publicized in the United States as 'the silent killer', a title which adds greatly to the discomfiture of the patient. Naturally, therefore, there are many books by doctors dealing with either the condition as a whole or aspects of it. This book by Dr Julian Tudor Hart is the only one I know written by a primary care physician or family doctor for his colleagues. Since this is essentially a malady for family doctors this is a timely work.

The reader would expect the author to deal with the intellectual and technical aspects, such as causes, measurement of blood pressure and treatment. These things he will also find in other books, although perhaps not so lucidly expressed or so well balanced as here. What is, however, unique about this book is the account of how to manage the condition by a practitioner who is responsible for the whole field of human disease. In other words, how a generalist (be he physician or family doctor) can organize himself, his staff and his patients so that medical care can be of the highest efficiency and greatest efficacy. In doing this, Dr Tudor Hart shows unusual insight into patient behaviour. It is, of course, on such doctor-patient relationships that effective management depends. For the essential cause of failure of treatment is that in the early stages the patient feels perfectly well, and resents the nuisance of a regime which often makes him feel unwell. Avoidance of unnecessary restrictions, the choice by the doctor of the least unpleasant pills and an understanding by the patient of what the issue is for him are essential components of successful compliance.

Some years ago I wrote an obituary of that great Wensleydale practitioner, William Pickles. I quoted this from his work:

> And as I watched the evening train creeping up the valley with its pauses at our three stations, a quaint thought came into my head and it was that there was hardly a man, woman or child in all those villages of whom I did not know the Christian name and with whom I was not on terms of intimate

friendship. My wife and I say that we know most of the dogs and, indeed, some of the cats.

I would like to quote this from Dr Tudor Hart's book:

For the past 18 years I have given day to day care to, and lived my own life among, a stable community of 1400 men and women of 20 years and over, for every one of whom I have known the mean of two or more casual pressures. From this I have learned that there is no feature of personality, physique, or other outward sign, that gives any clue to the pressures found on measurement. If psychosocial factors are important in determining blood pressure (and they probably are) they are too complex or remote in time from their consequences to be evident to observation alone. Such experience makes one impatient with simplistic hypotheses and single causes.

One of the most encouraging features of contemporary medicine in Britain is that the leaders of family doctors exhibit such wisdom and affection for their patients. It is a pleasure for an elderly physician like me to welcome younger men of such promise as Dr Julian Tudor Hart.

Sir George Pickering
1980

Foreword to the Third Edition

As you will have read, my old chief George Pickering was very generous in his Foreword to the first edition, for it has to be said that this book was then in its way a real rival to George Pickering's own book *High Blood Pressure*. Both were written by a single author, both used good English and both authors knew what they were talking about.

This new edition, like that first edition, is a very good read. As well as GWP's book it reminds me of Paul Wood's cardiology classic. All three are based, not on a re-hash of what went before, but on carefully gathered observations of well-organized practice, tempered by wide knowledge of the literature. Dr Tudor Hart's book is a truly scholarly work. In his Preface he says that this will be his final edition, since he has now retired. Personally, I doubt this. I hope that in a few years' time he will be able to give us a perspective on what is happening now in the newly re-organized National Health Service, since his book is full of sound common sense about how the health service should be organized, and I sense that, although he may approve of some of the new developments, he by no means approves of all. This is a very personal book, and well up-to-date with accounts of the recent big trials particularly in elderly patients – the SHEP, STOP and MRC elderly trials.

It is appropriate that a book on hypertension should be written by a GP, for they have a much more balanced and general view about how to treat this common and far from benign condition. We in hospital practice get a rather distorted view of what is happening to the totality of hypertensive patients. However, hospital practice cannot be all bad, for I found very little to quarrel with in this book. There are very good reviews on diagnosis, aetiology – particularly environmental influences – and on treatment. All the references to others' work are peppered with personal experience and numerical data from his remarkable 20 year studies on his own practice. George Pickering compares him to the Yorkshireman, William Pickles. In the same manner, Julian Tudor Hart's love and concern for his patients in Glyncorrwg, over the whole of his professional lifetime, is an inspiration to everyone in the National Health Service.

The book finishes with practical appendices which will be particularly helpful to the new generation of GPs, many of whom have the same ethos, and desire to run a well organized practice, as Dr Tudor Hart.

It would be a mistake to assume that because this is written by a GP it is a book for GPs. It is a book for all doctors and not just for those who are interested in hypertension. In these days of monster multi-contributor works, students, GPs, and hospital physicians should have this book on their shelves.

Peter Sleight
Field-Marshal Alexander, Professor of Cardiovascular Medicine
University of Oxford

Preface

I am grateful to Radcliffe Medical Press for undertaking a third edition, 13 years after the first. As I have now retired from responsibility for day to day patient care, it will be the last. It has again been completely rewritten, incorporating much more practical material from experience of caring for a defined population from 1961–87, with virtually complete ascertainment and follow-up from 1968–92.[1]

I hope it will be useful to a wide range of people concerned with primary care, including medical students and general practice trainees, as well as established practitioners, practice nurses running hypertension follow-up clinics, practice managers, consultants concerned with the interface between primary and secondary care, and Family Health Service Authority administration staff with responsibility for developing 'health promotion'. This may seem an impossibly wide audience, but because this book deals with real experience of patient care, I think most of it will be useful and accessible to them all. If we believe in team care, based not on blind obedience to either doctors or managers but on all members learning from one another, why not team books? This has required more comprehensive treatment, so that each chapter can be read on its own. A practice manager, for example, might want to read only the chapters on screening and records, and Appendix 1 (educational leaflet for patients). This means that some points have had to be repeated, although most require some reinforcement. This has made this edition much longer than the last, although I hope a much better work of reference.

Clinical management in primary care requires different skills, deployed in different circumstances from those in hospitals, particularly teaching hospitals. All family doctors have experience of work in hospitals, but few consultants have had responsibility in general practice. As Dr Gareth Beevers rightly observed in his review of the first edition, clinical medicine comprises one single and consistent body of knowledge. From this he wrongly concluded that there was no need for books by and for GPs, although he generously noted that any consultants who read mine 'would, secretly, learn something'. There is indeed only one mountain of knowledge, but the belief that everything can be seen and understood from the top of it is illusory; the view from above differs from the view from below, and the two approaches require different guides.

The first edition had a short section on high blood pressure in pregnancy, which was dropped from the second edition. There have been important developments in understanding and treatment of this disorder, key references to which are given below.[2-7] It still seemed sensible to exclude this topic, of which I have little experience.

Julian Tudor Hart
Gelli Deg
Penmaen
Swansea

References

1. Hart JT, Thomas C, Gibbons B *et al*. (1991) Twenty five years of audited screening in a socially deprived community. *Br Med J* **302**: 1509–13.

2. (1991) Practice imperfect [editorial]. *Lancet* **337**: 1195–6.

3. (1992) Bed rest and non-proteinuric hypertension in pregnancy [editorial]. *Lancet* **339**: 1023–4.

4. Chamberlain G. (1991) Raised blood pressure in pregnancy. *Br Med J* **302**: 145–8.

5. McParland P, Pearce JM, Chamberlain GVP (1990) Doppler ultrasound and aspirin in recognition and prevention of pregnancy-induced hypertension. *Lancet* **335**: 1552–4.

6. Tufnell DJ, Lilford RJ, Buchan PC *et al*. (1992) Randomised controlled trial of day care for hypertension in pregnancy. *Lancet* **339**: 224–7.

7. Uzan S, Beaufils M, Breart G, *et al*. (1991) Prevention of fetal growth retardation with low-dose aspirin: Findings of the EPREDA trial. *Lancet* **337**: 1427–31.

Size and Shape of the Task

1

The Rule of Halves ■ NHS 'reform' and the 1990 Contract ■ Anglo-American contrasts ■ Means and ends ■ Size and sign of the gross medical product ■ Constructive doubt ■ Blood pressure control as a model for continuing population care

Neither treatment nor understanding of the causes of high blood pressure have changed fundamentally since the first edition of this book in 1979. There have been incremental advances on most fronts, but nothing dramatic. What really has changed is appreciation of the size of the task, and the impossibility of dealing with it only through hospital based specialists. Because high blood pressure is normally an asymptomatic condition, some form of systematic population wide screening or case finding with follow-up is essential.

It is now generally accepted that management of uncomplicated high blood pressure implies continuing care of some sort (with or without medication) for between 10 and 30% of the adult population. The problem is greater in older and poorer populations, and less in the younger or more affluent. The sheer size of the problem precludes routine management in hospital clinics.

Continuity and a personal approach are now generally recognized as essential for good control and minimal drop-out, and these should be easier to provide at the centre of a community than at its periphery. We have come to accept a curiously inverted terminology in this respect, regarding district hospitals as more central than primary care, and tertiary super-specialist hospitals as more central still, and may ask: central to what and to whom? That depends on where we think life really goes on.

It is now also generally accepted that high blood pressure is rarely an isolated risk, and cannot be effectively managed as though it were. It is nonsensical to ignore or refer outside the primary care team the routine management of associated cardiovascular risks such as smoking or glucose intolerance, which also require generalist rather than specialist skills.

Finally, there is consensus agreement, at least in theory, that management of high blood pressure should begin, not with antihypertensive drugs, but with other measures to reduce either blood pressure itself, or its consequent risks.

I say these advances are 'generally accepted', but what does this actually mean?

Just as most people are content to celebrate on the sabbath a code of ethical behaviour they ignore for the rest of the week, advances in whole population care may be used more as a guide to right answers for examinations than as useful and necessary standard medical practice. When Whitfield and Bucks[1] asked GPs in the Bristol area, only 45% said they would always accept responsibility for management of moderately high blood pressure in the diastolic range 110–120 mmHg. Full acceptance of responsibility was not associated with age, so it was not just a matter of replacing tired old men with energetic young ones.

The Rule of Halves

Studies of what general practitioners (GP)s actually do, as opposed to what they say or know, have been even more damning. The Rule of Halves[2, 3] is alive and well, at least in the UK.

- Half the people with high blood pressure are not known.
- Half those known are not treated.
- Half those treated are not controlled.

As an order of magnitude, the Rule still held in the North East of Scotland in 1984–6 for men aged 40–59 years[4].

Figure 1.1 maps the consequences of hypertension, and of its still frequently neglected control, in England and Wales[5] and in Scotland. It shows a roughly threefold variation in the burden on both patients and health workers, which broadly parallels every other kind of social and economic disadvantage. Between 1961 and 1981, professional men in England and Wales enjoyed falls in mortality of 79% for hypertensive disease, and 60% for cerebrovascular disease. In contrast, the mean falls for semiskilled and unskilled men were 56% and 15% respectively[6] Ascertainment and management of high blood pressure evidently improved, but advance was, as usual, greatest where needs were least and care was most comfortable[7]. The Glasgow Western Infirmary's acute stroke unit admits about 300 unselected patients a year from a catchment population of 220 000. In 1992, of 351 patients with information on antecedent diagnosis and treatment, 132 had previously diagnosed hypertension but only 62 of these (47%) were receiving antihypertensive medication: of 58 aged under 70 years, only 27 (also 47%) were medicated[8].

Ascertainment and management have improved. The situation was worse when I reviewed it in 1987 for the second edition, and worse still in 1979 when I wrote the first. Throughout those years the average number of staff employed by UK GPs remained virtually unchanged, at 1.2 whole time equivalent staff per principal[9]. Teamwork, the key to effective care of populations, remained sabbath rhetoric, not everyday practice.

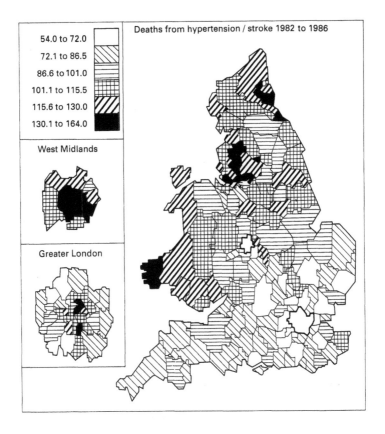

Figure 1.1: Deaths directly attributed to hypertension and/or stroke in England and Wales 1982–6. Standardized mortality ratios, England and Wales = 100[5]. (Reproduced with permission from the Controller of Her Majesty's Stationery Office.)

NHS 'Reform' and the 1990 Contract

The recent 'reform' of the UK National Health Service is typical of a worldwide abdication from co-operative public service and retreat to competitive marketed care, masked by accelerated advance toward rational health promotion[10]. The 1990 GP Contract, by linking practice income with 'health promotion' clinics and 3-yearly 'health checks', pushed many practices into activity. In West Glamorgan, before the 1990 Contract there were only about 10 'health promotion' clinics a week, other than antenatal or children's clinics; less than a year later there were 315, roughly one for each GP. In England, 94% of practices were running health promotion clinics by the end of the first year of the contract, and by 1991 the average was about two per practice. For all of these, high blood pressure was the favourite target.

The 1990 Contract paid for the first time for proactive care of populations, requiring a population approach, with more staff and more delegation of work. By 1991, three out of four practices had a practice manager, and 88% employed one or more practice nurses.

Before the 1990 Contract, a study of 14 training practices[11], of which nine employed a practice nurse and five did not, showed no difference between the with-nurse and without-nurse practices in the proportion of patients over 40 years with blood pressures recorded during the preceding 5 years (about 50% in both). This showed that measurements were not being delegated. Numerous studies have established that nurses, after suitable training, are usually able to measure blood pressures more accurately than doctors[12].

The many GPs I know who shared this passivity all had the same excuses; they hadn't enough time to read books or original papers, or to reorganize their practices to make full use of available skills. Many doubted the capacity of nurses to perform simple diagnostic tasks or to take clinical decisions, and most denied the value of standard protocols or algorithms for management of uncomplicated cases. Now the Contract appears not only to have solved all these problems of undertreatment at one stroke, but replaced them with new problems of reckless intervention, already familiar in the USA. Many 'health promotion' clinics now seem to be supervised almost wholly by practice nurses, with hardly a doctor in sight, although serious in-service education of these nurses for more or less autonomous decision making has (at the time of writing) scarcely begun in most areas.

Anglo-American Contrasts

The Rule of Halves, first described in the USA in the early 1970s, had disappeared there by the 1980s, at least in insured populations, for two reasons.

First, there was an energetic national campaign of professional and public education, led by outstanding, nationally known specialists and backed by campaigning public organizations. American cardiologists, for example Oglesby Paul, Paul Dudley White and Jerry Stamler, had a long and honourable tradition of public leadership. Their popular approach still seems inconceivable to most of their peers in the UK. Our gentlemanly tradition seems to have led to disbelief in the intelligence and educability of ordinary people.

Secondly, in the USA activism was accelerated by dollars. In their system of state subsidized private insurance, medical activity generated fees; in our salary and capitation based National Health Service, it generated taxes. Excessive displays of clinical energy were expensive to the exchequer, and difficult for family doctors who were unwilling either to employ a full team or to share responsibility with it. Restrained by capitation rather than spurred on by fees, UK GPs tended to maintain income through permanently excessive work-loads, so that consultations were too short to get beyond satisfaction of wants, towards an active search for needs.

Means and Ends

Encouraged by this evidence that incentives do motivate, policy planners have pushed NHS practice towards that in the USA. If process is paid for, process will be obtained. The trouble is, medical science ultimately concerns not process but outcome, not means but ends. Will more health promotion clinics or health checks mean better care, and therefore fewer heart failures, strokes, myocardial infarctions, and premature deaths?

We do have some evidence that process can safely be used in this way as a proxy for outcome. In all industrialized countries, even with the generally inadequate care provided since large scale treatment of high blood pressure became possible in the late 1950s, first malignant hypertension, then acute left ventricular failure, once fairly common events, became rarities. Both were usually consequences of years rather than months of neglect of severe but often asymptomatic high blood pressure. Neglect on that scale is now unusual. One way or another, most severe cases get recognized, by accident if not by design, because arterial pressures are measured more often, not only by GPs, but by insurance doctors, hospital staff, in antenatal clinics, in chemist's shops and even in airport waiting lounges. In a fumbling way, most of these worst cases get treatment somehow or other, before an artery blows or a kidney fails.

This suggests that the saturation approach popular in the USA may work; if enough blood pressures are measured, however indiscriminately, most potential patients will eventually be identified. From 90 mmHg of diastolic pressure upwards, American doctors have established a threshold for treatment. Not surprisingly, this not only reveals more high blood pressure, but generates a larger clientele.

At least one-third of American 60-year-olds with access to medical care are currently treated with antihypertensive drugs[13]. Using consensus American criteria (diastolic 90 mmHg) for mandatory medication of high blood pressure, between 15 and 30% of the adult population actually need antihypertensive drugs, continuously maintained over remaining lifetimes of 20–50 years. Using consensus UK criteria (diastolic 100 mmHg), this proportion falls to about 10%. Using the conservative interpretation of the original Veterans' Administration (VA) criteria[14] still advocated in this book (diastolic 105 mmHg in the absence of other major risks), it falls further to about 7%, rising again to about 10% if you add diabetics and others with specific indications for treatment at lower levels. In poorer or older inner city populations these proportions are all much higher.

All controlled trials have shown reductions in cardiovascular deaths for treated hypertension, even at moderate or borderline levels of pressure, but reductions in deaths from all causes have been shown only for more severe hypertension, in the diastolic range 110 mmHg upwards, and in the elderly. A simple conclusion follows; that treatment of mild to moderate hypertension in middle age, with the antihypertensive drugs available when these trials were done (no large trials have yet included calcium channel blockers or ACE inhibitors) was, directly or indirectly, causing as many deaths as it prevented.

Is iatrogenic damage on this scale really possible? The sad truth is that even major side effects from commonly prescribed medication are easily missed if they are neither imagined nor looked for. For example, although thiazide diuretics were in mass use all over the world from the late 1950s, the first suggestion that they might cause erectile failure in men was not published until 1975; even then it was not generally noticed or believed. The effect was not confirmed or measured until 1981, when 16% of men in the MRC mild hypertension trial[15] dropped out because of impotence in the first 12 weeks of treatment. Sexual failure has consequences contributing to chains of events which can easily end in death through accidents, violence, or the effects of depression on other otherwise non-fatal illness. This was a major, and occasionally lethal, side effect, following social rather than biological paths of causation, and therefore ignored by conventional clinical wisdom. We have been warned, but to little avail; as I write this, there has still been no published research into the effects of thiazide diuretics on sexual experience in women.

A further example comes from attempts to control blood cholesterol levels by medication rather than dietary change, a subject closely linked with blood pressure control because there are usually associated risks for coronary disease.

Subjects randomized to cholestyramine in the American Lipid Research Clinics Program trial[16] had 38% fewer fatal and non-fatal cardiovascular events than those randomized to placebo. This result was quickly made known and almost universally accepted as significant. Little attention was paid to a simultaneous 175% increase in non-cardiovascular deaths in the treated group, mainly from accidents, violence, and homicide. As in the MRC trial[17], there was no net reduction in deaths from all causes. These deaths appear to have been related to medication rather than cholesterol level itself[18]. In the absence of further evidence, we can account for these results only by accumulation of perhaps small impairments in concentration, reaction time, or emotional control, applied to large numbers over prolonged time.

Size and Sign of the Gross Medical Product

On present evidence, we should assume that similar results are likely for other attempts at indiscriminate mass chemical engineering, unless and until proved otherwise by large scale randomized trials, with suitable attention to effects on all causes of mortality, not just cardiovascular mortality. According to a *Lancet* editorial[19] which has not been challenged, medication side effects are undetectable by the usual premarketing trials if they occur in less than 1% of cases. Only very large trials in free living populations, using medication in the ways that are probable under ordinary conditions of practice, can even begin to answer these questions. As these and many other examples[20] show, even then we tend to see and hear not what is there, but what we, or more importantly, what shareholders in the pharmaceutical industry, want to see. In the absence of evidence, our default mode remains chemical intervention, not behavioural change.

Doctors and nurses in primary care should and do worry about reckless development and promotion of mass medication. Most people in the generally well fed and housed populations (at least by world standards) of developed economies reach old age before they die. There is therefore little scope in these areas now for large effects on mortality through advances in medical care. For mortality, but not for morbidity, the entire medical enterprise cannot have a large positive net product, although that is not to say that the small advances actually possible are not worthwhile.

From this it follows that if clinical processes are applied on a mass scale by numerous small units which cannot pool their experience, small risks multiplied by large populations, and multiplied further by years of sustained medication, may easily and imperceptibly transform marginal net gain to marginal net loss. In terms of mortality at least, the gross medical product may be not just small, but negative.

Constructive Doubt

People reading this book are actual or potential innovators. To change the still generally bad situation they are likely to find in all but the most affluent practice (and even there I am suspicious), they need all the motivation, optimism and enthusiasm they can honestly get, and this enthusiasm needs to be shared by their patients. Primary care for ordinary people is hard, time consuming, and physically and emotionally exhausing work, which cannot be sustained on romantic illusion.

With experience, clinical activism is sustainable only in one of two diametrically opposed ways. One is to seek, and eventually find, evidence of real benefit to patients' health. If no such evidence can be found, processes must be changed, even if this means recognizing previously valued skills as obsolete, and undertaking even more work to acquire new skills that are relevant. It is a hard road of permanent scholarship and experimental science through the cycle of audit, without the social resources usually considered essential for disciplined academic work.

The other way is to assume that clinical processes are safe proxies for health outcomes, and then ensure that they are performed as often and efficiently as the market will stand. So long as we always do what everyone else does, and never do anything that everyone else does not do[21], what can usually still pass for clinical conscience is satisfied, and rewards may be high.

In clinical medicine, economic motivation is worse than none at all, because means then become ends[10]. Tinkering with human machinery is difficult and dangerous enough in any circumstances; entangled with economic motives, we can neither be trusted nor trust ourselves.

Blood Pressure Control as a Model for Continuing Population Care

Previous editions of this book have encouraged practice teams to view control of high blood pressure in whole registered populations as a pilot model for continuing care of other chronic or recurrent problems. Experience has confirmed that this was useful.

Blood pressure control in the community, although not easy, is a much simpler task than (for example) control of nicotine or alcohol dependence, diabetes, schizophrenia, epilepsy, or airways obstruction. All effective primary care is essentially continuing rather than episodic, requiring thought not only about immediate symptoms and presented problems, but for anticipatory care. Not only the management of high blood pressure, but all effective primary care, depends on continuing personal relationships between patients and professionals, through which patients need help to move from roles as passive consumers to active producers of their own health.

References

1. Whitfield M and Bucks R (1988) General practitioners' responsibilities to their patients. *Br Med J* **297**: 398–400.

2. Wilber JA and Barrow JG (1972) Hypertension – a community problem. *Am J Med* **52**: 653–63.

3. Hart JT (1992) Rule of Halves: Implications of under-diagnosis and dropout for future workload and prescribing costs in primary care. *Br J Gen Pract* **42**: 116–19.

4. Smith WCS, Lee AJ, Crombie IK *et al.* (1990). Control of blood pressure in Scotland: The Rule of Halves. *Br Med J* **300**: 981–3.

5. Acheson D (1988) *On the state of the public health for the year 1987*. HMSO, London.

6. Mackenbach JP, Stronks K and Kunst AE (1989) The contribution of medical care to inequalities in health: Differences between socio-economic groups in decline of mortality from conditions amenable to medical intervention. *Soc Sci Med* **29**: 369–76.

7. Hart JT (1971) The inverse care law. *Lancet*, **i**: 405–12.

8. Lees KR, McInnes GT, Reid JL *et al.* (1992) Managing hypertension. *Br Med J* **304**: 713.

9. Hart JT (1985) Practice nurses: An underused resource. *Br Med J* **290**: 1162–3.

10. Hart JT (1992) Two paths for medical practice. *Lancet* **340**: 772–5.

11. Grout P and Williams M (1986) Factors influencing the routine recording of blood pressure. *Br Med J* **293**: 488.

12. Richardson JF and Robinson D (1971) Variations in the measurement of blood pressure between doctors and nurses. *J R Coll Gen Pract* **21**: 698–704.

13. Najarian JS, Chavers BM, McHugh LE *et al.* (1992) 20 years or more of follow-up of living kidney donors. *Lancet* **340**: 807–10.

14. Veterans' Administration Co-operative Group on Antihypertensive Agents (1970) Effects of treatment on morbidity in hypertension. II: Results in patients with diastolic pressures averaging 90 through 114 mmHg. *JAMA* **213**: 1143–52.

15. Medical Research Council Working Party on Mild to Moderate Hypertension (1981) Adverse reactions to bendrofluazide and propranolol for the treatment of mild hypertension. *Lancet*, **ii**: 539–43.

16. Lipid Research Clinics Program. (1984) The lipid research clinics coronary primary prevention trial results. I: Reduction in incidence of coronary heart disease. *JAMA* **251**: 351–64.

17. Medical Research Council Working Party (1985) MRC trial of treatment of mild hypertension: principal results. *Br Med J* **291**: 97–104.

18. Davey-Smith G, Shipley MJ, Marmot MG *et al.* (1990) Lowering cholesterol concentrations and mortality. *Br Med J* **301**: 552.

19. Measuring therapeutic risk [editorial]. (1989) *Lancet* **ii**: 139–40.

20. Medawar C (1992) *Power and dependence: social audit on the safety of medicines.* Social Audit, London.

21. Shaw GB (1907) The doctor's dilemma [Preface]. John Constable, London.

2

Nature, Mechanisms and Causes of Primary High Blood Pressure

The predictive power of a single measurement of arterial pressure for future cardiovascular risk in young men was first recognized around 1910, not by doctors but by actuaries seeking profitable forecasts for insurance[1]. Doctors, then as now, found it difficult to reconcile their traditionally absolute, qualitative disease labelling with quantified relative risks to health, but the insurance business had to act rationally.

Despite this remarkable predictive power, a signal in large populations so powerful that it penetrates all its surrounding noise of measurement error and variability, arterial pressure is not itself a fundamental biological value. Variations in pressure reflect varying circumstances within which perfusion pressure through the terminal capillary loop must be maintained. Capillary perfusion pressure is one of the great constants of Claude Bernard's *milieu intérieure* with an inflow pressure of 32 mmHg (a little more than the colloid osmotic pressure of plasma) and an outflow pressure of 15 mmHg (a little less than the colloid osmotic pressure of plasma). The variability of arterial pressure is the means of maintaining this internal constancy in wildly fluctuating external circumstances.

This pressure gradient must be maintained by arteriolar control throughout an extraordinarily variable capillary network. Total blood flow at rest is about 6 litres a minute, of which 13% goes to the brain, 24% to the gut, 19% to the kidneys, 4% to heart muscle, and 21% to voluntary muscle. During maximal exercise brain blood-flow remains constant, but total blood flow increases more than fourfold to 25 litres a minute. Flow through heart muscle increases fourfold, and through voluntary muscle 18-fold. Simultaneously, flow falls fourfold through the kidneys, and nearly fivefold through the gut. These changes are no different in people with high blood pressure, until they go into heart failure, when output begins to fall.

Causes of Primary High Blood Pressure

Traditionally, high blood pressure has been divided into secondary hypertension—caused by other named diseases and whose cause was, therefore, in that limited sense known—and essential hypertension, whose cause was not known. Secondary hypertension was rare but at least theoretically treatable through its known causes; essential hypertension was common but untreatable because we did not know its cause.

The advent of effective and tolerable antihypertensive drugs in the late 1950s, and later recognition that virtually nothing in medicine has a single cause, made this terminology obsolete, but we still use it. Primary hypertension was 'essential', not because patients couldn't do without it, but because it was 'of the essence'; to the wise child's question 'why is high blood pressure high?', ignorant but cocksure medicine replied, 'Because it is so'.

In the most general terms, biological control systems operate at three levels: rapid responses through the nervous system, delayed responses through hormonal systems, and long term adaptations through changes in the structure and behaviour of any or all systems, organs and tissues. Again, in the most general terms, each of these three has its own sequence of control systems, so that if one fails, a back-up system operates at a more primitive level.

By the nature of its techniques, experimental physiology first revealed the crudest and most primitive systems, which were least relevant to intact patients as they actually live in society, at an early stage of disorder. It is easier to study short term, rapidly reversible mechanisms in individuals than long term adaptations in groups, so we tend to know most about what is ultimately least important, and to know so much of this that we are more conscious of the vastness of published knowledge than of our far greater remaining ignorance.

Discussing causes of primary hypertension in 1954, Pickering concluded:

'. . . what has been called essential hypertension is a purely arbitrary segregation of those having arterial pressures in the higher ranges and having no disease to which these high pressures can be attributed. The factors concerned in the pathogenesis of so-called essential hypertension are thus those concerned in determining the arterial pressure in the population at large.'[2]

This revolutionary statement, and the debate with Sir Robert Platt to which it led[3], deserve serious thought. Pickering, who had spent his life looking for the cause of the disease 'hypertension', was by logic compelled to conclude that it was not a disease which some had and others had not, but a continuously distributed risk, affecting everyone to some measurable extent. All subsequent evidence has confirmed that there is no level of systolic or diastolic blood pressure, low or high, at which lower pressures are not associated with reduced risk, and higher pressures are not associated with increased risk of premature death.

Pickering had more courage than most of his successors, who continue to talk about hypertensive and normotensive populations, and real or fixed hypertension as opposed to spurious or labile hypertension. The Platt-Pickering conflict was fundamentally not about the nature of hypertension, but the nature of medical practice; medical trade versus medical science.

We are therefore considering not the cause of a disease, but all the factors that raise or lower blood pressure, not transiently but as a mean value over periods of days, weeks, months or years (all of which may be different, just as the causes of transient rises over seconds, minutes, or hours are different). It is not necessary to assume a single or even a dominant cause, although the latter is at least possible.

Group mean blood pressure rises with age in all post-Stone Age cultures. Even in childhood, age has a closer positive association with arterial pressure than weight or height, but this association is not causal. Inevitably and inextricably, age includes both time and experience; evidently it is experience, rather than lapsed time, which interacts with polygenic inheritance to determine the distribution of adult blood pressure.

A typical example of the distribution of blood pressures in the general population of a developed economy is shown in Figure 2.1[4]. Wherever total populations are studied in industrialized societies, similar distributions are found, unimodal and skewed to the right (more highs than lows). They also show a consistent rise in group mean pressure and increasing skewness with age (Figures 2.2, 2.3)[2]

The search for causes of high blood pressure should begin with the study of these differences throughout their range, throughout life, and in different environments and societies. Then we can ask two important questions.

■ Why are there differences between populations? Why, in some populations but not others, is there a positively skewed distribution within age groups and a rise with age?
■ Why are there differences within populations? Why, within national populations with the usual positively skewed and age related distribution, do mean pressures vary so much from one person to another?

We may then begin to identify external, and therefore avoidable, causes, as well as internal and possibly treatable mechanisms, both of which can be experimentally verified.

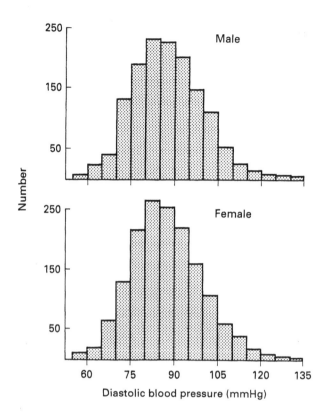

Figure 2.1: Distribution of diastolic blood pressure in 45 000 men and women aged 45–64 years in Renfrew, Scotland[4]. (Reproduced with permission from the authors.)

Crude Models

As every student knows:

arterial pressure = heart output × peripheral resistance

Both heart output and arteriolar constriction are under autonomic control, with connections to the cerebral cortex and therefore to mind and experience. The effects of alarm on heart rate and stroke volume, and its much smaller effects on arterial pressure, are well known, but these are short term effects which are not necessarily relevant to continuing high blood pressure.

It has been widely believed that primary high blood pressure starts with a sustained rise in heart output, possibly initiated by states of chronic alarm. The idea is reinforced by the term 'hypertension', which seems to imply that high blood pressure has something to do with 'tension' as that word is usually under-

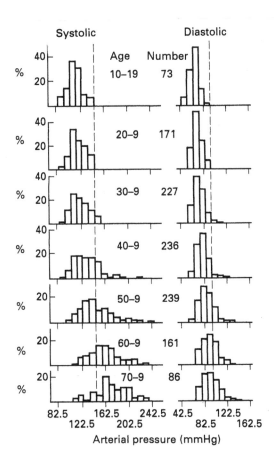

Figure 2.2: Distribution of female systolic and diastolic pressures in Pickering's pioneer study (1951), showing unimodal distribution and increasing skewness with age. Then current distinctions between normal and high blood pressures are indicated by vertical dashed lines[2]. (Reproduced with permission.[1])

stood: a state of stretched nerves and alertness for combat. In fact the term 'hypertension' was originally derived from stretched arteries. The word implies knowledge of causes where all we have are assumptions. It is therefore thoroughly misleading and should be replaced by the older, simpler and less pretentious term 'high blood pressure', as it will be throughout the rest of this book; the title is attributable to the publisher, not the author.

By the time high blood pressure is clinically recognizable, both this supposed high output and the chronic alarm that may have initiated it may no longer be present. In this second phase, the immediate mechanism of high blood pressure is raised peripheral resistance, sustained initially by fully reversible arteriolar constriction. Whatever else may be doubtful, this is not: high blood pressure is

15

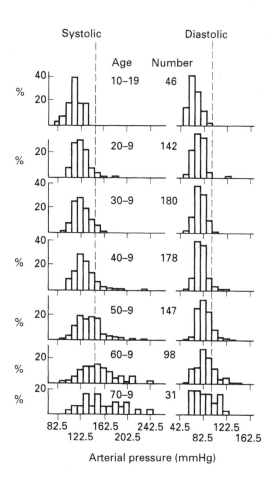

Figure 2.3: Distribution of male systolic and diastolic pressures in Pickering's pioneer study (1954), showing unimodal distribution and increasing skewness with age. Then current distinctions between normal and high blood pressures are indicated by vertical dashed lines[2]. (Reproduced with permission.[1])

maintained not by high output, but by raised arteriolar resistance. Later arterial constriction may in part be maintained by less easily reversible structural changes in the more proximal arterial tree, with deposition of fibrin, later organized to cholesterol plaque.

The growth and extent of these processes seem to depend on the level of arterial pressure already attained, so that high blood pressure becomes a cause of higher pressure, a self-accelerating cycle. In malignant hypertension this rise becomes exponential, a clinical emergency which the mundane nature of most primary high blood pressure should on no account obscure. The rate of rise also depends on levels of blood cholesterol and fibrinogen, both of which accelerate structural change in the arterial tree through deposition of atheromatous plaque.

Atheroma is not always a necessary part of this process, because severe hypertension is common in, for example, Shanghai Chinese with mean population cholesterol levels of 4.2 mmol/dl, in whom strokes account for about 25% of all deaths, but coronary disease is as yet much less common than in fully developed economies[5]. In a fully industrialized culture, atheroma usually modifies the course of hypertension, often acting together with raised pressure to cause heart failure with falling output. Arterial pressure consequently falls, so that the contribution of high blood pressure to this 'ischaemic heart failure' may not be recognized.

So there is evidence, by no means consistent, that primary hypertension may conform to the following crude sequential model:

- rising heart output
- → functionally raised peripheral resistance
- → structurally raised peripheral resistance
- → either falling output and heart failure and/or arterial thrombosis or haemorrhage, with organ failure.

The biggest problem with the first stage of this hypothesis is that attempts to observe transition from initial high output to subsequent raised peripheral resistance have failed, at least over a period of 5 years in young men[6].

Initiating Mechanisms

However, suspending justified doubts, let us accept that a sustained rise in blood pressure may be preceded by raised heart output; what might initiate this sequence?

Until recently there were two well defined schools of thought: stressites and saltites. Few deny that at least some kinds of stress, and some levels of dietary sodium, have some effect on hypertension at some point in its development, and are possible or probable external causes.

Stress and Enhanced Positive Autonomic Feedback

Until about 15 years ago, this was the most favoured theory of causation for what was then called essential hypertension. Depending mainly on differences in personality and life experience, it was suggested that some people were more liable than others to convert normal, transient hypertensive responses to current stress into sustained hypertensive responses to stress no longer present, perhaps through some intermediate process whereby structural changes in the kidney or arterioles made the process self-accelerating and irreversible. This was translated clinically into early labile and later fixed hypertension, still a popular concept in continental Europe.

Pain, anger, curiosity, fear, excitement and embarrassment all cause transient rises in blood pressure in all people. It is reasonable to suppose that sustained repetition of these feelings, or the circumstances that give rise to them, might cause sustained high blood pressure in some people. However, consistent and controlled evidence to support this idea, at least in this simplistic form, has been hard to find.

Such evidence could be of two kinds: prospective evidence of more pressor events, and/or evidence of greater pressor response to an equal burden of events, in early hypertensives than in normotensive controls. At the rather crude level at which these ideas were originally expressed (and which still dominate the imaginations of nearly all patients and most doctors), there is little hard evidence to support either of them; however, subtler forms of internalized stress remain likely, although difficult to test.

It is perhaps surprising that the aggressive Type A personality of Rosenman and Friedman, shown to be an important predictor for coronary heart disease in white collar but not blue collar workers in the USA (but not Britain), shows no association with blood pressure in population samples.[7, 8].

A beautifully designed and conducted study of self-reported stress in 1428 San Francisco bus drivers[9] found a highly significant inverse association between blood pressure and perceived psychosocial stress; the higher the stress, the lower the blood pressure. This negative association remained significant even after adjustment for 12 potentially confounding variables, although associations in the opposite and expected direction were confirmed for other gastrointestinal, respiratory and musculoskeletal problems. The authors' interpretation was that this suggested a link with objective stresses subjectively denied or contained, rather than with objective stress itself. Another, I think more attractive interpretation, is that stress has no sustained hypertensive effect in people whose personal philosophies accept, and within wide limits enjoy, the necessity of struggle as central to life in the real world.[10].

The fact that any relationship between psychosocial stress and blood pressure is not simple does not prove there is no such relationship. On the contrary, there is a wealth of generally neglected evidence that particular kinds of stress, measured in terms of both objective stressors and the ways these have meaning for stressees, are important for high blood pressure[11, 12], and much more so for coronary heart disease[13–15]. Perhaps we should concern ourselves less with stress and more with distress, which is a wider, less ambiguous, and more meaningful concept.

A third kind of evidence would be controlled trials of stress reduction in hypertensives, as a method of treatment. Such trials are extremely difficult to carry out, and although some results are persuasive, they have not proved easily replicable. These are discussed at length in Chapter 15.

The internal mechanism proposed for the stress hypothesis is autonomic response to signals from the brain cortex, leading to increased arteriolar tone. An apparently good animal model has been found in Wistar rats, which become hypertensive when overcrowded or tormented in various ways, unless they are protected before maturity by blockade of their autonomic beta-receptors. Beta-blockade was the natural human counterpart of this experiment, and at the birth of this group of antihypertensive drugs there were high hopes that they would prove uniquely successful by breaking this causal sequence closer to its origin. These hopes have not been fulfilled.

Although still attractive and commanding a large following, this theory in its original simplistic form has not withstood critical experiment with human subjects, nor does it provide consistent explanations for epidemiological findings.

Sodium Overload

This theory postulates that hypertension is caused by dietary sodium overload, leading to a raised output of renin, a raised renal threshold for diuresis, and thus to raised blood volume. This is a credible hypothesis because dietary sodium, at a daily intake of 130–400 mmol in industrialized societies, is vastly greater than the minimum physiological intake of 10 mmol/day. Neither high blood pressure nor a rise in blood pressure with age exist where sodium intakes are less than 30 mmol daily.

Stroke, a common consequence of severe hypertension, is exceptionally common in countries like Portugal and northern Japan, where sodium intakes commonly reach over 400 mmol/day. Sodium intakes in Britain are generally around 130–160 mmol/day, rather less than Australia and the USA with average daily intakes around 200 mmol, but penetration by the international fast food market is probably raising intake now.

In 1954 Dahl bred a strain of rats that became hypertensive when they were compelled to eat enormous quantities of salt, and another strain which did not become hypertensive no matter how much salt they ate. He thought there was a similar genetic difference in humans, and that the principal cause of primary hypertension was the sodium rich diet of all developed economies[16]. There is now yet another strain of rat which shows a fall in blood pressure when overfed with salt to the same improbable extent as Dahl's strain. Non-ratologists may be forgiven for sometimes wondering whether any hypothesis lacks some genetic strain of rats to endorse it; like humans, rats are omnivores outside the laboratory, with rich genetic reserves of variability permitting group survival on the most unlikely diets.

However, there is powerful circumstantial evidence in favour of sodium overload as an initiating cause. There are many other differences between generally underfed populations, and those who migrate from them to more developed economies; a notable example is the marked obesity of high salt migrant Polynesians in New Zealand, compared with thin, low salt Pacific islanders. However, only increased sodium load, and more doubtfully stress or social disorganization, can account for the very rapid shift that occurs with urbanization from remote cultures. For example, highlanders in Papua New Guinea, with a habitual daily intake of about 30 mmol sodium, showed increased blood pressures within 10 days of increasing their sodium load with an urban diet[17]. Kenyan Luo migrants from the country-side to Nairobi showed increased blood pressures within one month[18].

Dietary sodium overload is therefore a credible cause for the very existence of high blood pressure as a clinical problem; if we all ate like native Papuans, the problem might disappear. Food is an important part of all national cultures. No national cuisine in any developed economy would be recognizable at a daily sodium intake of 30 mmol or less. This is true not only of industrialized countries, but even more so of peasant cultures with traditional food storage methods based on salt; the sodium load in Chinese and Indian food is much higher than in the present western European cuisine. No very low sodium culture is associated with an average life span more than about half as long as our own. Although obviously most of these early deaths are not caused by low sodium intakes, we have yet to see longevity combined with very low sodium diet on a mass scale.

Dietary Sodium in Developed Economies

Dietary sodium overload is much less credible as an explanation of why, within the more usual range of daily sodium intake from 100–200 mmol, some people have much higher blood pressures than others, and much greater rises with age.

Day to day variability of sodium intake, in developed societies at least, is so great that within-subject variability is greater than between-subject variability for 24-hour urine collections[19]. Reliable characterization of habitual individual intake therefore requires continuous and complete collections of urine over at least 7 days. Few studies have met these exacting criteria[20] but those which do have generally confirmed two conclusions: first that, as we have seen, high blood pressure does not exist below a daily intake threshold of about 30 mmol sodium, and secondly, that very high levels of intake, at 300 mmol or more daily, are associated with a substantial upward shift of the entire distribution of blood pressure, as in Portugal and northern Japan.

Between these extremes, evidence of a close association between dietary sodium intake and arterial pressure remains convincing to believers but unconvincing to doubters[21]. Aiming to settle the question once and for all, the Intersalt Study applied a strictly standardized protocol, including 24-hour urine collections, to 200 men and women aged 20–59 years at each of 52 centres in 32 countries, with group mean daily sodium intakes ranging from 0.2 mmol (Yanomamo Indians) to 242 mmol (north China). The study concluded that a reduction of 100 mmol in daily sodium load should be associated with falls of 2.2 mmHg in mean systolic and 0.1 mmHg in mean diastolic pressure[22].

This reduction would be insignificant for individual clinical cases. Applied to whole populations through global shifts in national diet, Rose [23] argued convincingly that a reduction of 2–3 mmHg in diastolic pressure would have an effect on mortality equal to the entire current effort with antihypertensive drugs, but the fall demonstrated by Intersalt was almost wholly confined to systolic pressure, and did not in fact meet his target.

For the time being, the argument has been effectively ended by Law, Frost and Wald's meta-analysis of all important published between population studies[24]. They suggested that variability and consequent sampling error for both blood pressure and sodium output had led to underestimation of their association, so that only very large or aggregated trials could produce a meaningful result.

They concluded:

' . . . the association of blood pressure with sodium intake is substantially larger than is generally appreciated and increases with age and initial blood pressure . . . The variation among individuals in the response or susceptibility of blood pressure to sodium intake found in these results is similar in nature to Dahl's experiments on rats. Dahl showed that the variation in response was normally distributed and genetically determined, and human evidence also suggests this.'

The same authors conducted another meta-analysis of all within-population studies[25], reaching the same conclusion. However, it remains odd that although predicted relationships between blood pressure and sodium appear so slowly and have been so difficult to demonstrate, unexpected relationships with calcium[26], potassium[27] and dietary saturated fat[28] have all been easily demonstrated and appeared quickly. It is difficult for any non-statistician to argue with meta-analysis, but construction of so great a whole from such unimpressive parts leaves many of us with reasonable doubt. Their final meta-analysis was of trials of salt reduction; these are discussed in Chapter 15.

Intake of Potassium, Fat and Vegetarian Diet

There is now fairly consistent evidence that an increase in potassium intake of about 30%, or a fall in the Na:K ratio of food (measured as 24-hour urine output) has a lowering effect on blood pressure, and that arterial pressure in populations correlates negatively with potassium output, and positively with Na:K ratio[27]. All very low sodium intake populations are also high potassium intake populations, reflecting diets based on cereals, fruit and vegetables, which may at least partly explain the generally lower pressures consistently found in vegetarians[29].

Precise dietary studies are extremely difficult, with numerous confounding factors both in the food itself, and in associated features such as religiosity or attitudes to alcohol, and it is usually impossible to do them blindly with valid controls. There is convincing evidence that animal fats raise blood pressure[28], probably faster than added sodium[30], and that their absence accounts for part of the vegetarian effect.

These studies fit in well with the wealth of evidence that reduction of animal fat and increase in vegetable fibre reduce total blood cholesterol and the risk of coronary disease in populations, whatever their effect on blood pressure, that a high carbohydrate leguminous fibre diet improves all aspects of diabetic control[31], and that all these are effective components of any weight reducing diet. The case for a much higher vegetable and lower meat content for all diets is now overwhelming, and much better than the evidence against dietary sodium alone.

Coffee

Coffee does not raise blood pressure in hypertensives, and abstinence from coffee causes no fall[32].

Alcohol

Although older epidemiological studies failed to show consistent associations of alcohol intake with blood pressure, more recent and more rigorous studies have shown a positive linear association between systolic and diastolic blood pressure and alcohol consumption[33].

In October 1985, an audit of 71 male hypertensives, identified by screening and currently being followed up in Glyncorrwg, showed 17 (24%) with recognized alcohol problems either past or present, compared with 69 of 580 (12%) for the adult male population as a whole. None of the 61 hypertensive women had a known alcohol problem, compared with 16 out of 606 adult women (3%). A separate study of Glyncorrwg hypertensives diagnosed under age 40, however, showed exactly equal burdens of ever-recognized alcohol problems in male hypertensives and in age matched non-hypertensive controls, 50% in both groups[34]. Mean stated intakes were higher in hypertensives than controls, but not impressively so. Refractory hypertension often comes under control when heavy drinking is recognized and reduced, but this probably derives as much from improved medication compliance as from a direct effect of alcohol on blood pressure.

Puritan zeal should be tempered by consistent evidence that people who drink not more than four units of alcohol daily (1 unit = 1 glass of wine, half a pint of beer, or one measure of spirits) have lower coronary risks than either teetotallers or heavier drinkers, probably because alcohol raises HDL cholesterol[35], reduces fibrinogen concentration, and reduces platelet aggregation[36].

Inheritance

Genetic theory has been used to plug some of the leaks in both dominant theories of causation, stress and sodium overload. If predictions made from intensive laboratory studies of small numbers of patients cannot be confirmed in large population samples, one explanation might be that hypertensive mechanisms apply only to a subset of genetically susceptible people.

High blood pressure certainly runs in families. The better you know your population, the more striking this truth becomes. I have not been able to find anyone in Glyncorrwg with severe high blood pressure (mean diastolic pressure >120 mmHg) and whose parents' blood pressures were known, in whom one or both parents were not hypertensive (mean diastolic pressure >100m mHg). It is now universally accepted that high blood pressure cannot be inherited through a single gene, but polygenic inheritance is the best single predictor of individual pressures in industrialized populations, showing a regression coefficient of 0.34 for first degree relatives of both sexes at all levels of pressure[37, 38]. Although the multiple gene loci are as yet unknown, epidemiological methods of discovering these have been devised[39], and a new era of rapid advance in this field can be anticipated.

It is conventionally said that about two-thirds of the variability of blood pressure within populations is accounted for by inheritance (nature), and one-third by current or past environment (nurture). A more practical conclusion is that inheritance determines internal mechanisms through which external causes can then selectively operate, but only if they exist. If, for example, hypertensive response to dietary sodium overload were both a sole cause and an inherited trait in 25% of all people, prevalence of hypertension would be 0% in a Yanomamo Indian population none of whom eat more than 15 mmol of sodium a day, and 25% in a Portuguese population none of whom eat less than 200 mmol of sodium a day.

In our own research studies in Glyncorrwg, we could find no difference either in salt avidity or blood pressure response to changes in dietary sodium between offspring both of whose parents were in the top third of the blood pressure distribution, and offspring both of whose parents were in the bottom third of the distribution[40, 41].

Gender

Published studies of high blood pressure derived from unplanned general practice consultations and from hospital clinic series have always shown a large excess of women. In contrast, epidemiological studies of whole populations (including screened or case-found general practice populations) have always shown an excess of male hypertensives up to 45–50 years of age, after which a female excess gradually builds up with increasing age. This is so consistently true, that the male:female ratio at ages 20–45 for high blood pressure can be used as a rough measure of completeness of ascertainment in any general practice population. Women consult more often than men, particularly in younger age groups, and blood pressure measurement is routine in pregnancy and for management of oral contraception, so hypertensive women are less likely to escape detection.

There is a large (roughly 40%) male excess in young hypertensives, which we have found consistently in the fully screened population of Glyncorrwg. This has been confirmed by the Medical Research Council (MRC) national birth cohort study, which showed that high blood pressure (>140/90 mmHg) was almost twice as common in young men as in young women[42].

The increasing female excess in each age group over 50 years must in part reflect preferential survival of female hypertensives, who were in the past much less likely than men to die early from coronary disease, although their stroke risks were about equal. This may change now that young women smoke more than young men.

Differences in Cell Membrane Ion Transport

The search for differences in transport of sodium ions across cell membranes, between hypertensive and normotensive subjects, began in the 1950s. It then developed slowly through immense methodological difficulties, but is now at last beginning to provide some consistent and comprehensible answers. The search began in renal and vascular tissues, and was later extended to all tissues including red blood cells, which were easier to sample and handle in the laboratory.

As usual, what at first promised to be a simple answer has since proved contradictory and confusing. Even the methodology is still in dispute, and early attempts to apply still unstandardized laboratory techniques to small, poorly defined samples with various alleged genetic characteristics failed to give replicable results. Attention has moved beyond the behaviour of sodium ions to studies of potassium and calcium ions, with attempts to link these with dietary and genetic differences.

Stamler's group in Chicago took the (as far as I know) unique step of applying ion transport measurements to adequately defined population samples[43]. They found convincing evidence of small but significant differences in sodium transport across cell membranes between hypertensive and normotensive subjects drawn from the same population. They also found evidence of systematic differences between adolescent offspring of hypertensive and normotensive parents[44].

There now seems to be no doubt that sodium–lithium counter-transport activity in red cells is a marker of risk for primary hypertension, and that it is also linked with risk for non–insulin dependent diabetes[45]. This is probably the most important current growth area for population based research, much of which could with advantage be sited in stable general practice, where several generations of subjects may be readily available.

Association of Blood Pressure with Central Obesity through Insulin Resistance

Several cohort studies have confirmed that obesity in childhood and youth is a predictor for future hypertension[42]. All adult studies consistently confirm that blood pressure is positively associated with obesity. These associations are real, not effects of the false high readings produced by short sphygmomanometer cuffs on fat arms.

There is therefore evidence of a fundamental link between obesity, high blood pressure, and non-insulin dependent diabetes. Reaven[46] suggested this was insulin resistance, raising blood pressure through effects on sodium and potassium ion transport across cell membranes[47]. Insulin resistance may also be independently promoted by cigarette smoking[48].

This now fashionable idea was challenged by Jarrett[49], who pointed out that evidence associating hyperinsulinaeimia with high blood pressure was inconsistent. However, the clinical overlap between non-insulin dependent diabetes, obesity and hypertension is obvious to any experienced clinician; we noticed in the early 1970s that more than half the diabetics in Glyncorrwg were hypertensive, even on a diastolic threshold criterion of 100 mmHg. Whether the underlying mechanism for this is hyperinsulinaemia and insulin resistance, or some other biochemical pathway, seems to me less important than recognition that we are probably dealing here with a clinical reality which although it as yet has no name, contains at least as much truth as the manifest falsehood of essential hypertension or maturity onset diabetes, apparently simple categories which are in fact heterogeneous both in their genetics, and in the environmental factors leading to their expression. When we name diseases, we are not recognizing independent species, but simply taking the first step in plans of action to change or contain potential human tragedy. The only justification for the names and categories is that they are useful. It seems increasingly likely that we need some way to describe a package of disorders, including youthful obesity, raised blood pressure, and glucose intolerance, which should be understood and addressed as a whole.

Evidence that weight reduction reduces blood pressure is not entirely consistent[50], but on balance it seems to be effective[51], although difficult to achieve and maintain. The effect is probably greater in younger patients. There is encouraging evidence that episodic weight loss may have a lasting effect on blood pressure, even if it is not maintained[52], perhaps through reduction in insulin resistance.

This suggests the important possibility that weight reduction in young people, perhaps in their early 20s, might prevent much high blood pressure and diabetes in middle age. The question could be answered by a multicentre trial in general practice, which would need a follow-up of at least 10 years; it seems an ideal subject for the MRC General Practice Research framework.

Exercise

Blood pressure rises rapidly during exercise, but there is fairly consistent evidence that people who take regular exercise tend to have lower pressures at rest than those who do not. In a careful study using ambulant intra-arterial recordings, pressure in mild hypertensives fell by a mean 9.7/6.8 mmHg in resting blood pressure after a 6-month fitness training programme, and rose after detraining[53]. Sustained strenuous exercise effects on blood pressure probably resemble similar beneficial effects on lipid profiles, fibrinogen levels and glucose tolerance, and may be exerted by raised energy throughput on insulin resistance and central obesity.

Skin Colour

Data from the USA have consistently shown higher blood pressure levels for blacks than whites, and much higher levels of mortality from stroke and heart failure. Differences between blacks and whites in plasma renin, response to diuretics and beta-blockers, and in cell membrane ion transport, have usually been interpreted as additional evidence in favour of racial differences in susceptibility to hypertension. Since, in evolutionary terms, a black skin implies remote origins in hot, dry, and often salt-deficient environments, some of these differences are biologically plausible[54].

However, again there are difficulties. Studies of black, white, and Asian populations in England[55], and comparison of native Jamaicans with whites in South Wales[56] showed no significant differences in population mean blood pressure. Although Asian immigrants to the UK have much higher coronary mortality, this is probably caused by huge differences in glucose tolerance and consequently raised plasma cholesterol, rather than small differences in blood pressure[57]. American studies which have standardized for social class have reduced or abolished 'racial' differences[58].

Comparing black with white north Americans, there is little difference when standardized for family income, and it is interesting to note that the divergence between poorer blacks and richer whites appears strongly in the third and fourth decades of life, more for systolic than for diastolic pressure, and then levels off, suggesting that what is in fact a social class rather than a racial difference becomes clearly established in youth and early middle age[59]. The reverse seems to be true in Nigeria, where excellent studies have shown a positive relationship between levels of education and blood pressure, despite a surprising absence of urban-rural gradients[60].

Social Class

Higher blood pressures have been consistently associated with lower social class in all studies since the 1960s[61-63], but in UK studies these differences were small, unlike large and important differences in coronary risk[64]. Social class differences in the same direction were apparent by age 36 in men in the national birth cohort study[42].

Barker has shown a small inverse association between placental size and later blood pressure in adults[65]. It seems most unlikely that social class differences in blood pressure could depend entirely on prenatal development, as Barker sometimes seems to imply[66], but there is increasing evidence that tracking both for raised blood pressure and insulin resistance does begin during gestation and infancy, is linked in some way with poor nutrition in both mothers and their children, and may then be maintained to age 64 years[67].

Social class remains a huge and neglected body of association and causation for coronary disease, with still insufficient plausible explanation in social or biological terms, although smoking, fibrinogen[68] and, to a small extent, blood pressure all provide independently associated mechanisms. Low social class is a more powerful independent predictor of risk from ischaemic heart disease than blood cholesterol, smoking, or hypertension[69] and seems to be the most consistent factor underlying the large between population differences found by Shaper *et al.*[70] in their study of coronary risk factors in British towns.

Conclusion

We still know too little about the causes of high blood pressure to justify any convincing national policy for mass prevention, or personal steps to prevent high blood pressure in young people, other than control of central obesity, and assurance of plentiful and varied diets for expectant mothers and young children. Food supplement policies which already existed for this last group have been steadily dismantled since 1979, together with increasing social polarization which is certainly likely to increase coronary risk, and may increase stroke risk.

Reduction of dietary sodium load below 30 mmol/day would probably abolish the problem, but is neither culturally feasible, nor supported by evidence that such a diet would reduce age-standardized mortality from all causes.

The causes of primary hypertension now seem likely to share common origins with the causes of central obesity, insulin resistance, and non-insulin dependent diabetes, powerfully modified by genetic factors. National policies which might address these rationally are discussed in relation to prevention of coronary disease and stroke in Chapter 7.

References

1. Pickering GW (1968) *High blood pressure.* (2nd edn.) Churchill, London, 203–5.

2. Hamilton M, Pickering GW, Roberts JAF *et al.* (1954) The aetiology of essential hypertension. I: The arterial pressure in the general population. *Clin Sci* **13**: 11–35.

3. Swales J (1985) *Platt versus Pickering: An episode in recent medical history.* Keynes & Cambridge University Press, London.

4. Hawthorne VM, Greaves DA and Beevers DG (1974) Blood pressure in a Scottish town. *Br Med J* iii: 600–3.

5. Chen Z, Peto R, Collins R *et al.* (1991) Serum cholesterol concentration and coronary heart disease in a population with low cholesterol concentrations. *Br Med J* **303**: 276–82.

6. Andersson OK, Beckman-Suurkula M, Sannerstedt R *et al.* (1989) Does hyperkinetic circulation constitute a prehypertensive stage? A 5-year follow-up of haemodynamics in young men with mild blood pressure elevation. *J Intern Med* **226**: 401–8.

7. Shekelle RB, Schoenberger JA and Stamler J (1976) Correlates of the JAS type A behaviour pattern score. *J Chron Dis* **29**: 381–94.

8. Haynes SG, Levine S, Scotch NA *et al.* (1978) The relationship of psychosocial factors to coronary heart disease in the Framingham study. I: Methods and risk factors. *Am J Epidemiol* **107**: 362–83.

9. Winkleby MA, Ragland DR and Syme SL (1988) Self-reported stressors and hypertension: Evidence of an inverse association. *Am J Epidemiol* **127**: 124–33.

10. Antonovsky A (1985) The life cycle, mental health and the sense of coherence. *Isr J Psychiatry Relat Sci* **22**: 273–80.

11. Schnall PL, Pieper C, Schwartz J *et al.* (1990) The relationship between 'job strain', workplace diastolic blood pressure, and left ventricular mass index. *JAMA* **263**: 1929–35.

12. Borhani NO and Borkman TS (1968) *The Alameda County blood pressure study.* State of California Department of Public Health, Berkeley CA.

13. Marmot MG and Syme SL (1976) Acculturation and coronary heart disease. *Am J Epidemiol* **104**: 225–47.

14. Alfredsson L, Karasek R and Theorell T (1982) Myocardial infarction risk and psycho-social work environment: an analysis of male Swedish working force. *Soc Sci Med* **16**: 463–7.

15. Mattiasson I, Lindgarde F, Nilsson JA *et al.* (1990) Threat of unemployment and cardiovascular risk factors: Longitudinal study of quality of sleep and serum cholesterol concentrations in men threatened with redundancy. *Br Med J* **301**: 461–6.

16. Dahl LK (1972) Salt and hypertension. *Am J Clin Nutr* **25**: 231–44.

17. Rikimaru T, Fujita Y, Okuda T *et al.* (1988) Responses of sodium balance, blood pressure and other variables to sodium loading in Papua New Guinea highlanders. *Am J Clin Nutr* **47**: 502–8.

18. Poulter NR, Khaw KT and Hopwood BEC (1990) The Kenyan Luo migration study: Observations on the initiation of a rise in blood pressure. *Br Med J* **300**: 967–72.

19. Liu K, Cooper R, McKeever J *et al.* (1979) Assessment of the association between habitual salt intake and high blood pressure: Methodological problems. *Am J Epidemiol* **110**: 219–26.

20. Watt GCM, and Foy CJW (1982) Dietary sodium and arterial pressure: problems of studies within a single population. *J Epidemiol Community Health* **36**: 197–201.

21. Swales JD (1988) Salt saga continued: Salt has only a small importance in hypertension. *Br Med J* **297**: 307–8.

22. Intersalt Cooperative Research Group (1988) Intersalt: an international study of electrolyte excretion and blood pressure. Results for 24-hour urinary sodium and potassium excretion. *Br Med J* **297**: 319–28.

23. Rose GA and Marmot MG (1981) Social class and coronary heart disease. *Br Heart J* **45**: 13–19.

24. Law MR, Frost CD and Wald NJ (1991) By how much does dietary salt reduction lower blood pressure? I: Analysis of observational data among populations. *Br Med J* **302**: 811–15.

25. Frost CD, Law MR and Wald NJ (1991) By how much does dietary salt

reduction lower blood pressure? II: Analysis of observational data within populations. *Br Med J* **302**: 815–18.

26. Kesteloot H and Geboers J (1982) Calcium and blood pressure. *Lancet* i: 813.

27. Langford H (1983) Electrolyte intake and excretion and its correlation with blood pressure: Studies in children and adults. In: Gross F and Strasser T (eds). *Mild hypertension: Recent advances.* Raven Press, New York.

28. Puska P, Iacono JM, Nissinen A *et al.* (1983) Controlled, randomised trial of the effect of dietary fat on blood pressure. *Lancet* i: 1–5.

29. Rouse IL and Beilin LJ (1984) Vegetarian diet and blood pressure. *J Hypertens* **2**: 231–40.

30. Quizilbash N (1987) Blood pressure and fat intake: A review. *J Soc Med* **80**: 225–8.

31. Mann JI (1981) A high carbohydrate leguminous fibre diet improves all aspects of diabetic control. *Lancet* i: 1–5.

32. MacDonald TM, Sharpe K, Fowler G *et al.* (1991) Caffeine restriction: Effect on mild hypertension. *Br Med J* **303**: 1235–8.

33. Arkwright PD, Beilin LJ, Rouse I *et al.* (1982) Effects of alcohol use and other aspects of lifestyle on blood pressure levels and prevalence of hypertension in a working population. *Circulation* **66**: 60–6.

34. Hart JT, Edwards C, Haines AP *et al.* (1993) High blood pressure under 40 in a general practice population followed for 21 years. *Br Med J* **306**: 437–40.

35. Jackson R, Scragg R and Beaglehole R (1991) Alcohol consumption and risk of coronary heart disease. *Br Med J* **303**: 211–16.

36. Renaud S and de Lorgeril M (1992) Wine, alcohol, platelets, and the French paradox for coronary heart disease. *Lancet* **339**: 1523–5.

37. Miall WE and Oldham PD (1955) A study of arterial blood pressure and its inheritance in a sample of the general population. *Clin Sci* **14**: 459–88.

38. Miall WE and Oldham PD (1958) Factors influencing arterial pressure in the general population. *Clin Sci* **17**: 409–44.

39. Watt GCM, Harrap SB, Foy CJW *et al*. (1992) Abnormalities of glucocorticoid metabolism and the renin–angiotensin system: a four corners approach to the identification of genetic determinants of blood pressure. *J Hypertens* **10**: 473–82.

40. Watt GCM, Foy CJW and Hart JT (1983) Comparison of blood pressure, sodium intake, and other variables in offspring with and without a family history of high blood pressure. *Lancet* i: 1245–8.

41. Watt GCM, Foy CJW, Hart JT *et al*. (1985) Dietary sodium and arterial blood pressure: Evidence against genetic susceptibility. *Br Med J* **291**: 1525–8.

42. Wadsworth MEJ, Cripps HA, Midwinter RE *et al*. (1985) Blood pressure in a national birth cohort at the age of 36 related to social and familial factors, smoking, and body mass. *Br Med J* **291**: 1534–8.

43. Cooper R, Trevisan M, Ostrow D *et al*. (1984) Blood pressure and sodium–lithium countertransport: findings in population-based surveys. *J Hypertens* **2**: 467–71.

44. Cooper R, Miller K, Trevisan M *et al*. (1983) Family history of hypertension and red cell cation transport in high school students. *J Hypertens* **1**: 145–52.

45. Walker JD, Tariq T and Viberti G (1990) Sodium–lithium countertransport activity in red cells of patients with insulin dependent diabetes and nephropathy, and their parents. *Br Med J* **301**: 635–8.

46. Reaven GM (1988) Role of insulin resistance in human disease. *Diabetes* **37**: 1595–1607.

47. Ferrannini E, Buzzigoli G, Bonadonna R. *et al*. (1987) Insulin resistance in essential hypertension. *N Engl J Med* **317**: 350–79.

48. Facchini FS, Hollenbeck CB, Jeppesen J *et al*. (1992) Insulin resistance and cigarette smoking. *Lancet* **339**: 1128–30.

49. Jarrett RJ (1992) In defence of insulin: A critique of syndrome X. *Lancet* **340**: 469–71.

50. Haynes RB, Harper AC, Costley SR *et al*. (1984) Failure of weight reduction to reduce mildly elevated blood pressure: A randomised trial. *J Hypertens* **2**: 535–9.

51. Hovell MF (1982) The experimental evidence for weight loss treatment of essential hypertension: a critical review. *Am J Public Health* **72**: 359–68.

52. Sonne-Holm S, Sorensen TIA, Jensen G *et al.* (1989) Independent effects of weight change and attained body weight on prevalence of arterial hypertension in obese and non-obese men. *Br Med J* **299**: 767–70.

53. Somers VK, Conway J, Johnston J *et al.* (1991). Effects of endurance training on baroreflex sensitivity and blood pressure in borderline hypertension. *Lancet* **337**: 1363–8.

54. (1992) Hypertension: In black and white [editorial]. *Lancet* **339**: 28–9.

55. Cruickshank JK, Jackson SHD, Beevers DG *et al.* (1985) Similarity of blood pressure in blacks, whites and Asians in England: The Birmingham factory study. *J Hypertens* **3**: 365–71.

56. Miall WE and Cochrane AL (1961) The distribution of blood pressure in Wales and Jamaica. *Pathol Microbiol* **24**: 690–7.

57. Cruickshank JK, Cooper J, Burnett M *et al.* (1991) Ethnic differences in fasting plasma C-peptide and insulin in relation to glucose tolerance and blood pressure. *Lancet* **338**: 842–7.

58. Langford H (1981) Is blood pressure different in black people? *Postgrad Med J* **57**: 749–54.

59. Himmelstein D, Levins R and Woolhandler S (1990) Beyond our means: Patterns of variability of physiological traits. *Int J Health Serv* **20**: 115–24.

60. Ogenlesi AO and Akinkugbe OO (1992) Hypertension in black and white. *Lancet* **339**: 680–1.

61. Dyer A, Stamler J, Shekelle R *et al.* (1976) The relationship of education to blood pressure: Findings on 40 000 Chicagoans. *Circulation* **54**: 987–92.

62. Burns M, Morrison J, Skhoury PR *et al.* Blood pressure in black and white inner city and suburban adolescents. *Prev Med* **9**: 41–50.

63. Hodgkins BJ, Manring E and Meyers M (1990) Demographic, social and stress correlates of hypertension among the urban poor. *Fam Pract* **7**: 261–6.

64. Marmot MG, Smith GD, Stansfield S *et al.* (1991) Health inequalities among British civil servants: the Whitehall II study. *Lancet* **337**: 1387–93.

65. Barker DJP, Bull AR, Osmond C *et al.* (1990) Fetal and placental size and risk of hypertension in adult life. *Br Med J* **301**: 259–62.

66. Ben-Shlomo Y and Davey Smith G (1991) Deprivation in infancy or in adult life: Which is more important for mortality risk? *Lancet* **337**: 530–4.

67. Hales CN, Barker DJP, Clark PMS (1991) Fetal and infant growth and impaired glucose tolerance at age 64. *Br Med J* **303**: 1019–22.

68. Markowe HLJ, Marmot MG, Shipley MJ *et al.* (1985) Fibrinogen: A possible link between social class and coronary heart disease. *Br Med J* **291**: 1312–14.

69. Rose GA (1981) Strategies of prevention: Lessons from cardiovascular disease. *Br Med J* **282**: 1847–52.

70. Shaper AG, Pocock SJ, Walker M *et al.* (1981) British Regional Heart Study: Cardiovascular risk factors in middle-aged men in 24 towns. *Br Med J* **283**: 179–86.

3

Secondary High Blood Pressure

Renal hypertension ■ Bilateral causes ■ Unilateral causes ■
Coarctation ■ Phaeochromocytoma ■ Primary hyperaldosteronism
■ Intracranial tumours ■ Cushing's syndrome and hypothyroidism

Historically, secondary hypertension dominated thought about the causes, mechanisms, and even treatment of all hypertension, because before the advent of effective and tolerable antihypertensive drugs in the late 1950s, it was almost the only area within which rational treatment seemed possible.

This has long ceased to be true. Certainly less than 2%, probably less than 1%, of high blood pressure as customarily defined is caused by other known disease. Most, even of this, is now best treated on the same lines as primary high blood pressure (essential hypertension), simply by lowering blood pressure by antihypertensive medication, whatever the cause. As blood pressure can now usually be lowered so easily, possible causes are often not even considered, and no search is made either for secondary high blood pressure, or (more importantly) for some of the known causes of primary high blood pressure discussed in Chapter 2.

The main clinical problem with these secondary causes is to remember that they exist, and look for them effectively and intelligently, with cost effective use of diagnostic resources. These are considered in Chapter 12. Here we are concerned with classic causes of secondary high blood pressure only as sometimes illuminating examples of internal mechanisms, some of which are relevant to those of high blood pressure in all its forms.

Renal Hypertension

Renal function critically depends on perfusion of glomeruli, so it is not surprising to find powerful feedback mechanisms to maintain renal blood flow when perfusion is obstructed. More than 90% of all classical secondary hypertension is renal in origin. Evidence on mechanisms for this is conflicting, but is on the whole consistent with the view that structural damage to the kidney, whatever its cause, raises arterial pressure through this sequence:

- renal ischaemia
- → secretion of renin
- → activation of plasma substrate
- → angiotensin (the most potent vasocontrictor substance known).

In the normal kidney, renin release is usually reactive to dietary sodium intake, not to ischaemia, but there is some evidence that, at an early stage in reduction of renal arterial flow, renin release is increased, perhaps initiating a rise in pressure maintained later by other mechanisms. Virtually all forms of renal damage may do this: obstructive, inflammatory, infective, neoplastic and traumatic. Experimental renovascular high blood pressure in rats does not lead to insulin resistance,[1] so the pathways of renal hypertension and at least one large subset of primary high blood pressure are distinct, but obviously in humans they may be mixed.

Bilateral Causes

In primary care, the most frequent problem of this kind is the diabetic kidney, which is associated with hypertension in 90% of cases. This is a common and, at an early stage, treatable cause of eventual renal failure. It seems to be relentlessly progressive by the time clinically detectable proteinuria is present,[2] but if blood glucose[3] and blood pressure[4] are both assiduously controlled, the rate of deterioration of renal function may be delayed sufficiently to allow a normal lifespan.

Bladder obstruction, acute or chronic, raises blood pressure dramatically. Acute retention of urine is a common cause of misdiagnosed, and often hastily and unnecessarily treated, severe hypertension. Chronic prostatic obstruction is an avoidable cause of renal failure,[5] usually accompanied by high blood pressure.[6] Relief of obstruction will usually reverse both the renal failure and the hypertension if it is not too long delayed.[7]

Another common form of renal damage, even in developed economies, is probably still chronic infection leading to scarring, usually bilateral. This is much more important in poor countries than rich, because of their high prevalence of childhood renal stones leading to chronic pyelonephritis. Infection without scarring, acute or chronic, has no effect on pressure. In girls in the UK aged 5–12, about 1% have chronic or recurrent bacteriuria detectable by dip-culture. Of these, about half have radiologically demonstrable abnormalities of the urinary tract, with vesicoureteric reflux in one half, and reflux plus scarring in the other. It is this last group with reflux plus scarring which may go on to develop chronic pyelonephritis with raised arterial pressure.[8] Prevalence in boys is still unknown, but certainly much less. Once the scarring process begins, it seems to be irreversible; long term antibiotic control of infection makes no difference. The treatable stage of vesicoureteric reflux lies probably between birth and 4 or 5 years of age, and diagnosis should concentrate on this age group. This means that GPs should systematically use dip-cultures in suspicious (usually minor and non-specific) illness, picking up occasional cases of surgically correctable obstructive uropathies at the same time.

Gouty nephropathy is another common cause of both hypertension and renal failure, important because it may present with recurrent stones, referred to surgeons rather than physicians. GPs may then find themselves the only physicians involved, and unless they show some clinical curiosity, nobody does. The underlying abnormality, usually easy to control with allopurinol, may then continue uncorrected.

Other bilateral secondary causes are acute and chronic glomerulonephritis, much rarer now in Europe than before the demise of the streptococcus after the Second World War, but still common in poor countries. Both are probably initiated by renal ischaemia caused by autoimmune vasculitis. Unless it is controlled, high blood pressure may then accelerate further renal damage, leading ultimately to end-stage renal failure.

The adult form of polycystic kidneys[9] runs in families as an autosomal dominant, and may therefore be locally common. The kidneys are radiologically normal until late childhood, but rapid and economical genetic analysis now allows reliable presymptomatic diagnosis.[10] High blood pressure develops in about 80% of cases, but is rarely severe. As always, high blood pressure accelerates deterioration in renal function and therefore needs assiduous control.

Systemic sclerosis (scleroderma) is uncommon, but not as rare as specialist centres imagine; most cases remain undiagnosed. It eventually causes high blood pressure in most cases through bilateral renal fibrosis and ischaemia. Young women presenting with otherwise unaccountable Reynaud's phenomenon and a typically pinched, beaky facies are prime suspects.

Unilateral Causes

Ever since the Goldblatt kidney, students have been loaded with simplistic physiology and warnings about the critical importance of detecting unilateral renal disease causing a secondary rise in blood pressure, the favourite model being unilateral renal artery stenosis. Other causes are renin secreting tumours, other renal tumours both benign and malignant, unilateral chronic pyelonephritis, hydronephrosis, and renal tuberculosis.

Stenosis or occlusion of a renal artery has been said to be the commonest form of unilateral renal disease causing secondary high blood pressure, possibly accounting for up to 4% of all hypertensives, about 200 000 people in the whole of Britain. As clinical autopsy studies show renal artery stenosis in up to 46% of normotensives, and 20–40% of patients having arteriography for peripheral vascular or coronary disease are shown to have previously unsuspected atherosclerotic renal artery stenosis,[11] it is difficult to guess what, if anything, these figures mean.[12] Angiographic study of 100 consecutive patients with peripheral arterial disease presenting with leg pain showed that most had either stenosis or occlusion of one or both renal arteries, but neither renal function nor blood pressure showed any association with perfusion.[13]

Renal artery stenoses do not behave in the relatively simple fashion found by Goldblatt in his dogs. Yet again, initiating causes and maintaining causes are different, so high blood pressure often persists even after stenosis is relieved. Even a prospective series of nephrectomies for unilateral chronic pyelonephritis before the onset of high blood pressure showed no prophylactic effect.[8] The main clinical significance of renal artery stenosis is as a contraindication to treatment with angiotensin converting enzyme (ACE) inhibitors, which may precipitate renal failure.[14]

Coarctation

This is a stricture of the aorta usually close to the entry point of the ductus arteriosus, but occasionally in the abdominal aorta above or below the renal arteries. It probably, but not certainly, starts with abnormal fetal development.

The mechanism of hypertension in this case seems obvious: mechanical obstruction to perfusion of the lower half of the body requires a large increase in left ventricular output, with high arterial pressure in the proximal segment perfusing upper limbs, and low pressure in the lower segment perfusing lower limbs. As usual, it is not so simple. High blood pressure often persists after reconstruction of the stricture. Yet again, initiating causes may not be the same as maintaining causes, which in this case is probably impaired renal perfusion leading to permanent renal ischaemia.

Phaeochromocytoma

These tumours are rare, but important to detect early because they are usually treatable, may cause disabling symptoms for many years, and are commonly missed; 85% of those seen at the Mayo Clinic from 1928 to 1977 were first diagnosed as necropsy.[15] Many of them are familial, with autosomal dominant inheritance and high penetrance. About 1% of patients with neurofibromatosis develop these tumours, of which 90% arise in the adrenal medulla, but they may arise anywhere where there is chromaffin tissue. All secrete noradrenaline (norepinephrine), which is the immediate cause of high blood pressure if and when this occurs; it is not invariable.

Phaeochromocytomas may also produce adrenaline (epinephrine), which reduces diastolic pressure, and both precursors and degradation products of catecholamines in various proportions, causing a wide variety of symptoms. The high blood pressure they cause is not always paroxysmal, and is rarely severe. Most of them are benign, but malignant tumours can occur which are aggressive and respond poorly to chemotherapy.

Primary Hyperaldosteronism

This has been said to account for between 0.1 and 1% of all cases of high blood pressure. In classic Conn's syndrome aldosterone is secreted from a benign tumour of the adrenal cortex. Similar effects on arterial pressure occur if there is autonomous hypersecretion from an apparently normal adrenal, or from adrenal or ovarian carcinoma. High blood pressure is always present, but seldom severe. It seems to be caused by the sequence:

- excess aldosterone
- → K depletion + Na retention
- → raised plasma volume, raised heart output, low renin.

Intracranial Tumours

Experientially, electric stimulation of the frontal and temporal cortex or the floor of the fourth ventricle all raise arterial pressure. Any cause of raised intracranial pressure may therefore present as fairly severe high blood pressure, often intermittent. Accompanying headache, papilloedema and central nervous system signs may then be attributed to high blood pressure itself, rather than to raised intracranial pressure. Posterior fossa tumours are particularly likely to raise arterial pressure, probably by distorting the brain stem.

Cushing's Syndrome and Hypothyroidism

High blood pressure occurs in about three-quarters of all cases of Cushing's syndrome, which seems to have roughly the same prevalence as phaeochromocytoma and hyperaldosteronism. The chief mechanism of this seems to be the sequence:

■ excess cortisol
■ → excess angiotensin substrate.

High blood pressure is 50–100% more common than in the general population in both symptomatic and biochemical hypothyroidism.[16] The mechanism is unknown. Hypothyroidism is usually associated with raised total serum cholesterol, but the large excess of coronary disease in these patients occurs almost entirely in those with high blood pressure. In about half of these, pressure returns to normal after correction of the thyroid deficiency.

References

1. Buchanan TA, Sipos GF, Gadalam S et al. (1991) Glucose tolerance and insulin action in rats with renovascular hypertension. *Hypertension* **18**: 341–7.

2. Viberti GC, Jarret RJ, Keen H et al. (1982) Microalbuminuria as a predictor of clinical nephropathy in insulin-dependent diabetes mellitus. *Lancet* i: 1430–2.

3. Viberti GC, Bilous RW, Mackintosh D et al. (1983) Long term correction of hyperglycaemia and progression of renal failure in insulin dependent diabetes. *Br Med J* **286**: 598–601.

4. Parving HH, Smidt U, Anderson AR et al. (1983) Early aggressive antihypertensive treatment reduces rate of decline in kidney function in diabetic nephropathy. *Lancet* i: 1175–8.

5. Sacks SA, Aparicio SAJR, Bevan A et al. (1989) Late renal failure due to prostatic outflow obstruction: A preventable disease. *Br Med J* **298**: 156–9.

6. Ghose RR and Harindra V (1989) Unrecognized high pressure chronic retention of urine presenting with systemic arterial hypertension. *Br Med J* **298**: 1626–8.

7. Ghose RR (1990) Prolonged recovery of renal function after prostatectomy for prostatic outflow obstruction. *Br Med J* **300**: 1376.

8. Asscher AW (1983) Urinary tract infection as a cause of hypertension in man. In: Robertson JIS (ed) *Handbook of hypertension. Vol 2: Clinical aspects of secondary hypertension*, pp 18–32. Elsevier, Oxford.

9. Milutinovic J, Fialkow PJ and Phillips LA (1980) Autosomal dominant polycystic kidney disease: Early diagnosis and data for genetic counselling. *Lancet* i: 1203–6.

10. Harris PC, Thomas S, Ratcliffe PJ *et al.* (1991) Rapid genetic analysis of families with polycystic disease 1 by means of a microsatellite marker. *Lancet* **338**: 1484–7.

11. Cairns HS (1992) Atherosclerotic renal artery stenosis. *Lancet* **340**: 298–9.

12. MacKay A, Brown JJ, Lever AF *et al.* (1983) Unilateral renal disease in hypertension. In: Robertson JIS (ed) *Handbook of hypertension. Vol. 2: Clinical aspects of secondary hypertension*, pp 33–79. Elsevier, Oxford.

13. Choudhri AH, Cleland JGF, Rowlands PC *et al.* (1990) Unsuspected renal artery stenosis in peripheral vascular disease. *Br Med J* **301**: 1197.

14. Hricik DE, Browning PJ, Kopelman R *et al.* (1983) Captopril induced functional renal insufficiency in patients with bilateral renal artery stenosis in a solitary kidney. *N Engl J Med* **308**: 373–6.

15. (1990) Phaeochromocytoma still surprises [editorial]. *Lancet* **335**: 1189–90.

16. Bing RF and Swales JD (1983) Thyroid disease and hypertension. In: Robertson JIS (ed) *Handbook of hypertension. Vol 2: Clinical aspects of secondary hypertension*, pp 276–90. Elsevier, Oxford.

4

Iatrogenesis

The most common iatrogenic cause of apparent high blood pressure is to detect and treat it when it isn't there, by hasty diagnosis, poor conditions and technique of measurement, or poorly organized follow-up, as dealt with in Chapters 8 and 10.

The most common iatrogenic causes of truly sustained high blood pressure or unexplained resistance to antihypertensive drugs are sympathomimetic amines, monoamine oxidase inhibitors (MAOIs), carbenoxolone, non-steroidal anti-inflammatory drugs (NSAIDs) and the contraceptive pill.

Sympathomimetic Amines

These are contained in cold remedies, appetite suppressants and stimulants related to amphetamine. Illegally produced and procured amphetamine, and its recent more dangerous variant 'Ecstasy', are common possibilities in young patients with unexpectedly high blood pressures. Wildly variable pressure values may reflect intermittent bingeing. Sympathomimetic amines usually cause psychiatric rather than cardiovascular symptoms, but forgotten use or unsuspected abuse of these drugs is an occasional cause of raised pressure, or of hypertension inexplicably resistant to treatment.

Phenylephrine eye-drops used in newborn infants have been found to raise blood pressure by 25%, and a persistent systolic pressure of 130–160 mmHg was caused in one 7-week-old baby by 6-hourly eye drops containing 10% phenylephrine and 0.25% pseudoephedrine.

All these drugs, including across-the-counter decongestant nasal drops and sprays, seem to create dependency in some people. Prescription of amphetamine related appetite suppressants can rarely be justified, but is still a common cause of moderately raised pressure.

Monoamine Oxidase Inhibitors

Monoamine oxidase inhibitors (MAOIs) are effective antidepressant drugs, useful because they act more quickly than tricyclic or quadricyclic antidepressants, do not cause the often troublesome anticholinergic side effects of tricyclics, and are less dangerous suicidal agents. For all these reasons they remain useful drugs despite a bad reputation, earned during the early years when their interactions with amine–containing foods and drugs were not fully understood, and reinforced by the usual promotional neglect suffered by all drugs as they lose patent protection and therefore become less profitable.

Patients on MAOIs, who are taking amines by self medication or prescription, or in foods such as cheese, yeast extracts like Marmite, red wine, stout, or any smoked or traditionally preserved food that may contain putrefactive elements, are liable to acute hypertensive crises which may precipitate stroke. This is even more likely in patients who are already hypertensive. MAOIs should never be used for people with known hypertension, or be initiated without checking blood pressure. Used in normotensives, these risks and their mechanism should be explained simply to patients, backed up by written material. Their medical records should be clearly marked, signifying a major risk of drug interaction.

Carbenoxolone

Carbenoxolone is an effective treatment for gastric ulcer, but rarely used since the advent of histamine H_2 antagonists and antibiotic control of *Helicobacter pylori*. Like liquorice, from which it is derived, it resembles deoxycorticosterone in its chemical structure and has mineralocorticoid activity. It causes water and sodium retention, and at daily doses of about 300 mg causes a rise of 15–30 mmHg systolic and 3–25 mmHg diastolic pressure.[1] Liquorice bingers undergo similar changes.

Non-Steroidal Anti-Inflammatory Drugs (NSAIDs)

Prostaglandin synthetase inhibitors, such as indomethacin and its innumerable descendants, cause sodium retention and antagonize the anthihypertensive effects of beta–blockers and diuretics.[2] Writers on the subject seem uncertain whether NSAIDs themselves cause a rise in pressure, or only antagonize the effects of antihypertensive medication. When I took indomethacin, my own untreated blood pressure rose from mean 130/65 to mean 145/90 mmHg, and the fact that

NSAIDs are promoted for treatment of so-called 'hypotension' in Germany suggests that they have a general blood pressure raising effect. Both possibilities are important because NSAIDs are so commonly prescribed. The fall in systolic pressure when they are stopped is often as much as 10 mmHg.

This is probably the most common important drug interaction in current practice, frequently ignored and responsible for poor control in many patients. All practice staff need to be aware of it. Some NSAIDs, for example dipropazone, are effective for some patients despite low prostaglandin synthetase inhibitory activity and probably have less hypertensive effect.

Oral Contraceptives: the low universal rise

Because of the massive scale on which they are used and the early age at which they are applied, any contribution of oral contraceptives to cardiovascular risk is important. This is a subject on which all GPs should be well informed, and should formulate responsible practice policies, known to the whole team and to patients themselves; if patients are well informed, some of them at least may help to enforce safe practice.

Figure 4.1 shows changes in systolic pressure after two years in 186 women aged 21–30 on combined oestrogen-progestogen oral contraceptives compared with 60 controls.[3] Oral contraceptives are associated with a mean rise of nearly 8 mmHg. Follow-up after another 3 years (5 years in all) showed a difference in the same direction of 12 mmHg systolic and 8 mmHg diastolic pressure.

This rise is not easily recognized in general practice, because oral contraceptives are taken by young women with systolic pressures so low, often around 100 mmHg, that even a rise of 10 or 20 mmHg of systolic pressure still remains well below levels that will attract attention from most doctors or nurses. Even if pressures are monitored regularly every 3 months or so, as they should be, the initial apparent fall caused by habituation may exceed and thus mask an underlying rise in mean ambulatory pressure.

This moderate rise seems to occur in nearly all women after about 6 months on oral contraceptives. The huge Royal College of General Practitioners' study[4] of long term risks showed a fivefold increase in cardiovascular deaths in oral contraceptive users (25.8/100 000 woman-years) compared with non-users (5.5/100 000 woman-years), rising to 10-fold after 5 years. Most of this added risk was from thromboembolism, but there was also increased risk of subarachnoid haemorrhage and coronary disease, much of which may have been related to rise in blood pressure.

These data refer to old oral contraceptive formulations with 50 μg oestrogen. With 30 μg or even less now generally preferred, risks are probably smaller, and later studies suggest that the cardiovascular risk of using oral contraceptives has indeed fallen substantially.[5]

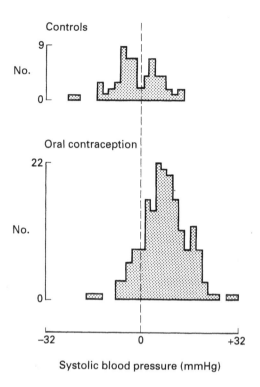

Systolic blood pressure (mmHg)

Figure 4.1: Changes in systolic pressure after two years in 186 women aged 21–30 on combined oestrogen-progestogen oral contraceptive compared with 60 controls[3]. (Reproduced with permission.)

The High Exceptional Rise

Figure 4.2* demonstrates this process in a Glyncorrwg woman of 18; it shows a rapid rise from 135/82 mmHg to 168/115 mmHg after 9 months on oral contraceptives, first monitored by daily readings, then a rapid fall after their use was stopped. Figure 4.3 shows pressures recorded for another Glyncorrwg woman started on oral contraception at age 35, before its potential effect on arterial pressure was known. Note that two readings before starting their use, at 180/120 and 170/100 mmHg, already showed high pressures. After starting oral contracep-

---

* Figure 4.2 and subsequent graphic blood pressure records have a variable time scale along the bottom line, to accommodate frequent measurements in some years and none in others, yet retain clarity. In many cases, pressures recorded before treatment, or in the early years of treatment before this was well organized, are compressed to a short space. From 1968, practice policy was to record pressures at least once every 5 years in all adults, every year in borderline hypertensives (diastolic 90–104 mmHg) and frank hypertensives who refused treatment, and every 3 months in treated hypertensives. Where pressures were poorly controlled, they were recorded daily or weekly.

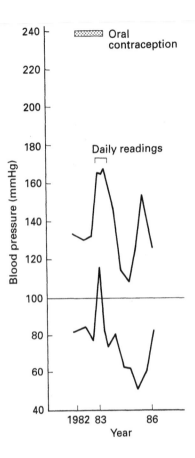

Figure 4.2: Blood pressure record of an 18-year-old Glyncorrwg woman who started oral contraception in 1982.

tives, pressure rose to 240/160 mmHg. She started antihypertensive medication, and the oral contraceptive was fortunately stopped, although I was still, like everyone else in 1966, unaware of the interaction. A year later she resumed using oral contraceptives, and after about 3 months pressure rose again to 185/110 mmHg, and again fell when oral contraception was stopped.

These are frightening pressures, and fear is well justified. In 1975 a case was reported of a 27-year-old woman, previously normotensive, who developed a systolic pressure of 180 mmHg on receiving an oestrogen-progestogen oral contraceptive.[6] Pressure fell to normal when the oral contraceptive was stopped, but after the next pregnancy it was resumed; blood pressure rose to 250/160 mmHg, she developed malignant hypertension and died of irreversible renal failure.

Unfortunately the RCGP study gathered no quantified blood pressure data, only qualitative diagnoses of 'hypertension', and Vessey's study related only to mortality. Even my very limited clinical experience shows that oral contraception

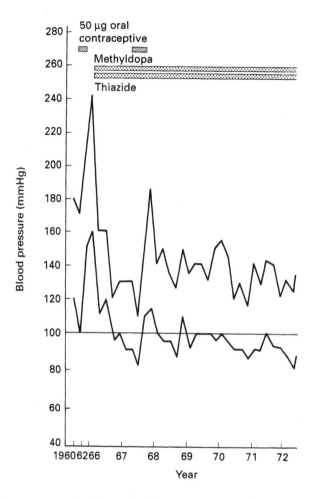

Figure 4.3: Pressures recorded for another Glyncorrwg woman who started oral contraception at age 35 in 1962.

was originally a common cause of serious hypertensive risk. Even at current lower formulations, this risk should still be taken more seriously than most authorities seem to do. Certainly it invalidates arguments in favour of across-the-counter availability of oral contraceptives, without medical advice or monitoring. The risk, particularly of malignant hypertension, seems to be much higher in oral contraceptive users who smoke cigarettes.[7]

Prescription of oral contraceptives carries with it a duty to ensure that blood pressure is checked regularly. Our practice has been to record it every 3 months, when prescriptions are renewed. The common practice of prescribing for 6 months is, in my opinion, unsafe. Every woman who starts on oral contraceptives should be informed of this risk, as well as the risk of smoking, and encouraged to insist that her blood pressure be measured whenever she renews her prescription. Nurses and office staff are busy people, and patients need encouragement to enforce safe practice on their own initiative.

Hormone Replacement Therapy

Hormone replacement therapy (HRT) is a controversial subject when related to blood pressure. This is because both oestrogens and progestogens can raise blood pressure in at least some younger women. For this reason many practice teams have avoided it for patients whose blood pressures are known to be high, or have blamed subsequent high pressures on this treatment.

There is impressive evidence that unopposed oestrogen supplements in postmenopausal women reduce their mortality from coronary heart disease and stroke by half compared with untreated women,[8] a much bigger difference than anyone has been able to demonstrate for antihypertensive drugs. The effect seems partly due to improved blood lipid profile, perhaps also partly to increased cardiac efficiency and peripheral perfusion, and partly through reduced atheroma in major arteries.[9] In women with a positive indication for treatment—severe flushes or sweats, slender bones (and therefore a high risk of osteoporosis), or a family history of osteoporosis or early coronary disease—borderline or high blood pressure is not a convincing contraindication to HRT.

Women who have had an early hysterectomy are in urgent need of HRT, but are often not offered it.[10] Conservation of ovaries is often poor, because their blood supply may be impaired even by hysterectomy alone.

Dogmatic statements in recent years, in the *British National Formulary*, that unopposed oestrogen should never be prescribed for women with an intact uterus because of increased risk from endometrial cancer, seem poorly supported by the balance of available evidence. Endometrial cancer is much rarer than coronary disease or stroke, and usually presents at an early stage, when it is easily and effectively treatable. The cardiovascular benefits of HRT are likely to be lost if only opposed oestrogens are prescribed.[11]

Equally there is no current evidence to support routine use of HRT in all women without menopausal symptoms or personal indications of high risk for coronary disease or osteoporosis. HRT has simply not been available long enough to measure its effects when sustained for postmenopausal lifetimes of 30 or 40 years, and there are good theoretical reasons for suspicion that this could increase the incidence of breast cancer, perhaps by around 12%. Consequent mortality losses might be much less than gains through reduced coronary deaths, but that is a choice women will want to make for themselves in the light of trials evidence of the kind that will start in the MRC GP Research Framework 1994.

Hypertensive women are certainly at high risk of coronary disease even if pressure is well controlled. They are also at higher risk of stroke, although most of this risk can be removed by assiduous control of blood pressure. Prudence suggests that most, if not all, of them should receive HRT for these reasons alone, even without other indications. Their blood pressures will, like those of other treated hypertensives, be closely monitored, and any individual patients whose pressures seem to escape control can have HRT withdrawn if this is the suspected cause; the important thing is to keep such a possibility in mind.

References

1. Nicholls MG and Espiner EA (1983) Liquorice, carbenoxolone and hypertension. In: Robertson JIS (ed) *Handbook of hypertension. Vol. 2: Clinical aspects of secondary hypertension*, p 189. Elsevier, Oxford.

2. Watkins J, Abbott EC, Hensby CN *et al.* (1980) Attenuation of hypotensive effect of propranolol and thiazide diurectics by indomethacin. *Br Med J* **281**: 702.

3. Weinberger MH and Weir RJ (1983) Oral contraceptives and hypertension. In: Robertson JIS (ed) *Handbook of hypertension. Vol. 2: Clinical aspects of secondary hypertension*, p 196. Elsevier, Oxford.

4. Royal College of General Practitioners Oral Contraception Study Group (1981) Further analyses of mortality in oral contraceptive users. *Lancet* **i**: 541–6.

5. Vessey, MP, Villard-Mackintosh L, McPherson K *et al.* (1989) Mortality among oral contraceptive users: 20-year follow up of women in a cohort study. *Br Med J* **299**: 1487–90.

6. Zech P, Rifle G, Lindner A *et al.* (1975) Malignant hypertension with irreversible renal failure due to oral contraceptives. *Br Med J* **iv**: 326.

7. Petitti DB and Klatsky AL (1983) Malignant hypertension in women aged 15 to 44 years and its relation to cigarette smoking and oral contraceptives. *Am J Cardiol* **52**: 297–8.

8. Stampfer MJ, Willet WC, Colditz JA *et al.* (1985) A prospective study of postmenopausal estrogen therapy and coronary heart disease. *N Engl J Med* **313**: 1044–9.

9. Gangar KF, Vyas S, Whitehead M *et al.* (1991) Pulsatility index in internal carotid artery in relation to transdermal oestradiol and time since menopause. *Lancet* **338**: 839–42.

10. Spector TD (1989) Use of oestrogen replacement therapy in high risk groups in the United Kingdom. *Br Med J* **299**: 1434–5.

11. Henderson BE, Ross RK, Lobo RA *et al.* (1988) Re-evaluating the role of progestogen therapy after the menopause. *Fertil Steril* **49**: 95–155.

5

Natural History and Complications

Changes in blood pressure over time ■ Does high blood pressure ever regress naturally without treatment? ■ High blood pressure is self-accelerating ■ Association of blood pressure with risk of stroke and coronary heart disease ■ Accelerated (malignant) hypertension and retinopathy ■ Symptoms of hypertension ■ Bursting effects and blocking effects ■ Stroke ■ Eye damage ■ Kidney damage ■ Heart failure ■ Ruptured aorta ■ Angina and claudication ■ Coronary thrombosis ■ Outcome of hypertension in developing countries ■ You have to die somehow

The natural history of high blood pressure falls into two parts:

■ quantitative development as a risk factor, without local organ damage or symptoms (Group 1)

■ qualitative shift to organ damage, symptoms and disease (Group 2).

Organ damage again subdivides into:

■ many cases of large artery atherothrombotic disease, in which high blood pressure is one of several causes, only slowly reversible by reduction in pressure (Group 2a)

■ a few cases of small artery necrosis, caused by severe or accelerated (malignant) hypertension, rapidly reversible by reduction in pressure (Group 2b).

Following this pattern of natural history, primary care teams need to think in terms of four rather different sets of problems and opportunities for effective intervention. The first two sets described below derive from Group 1 above, the second two from Groups 2a and 2b respectively.

■ Management of blood pressure as a continuously distributed risk throughout the whole registered population:
Monitoring of risk by screening or case-finding; community-wide reduction of risk through group effects on local patterns of eating, drinking, and

employment, availability and use of facilities for participative sport and exercise.

■ Management of treated hypertensives without evidence of organ damage:
These people differ from those in the first set only in that they have been found to have personal mean blood pressures above a threshold beyond which (on current evidence) medical intervention is likely to do substantially more good than harm. All of these need long term follow-up. There should be few urgent or dramatic clinical problems, symptoms will derive mainly from treatment, and the main problem will be to maintain high compliance and low drop-out in people who feel well, or would do so were it not for their treatment.

■ Management of treated hypertensives with evidence of large artery organ damage:
Most, but not all, of these patients will have symptoms. They are at high risk of coronary or stroke events, and care must be organized to anticipate these, as well as to avoid them as far as possible. Compliance and drop-out are smaller problems, because both patients and professionals are more strongly motivated, and the pattern of care begins to conform to the traditional model of sick people seeking professional help. Most people in the second set will eventually move into this third set; our aim is to delay this for as long as possible.

■ Initial management of treated hypertensives with accelerated (malignant) hypertension:
This uncommon but important clinical emergency arises entirely from people who have had severe high blood pressure for several months at least, usually several years. Initially they may be entirely free from symptoms, and will be detected only by examination of urine for protein, and of optic fundi for retinal oedema, haemorrhages, and papilloedema, prompted by detection of uncontrolled severe high blood pressure (diastolic pressure 120 mmHg+).

These categories assume good management of the entire population, starting from measurement of blood pressure at least once every 5 years in all adults. Without this, new cases may be detected at any stage, and are already likely to have organ damage, some of which may be irreversible.

Changes in Blood Pressure Over Time

Changes with time are changes with both age and cumulative environmental effects (experience). Figure 5.1 and 5.2 show trends in mean blood pressure in 1661 men and women randomly sampled from the general population of the Rhondda Fach and Vale of Glamorgan, and followed up four times over the next 10 years.[1] None of these people were on antihypertensive medication. Most

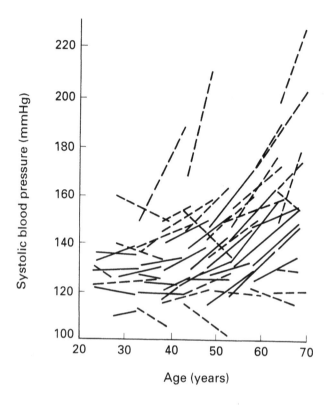

Figure 5.1: Trends of mean systolic pressure for men randomly sampled from the general population of the Rhondda Fach and Vale of Glamorgan, and followed up four times over the next 10 years. Lines represent groups divided by age and systolic pressure at entry. Continuous lines = groups with 10 or more subjects, dashed lines = groups with less than 10 subjects[1]. (Reproduced with permission from the authors.)

pressures, although not all, rose with age. Steep rises and falls were shown from low and high initial levels respectively (regression to the mean).

Does High Blood Pressure Ever Regress Naturally Without Treatment?

Despite general tendencies for all blood pressures to rise with time and experience in industrialized societies, and for high pressures to rise faster than low ones, these generalizations cannot be applied to individual patients.

This is partly because arterial pressure is a relatively unstable variable, and one, two or even three pressures recorded on separate days may not always

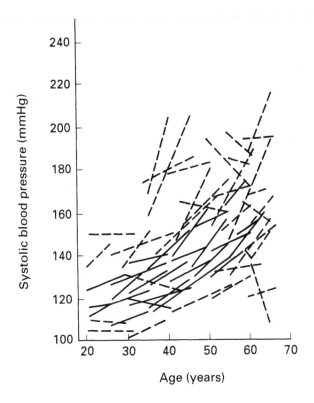

Figure 5.2: Trends of mean systolic pressure for women randomly sampled from the general population of the Rhondda Fach and Vale of Glamorgan, and followed up four times over the next 10 years. Lines represent groups divided by age and systolic pressure at entry. Continuous lines = groups with 10 or more subjects, dashed lines = groups with less than 10 subjects[1]. (Reproduced with permission from the authors.)

characterize mean pressure over days or weeks. Blood pressure may also fall without treatment in people with failing hearts.

Obviously it is also possible that in some people the still incompletely understood hypertensive process may be transient rather than permanent, and that after a few months or years, even a sustained and well documented high pressure may fall without treatment. Despite long initial run-in periods to eliminate regression to the mean, such falls seem to have occurred in both the Australian (ANBPS)[2] and the Medical Research Council (MRC)[3] trials in many of the untreated or placebo treated controls, and also in the Framingham study.[4] In the ANBPS trial nearly 2000 untreated mild hypertensives were followed up. Mean pressure (three readings) fell from 158/120 mmHg at entry to 144/91 mmHg; 3 years later 9% rose by more than 10 mmHg, 22% fell by more than 10 mmHg, and 69% remained within 10 mmHg of the original readings. In the MRC trial more than 7000 placebo treated hypertensives were followed up, with

53

mean entry pressures (four readings) of 158/96 mmHg. Over the next 3 years of follow-up 18% had diastolic pressures less than 90 mmHg at all anniversary visits.

Despite this evidence from large trials, in my experience, if the original diagnosis of hypertension is supported by three or more readings, each a week or more apart, misclassification seems to be rare, although it may occasionally occur. In preparing the second edition of this book and in the light of trials evidence, I was sure I would find in the Glyncorrwg population several examples of people with originally high and sustained pressures, who for one reason or another had not been treated but whose pressures nevertheless fell, and who then lived happily ever after. A careful search through the records of all apparent candidates revealed not one valid example of this process; those whose blood pressures fell in subsequent years all either had erratic readings when first detected, or were later found to have either heart failure or other serious underlying disease causing falls in pressure.

However, studying GP records in Scotland, Parkin[5] found that antihypertensive medication was started after a single reading in more than a third of all cases, and there is no reason to think the results would have been different elsewhere in Britain. The potential for misclassification and unnecessary treatment resulting from this are obvious; a clinical example of the consequences of uncritical diagnosis is given in Table 10.3 (*see* page 151).

To start antihypertensive treatment after only one measurement of blood pressure is a clinical crime. Even at very high pressures (diastolic 150 mmHg or more), the reading should be replicated over at least a few minutes, before intervention.

High Blood Pressure Is Self-Accelerating

In general, blood pressures rise with time, and rise fastest in those with the highest pressures, probably because of structural change in large arteries. High blood pressure is therefore usually self-accelerating unless and until it is controlled by medical intervention of some kind, but rapid acceleration rarely occurs from diastolic pressures below 90 mmHg over 10 years of follow-up.[6]

Association Of Blood Pressure With Risk Of Stroke And Coronary Heart Disease

By 1990 there had been nine prolonged prospective observational studies of large, virtually untreated, middle-aged populations totalling 4 200 000 person-years of observation, including 843 strokes and 4856 coronary events observed over 6–25 years of follow-up (mean 10 years).[7] All these confirmed positive, continuous, independent association of stroke and coronary risk with blood pressure throughout its range. There was no evidence of a threshold between 'normal' blood pressure and disease, as shown in Figure 5.3. There was also little evidence in these untreated populations of a 'J-curve', a rise in risk with fall in pressure at any critical threshold. Populations studied were all middle aged, from North America, Europe, Puerto Rico and Hawaii (largely Asians), and 96% were men; there are therefore still some big questions to be answered about the extent to which these asssociations hold for women, and for Africans.

This association is inevitably understated in each individual study, because each depended on initial readings subject to sampling error. Corrected for this 'regression dilution' bias, prolonged differences in diastolic pressure of 5, 7.5 and 10 mmHg were respectively associated with shifts of at least 34%, 46% and 56% in stroke risk, and 21%, 29% and 37% in coronary risk. These figures refer to association with entry pressures, not treatment pressures.

Accelerated (Malignant) Hypertension And Retinopathy

At any age, in people with diastolic pressures sustained over about 120 mmHg, pressure may suddenly begin to rise exponentially over weeks, days or hours, rather than the years of steady increment for primary ('benign' or 'essential') high blood pressure. This is accelerated, or malignant, hypertension, with destruction of arteriolar networks in the brain, retina and kidney causing sometimes irreversible damage even before alerting symptoms occur.

The classic criteria for diagnosis of malignant hypertension are high pressure and neuroretinopathy: fluffy white patches usually close to the disc, often radiating fanwise towards the macula, usually accompanied by retinal haemorrhages, often with papilloedema, and almost always with proteinuria. Without papilloedema, purists have insisted that this is only 'accelerated hypertension'. The other clinical features and survival rate of accelerated and malignant hypertension are identical,[8] so the distinction seems meaningless.

Fluffy white exudates (actually oedema of the retinal capillary bed) and papilloedema are unique to the malignant phase. They are evidence of its characteristic small artery disease, with arteriolar necrosis and multiple small infarcts.

Similar arteriolar necrosis occurs in the brain, sometimes causing hypertensive encephalopathy with headache, transient symptoms and signs of brain injury from multiple small infarcts, sometimes causing frank haemorrhage and stroke. If these do not leave a gross neurological deficit, they may be misdiagnosed as fully reversible transient ischaemic attacks (TIAs).

Renal damage is invariable, but often asymptomatic, and is caused by the same process of arteriolar necrosis with multiple small infarcts. There is proteinuria, and rising serum urea and creatinine. Even without symptoms, renal damage may become progressive and irreversible if pressure remains uncontrolled.

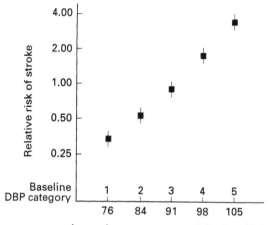

Stroke and usual DBP (in 5 categories
defined by baseline DBP)
7 prospective observational studies:
843 events

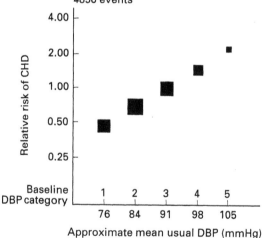

Coronary heart disease and usual DBP
(in 5 categories defined by baseline DBP)
9 prospective observational studies:
4856 events

Figure 5.3: Relative risks of stroke and of coronary heart disease, estimated from combined results: solid squares represent disease risks in each category relative to risk in the whole population; sizes of squares are proportional to number of events in each diastolic blood pressure (DBP) category; 95% confidence limits are indicated by vertical lines. (Reproduced with permission from Clinical Trial Service Unit, Oxford.)

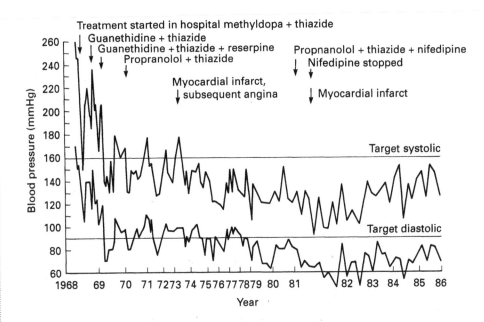

Figure 5.4: Blood pressure record of a Glyncorrwg man over a period of 17 years, starting at age 43 when his blood pressure was measured for the first time at screening in 1968. His initial pressure was 300+/170 mmHg (systolic pressure was beyond the range of the manometer), and blood urea had already reached 80mg/dl.

Malignant hypertension in young women seems usually to be associated with underlying renal disease, cigarette smoking, oral contraception, or all three.[9]

Figure 5.4 shows pressures recorded in a Glyncorrwg man over a period of 17 years, starting at age 43, when his blood pressure was measured for the first time at screening in 1968. His initial pressure was 300+/170 mmHg (systolic pressure was beyond the range of the manometer), and blood urea had already reached 80mg/dl. He had no symptoms, and I was surprised to find no retinopathy. His impaired kidney function quickly returned to normal after the blood pressure was controlled. Although space limits follow-up in Figure 5.4 to 1986, in 1992 he remains in good health with a well controlled blood pressure at age 67, despite three small myocardial infarcts. He is a lucky man; without screening, he would almost certainly have died 20 or more years ago. He was in the presymptomatic phase of malignant hypertension, with an untreated mortality of 50% at 6 months and 99% at 5 years after diagnosis.[10]

Figure 5.5 shows pressures recorded for another man from an adjoining village, which was not included in the 1968 screen. Because of poor practice organization, several measurements of very high pressures were recorded at age 51 before his retinopathy was recognized and pressure was controlled. The delay was fortunately not fatal, but might easily have been. He also is now in good health with a well controlled blood pressure.

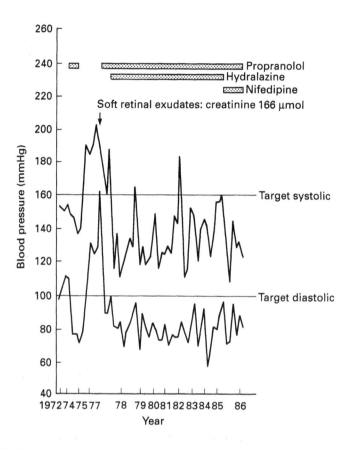

Figure 5.5: Blood pressures recorded for a man who was not included in the 1968 screen. The record begins in 1972, when he was 46 years old.

Neither of these men had headache or other alerting symptoms; both were on the brink of brain infarction or irreversible kidney failure. There is no way of looking for these uncommon but extremely dangerous and urgent cases, which does not entail measurement of all blood pressures in the whole adult population—in other words, some form of screening. They may be rare, but they are not rare enough to remain outside the experience of most GPs; in two consecutive populations of about 2000, I saw one case in 5 years in the first practice, and three more in 27 years in the second.

Annual reports of medical insurance societies continue to record cases of indefensible neglect or ignorance, in which patients with gross symptoms of headache, visual disturbance, or unexpected bleeding from any site, have not had their blood pressures measured, sometimes even after an optician has reported disc changes.[11] It is only a matter of time before malpractice will be rightly extended to include failure to record blood pressure routinely in patients without symptoms. The malignant phase is usually preceded by a substantial rise in pressure for at least 5 years without symptoms, so if screening or case finding systems operate efficiently on a 5-year cycle, few will be missed.

Symptoms of Hypertension

There are two sets of hypertensive symptoms: symptoms *of* hypertension, and symptoms *with* hypertension.

Violent headache is an important and imminently dangerous symptom of severe hypertension, at all ages including childhood. A doctor who does not measure blood pressure in a patient complaining of headache, and without a recently recorded previous value, is certainly foolish and may be blameworthy. However, headache is not a symptom of moderate or mild hypertension. From a diastolic threshold of 130 mmHg, headaches become commoner in hypertensives than in normotensive controls,[12] but below this level there is no difference from the prevalence of headache in random samples of the general population.[13]

Robinson[14] studied the relation of supposedly classic hypertensive symptoms (headache, dizziness, breathlessness, fatigue, palpitations, insomnia, anxiety, and depression) to levels of blood pressure, decisions of patients to consult doctors, and of doctors (in the 1960s) to measure blood pressure. The only symptom showing any significant association with pressure was breathlessness, and this was related more to obesity than to blood pressure.

In the early 1950s, when tuberculosis was still common, the main rational indication for requesting a chest radiograph was not chronic cough, night sweats, weight loss, or haemoptysis, but simply the absence of a previous examination during the last 10 years. If it was to be fully ascertained before causing irreversible damage, tuberculosis had to be actively sought everywhere, not only in those with symptoms. The same applies to measurement of blood pressure today; the main indication for measuring blood pressure should be that no such measurement has been recorded during the previous 5 years. For too many patients, the first symptom of high blood pressure is still stroke, heart failure, retinal artery occlusion, or myocardial infarction.

Bursting Effects And Blocking Effects

Damage from high blood pressure can be crudely but usefully divided into bursting effects, which are closely, directly, and reversibly related to high blood pressure, and blocking effects, whose relation to blood pressure is much more complex.

Bursting effects are: brain haemorrhages and capsular infarcts, arteriolar necrosis in the brain, retina and kidney, ruptured aorta, and left ventricular heart failure. They are caused directly by pressure alone, and rarely occur below a diastolic threshold of about 120 mmHg. They are therefore most evident in accelerated (malignant) hypertension, and in the upper range of severe high blood pressure. They are fully and rapidly preventable by assiduous control of blood pressure.

Blocking effects are: atherothrombotic plaque in large and middle sized arteries resulting in angina, claudication, carotid embolism, and thrombosis in the brain and coronary arteries. They are causally related to blood pressure at all levels; at any level, however low, higher pressure implies higher risk, so that (for example) risk of coronary thrombosis is higher at 150/85 than at 140/80 mmHg, although both of these are below any current clinical definition of hypertension. However, they are also causally related to smoking, blood cholesterol, and fibrinogen, generally more closely than to blood pressure. There is little evidence that they are reversible by reduction in blood pressure alone over periods of about 5 years, but there is good evidence that they are at least partially reversible over much shorter periods by stopping smoking, and by reducing blood cholesterol and fibrinogen.

Stroke

Strokes can be defined clinically as any acute loss of brain function (focal, or occasionally global) lasting more than 24 hours or leading to death, without an apparent non-vascular cause. Persistent minor loss of function after 24 hours may be difficult for non-specialists to demonstrate, but careful evaluation of the opinion of other members of the family often reveal more than neurological signs. Without computerized tomography (CT) diagnosis is uncertain; 1.5% of 325 consecutive cases of apparent stroke, so diagnosed by experienced neurologists before CT, proved after CT to have other causes (two primary and one metastatic brain tumour and two subdural haematomas).[15]

All kinds of interrrupted arterial blood supply to the brain, and thereby all forms of brain infarction, are increased by high blood pressure. There is a closer association with haemorrhage than with thrombosis or embolism, but all these mechanisms of brain infarction are positively associated with arterial pressure. More importantly, they are associated reversibly; if pressure is reduced, so is the risk, and quickly.

The mechanisms of stroke are:

- ruptures of large berry aneurysms, usually resulting in subarachnoid haemorrhage
- ruptures of Charcot-Bouchard microaneurysms, usually resulting in intracerebral haemorrhage
- emboli of mural thrombi from atherosclerotic carotid arteries, usually pre-

ceded by warning TIAs; emboli may also come from the heart after myocardial infarction, or from the left atrium after weeks or months of heart failure, especially with valvular disease; all of these (including valvular disease) are commonly associated with high blood pressure

■ intracerebral infarcts, usually capsular or cerebellar, often with histological evidence of arteriolar necrosis despite absence of other features of malignant hypertension in life; peceding pressures have usually been very high.

Non-fatal strokes outnumber fatal strokes by about five to one, so disability is a much bigger problem than mortality. Stroke risk is more closely associated with blood pressure than coronary risk. In the UK, it is estimated that about 40% of all strokes are attributable to systolic pressures of 140 mmHg or more.[16] After standardizing for age, men aged 40–59 with systolic pressures at 160–180 mmHg have a roughly four times higher risk of stroke during the next 8 years, compared with men with systolic pressures at 140–159 mmHg, and there is a similar but smaller relation to diastolic pressure.[17]

Although both stroke and coronary disease risks are related to blood pressure, other risk factors for stroke differ from those for coronary disease.[18] There is no relationship with blood cholesterol in UK studies, and the independent association with smoking is much less than for blood pressure. Male smokers had a more than twofold risk of stroke in the same study, but there was no relationship to the amount smoked, and those who stopped smoking did not reduce their stroke risk significantly. However, there seems to be a synergistic relationship with high blood pressure, so that the combination of smoking with systolic pressure of 160–180 mmHg increases stroke risk more than 10-fold. Frank diabetes doubled stroke risk in both sexes over 16 years of follow-up in the Framingham study.[19]

There are other undiscovered major determinants which must account for the steep decline in stroke mortality, mainly for haemorrhagic stroke,[20] observed in most countries for at least the last 35 years.[21] For example, in North American women over 65, reduction by one standard deviation (SD) in bone mineral density predicts a roughly 300% increase in stroke mortality, compared with only a 70% increase with one SD rise in systolic pressure,[22] and ventilatory function is also a powerful indicator for fatal stroke.[23] A directly causal relationship is unlikely; diminished bone mass seems to be a good general marker for poor health, poor diet, and reduced activity. This example emphasizes how much we still don't know, even for an outcome of high blood pressure which seems much more straightforward than coronary disease.

However, Figure 5.6 is a reminder of how effective treatment of severe high blood pressure can be in preventing stroke in these very high risk patients, and how important it is to keep trying. In 162 hypertensive patients who had already survived one stroke, Beevers[24] compared subsequent cardiovascular events in three groups: those with good control (mean diastolic pressure <100 mmHg), fair control (mean diastolic pressure 100–109 mmHg), and poor control (mean diastolic pressure >110 mmHg). All were followed up for an average of 4 years. There is an obvious difference in the amount of stroke and heart failure according

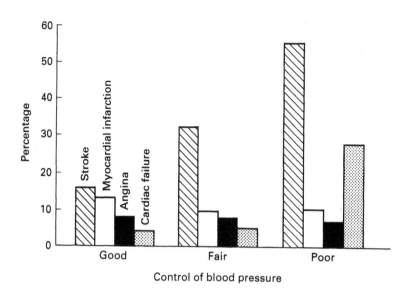

Figure 5.6: Frequency of cardiovascular and cerebrovascular disease in relation to control of blood pressure[24]. (Reproduced with permission from *The Lancet*.)

to quality of control, but little difference (and that in the wrong direction) for myocardial infarction.

Strokes account for about 12% of all deaths. About 25% of all strokes, and about 8% of fatal strokes, occur under 65 years of age. Numerous controlled trials of treatment for high blood pressure have confirmed reductions of around 45% in stroke mortality. This reduction would probably be inceased by wider use of low dose aspirin in this high risk group, and certainly by aspirin use in those with a history of TIAs. If all moderate to severe high blood pressure were controlled by treatment with antihypertensive medication and all patients with TIAs were treated with aspirin, stroke mortality would be reduced by an estimated 17% in the whole population.[25]

Risks from cerebral haemorrhage are probably increased by aspirin. Cerebral haemorrhage can be diagnosed reliably only by CT scanning (still not available in about half of all UK health districts), but because thrombotic and embolic strokes occur about five times more often than haemorrhagic strokes,[15] unselective use of aspirin still seems justified by improved outcome overall, at least until CT scanning becomes routinely available throughout the UK. Although increased risk from gastric erosion is small, it is nevertheless real. It is probably reduced by use of enteric coated aspirin.[25] Dosage remains controversial, with some experts still advocating 300 mg daily, and others 75 mg daily. Aspirin has a powerful and remarkably sustained effect on platelet adhesiveness, still measurable 4 weeks after a single dose. As gastrointestinal haemorrhage is measurably increased even at a dose of 75 mg daily, the larger dose of 300 mg daily may be optimal until the experts agree.

Eye Damage

Subconjunctival arteriolar haemorrhage is common at all levels of increased blood pressure, but more so at higher pressures.[27] Therefore, like headache, it is an obvious although non-specific indication for checking pressure.

Nearly all forms of retinal damage are commoner in people with high blood pressure: retinal haemorrhage, retinal detachment, and both venous and arterial central retinal occlusion, all of which may lead to blindness. Again the association is causal and reversible, and all these occur at all levels of hypertension.

Kidney Damage

Kidney damage in high blood pressure occurs in three circumstances. First, preceding kidney disease may raise blood pressure. Secondly, high blood pressure may cause kidney damage, by thrombotic occlusion of an atherosclerotic renal artery or by bilateral renal arteriolar necrosis in malignant hypertension. Even in a symptomless patient, renal damage in malignant hypertension may already be irreversibly and relentlessly progressive, even if blood pressure is controlled. Before the days of dialysis and transplant, late diagnosis of these symptomless patients meant certain death. Finally, kidney damage may coexist with high blood pressure, neither causing it nor initiated by it, but always likely to deteriorate faster if pressure is uncontrolled.

It is a good rule that, except in the malignant phase, high blood pressure is rarely if ever the principal cause of renal failure. Seriously impaired kidney function should never be attributed to uncomplicated high blood pressure alone, except in the malignant phase, although it may well result from a complication such as renal infarction. A second good rule is that in all states of impaired renal function, however caused, good control of even moderately raised pressure preserves renal function and delays end-stage failure. This is particularly important in diabetics, for whom early renal damage should always be assumed even in the absence of proteinuria.

Heart Failure

Like stroke and retinal damage, heart failure may be caused by high arterial pressure, and prevented by its control. Unlike them, it is often ignored or misdiagnosed. It is still necessary to teach many trainees that chronic cough is commonly the main presenting symptom of heart failure, and that breathlessness, lung crackles, and impaired peak expiratory flow rates may represent heart disease as well as, or instead of, lung disease.

Heart failure remains grossly underestimated as a major preventable and treatable cause of death, accounting for about 5% of all adult hospital admissions.[28, 29] The Framingham Study[30] showed that high blood pressure is now its principal cause. Later studies in Framingham showed that about half of all patients died within 5 years of diagnosis despite traditional treatment with diuretics and digoxin, a prognosis similar to State II squamous cell lung cancer and worse than Stage II breast cancer. Modern treatment with ACE inhibitors has reduced mortality substantially, but McMurray and Dargie[31] estimate that in the UK only one in five patients receive them.

Hypertensive heart failure is easy to recognize when it presents as acute left ventricular failure, with paroxysmal nocturnal dyspnoea, wheezing, triple rhythm, crackles all over the lungs and high blood pressure. It is not so easy to recognize in the form of untreated hypertension over many years, slowly replaced by 'normal' blood pressure as the left ventricle fails. These are the women with 'ischaemic heart failure', so-called because they are seen by specialist or junior hospital staff without past evidence from GP records; their male counterparts have mostly already died from coronary disease.

A lot of heart failure is therefore preventable, and as high blood pressure in middle age becomes more fully diagnosed and treated, it should decline in incidence, as we have already seen for emergency night calls for left ventricular failure. As every elderly GP knows, these were once an almost weekly event; now they are seen once or twice a year, if that. It seems a good subject for audit.

Ruptured Aorta

Ruptured aortic aneurysm is a common and probably increasing[32] cause of sudden or rapid death (3 in 25 years in the Glyncorrwg population of roughly 2000). It usually follows long standing hypertension. Abdominal aneurysms sometimes give warning symptoms and may be suspected clinically and confirmed radiologically by their calcified outline, as atheroma is always severe. They are now easily measured by ultrasound, and there is now a good case for systematic screening.[33]

Above a critical diameter of 6 cm, half of them rupture within a year; below this threshold, about one-fifth rupture within a year. Patients are usually elderly, and these risks should be discussed with patients and relatives against the risks and personal costs of a Teflon graft.

Angina and Claudication

In unscreened populations, angina and claudication are common presenting symptoms of long standing high blood pressure. As high arterial pressure speeds the deposition of atheroma in large and medium arteries, angina and claudication tend to occur sooner in hypertensives than in normotensives, but this also depends on serum cholesterol levels, fibrinogen levels, and smoking. Both symptoms usually improve when pressure is reduced, showing that simple arguments by analogy with plumbing can be misleading.

Coronary Thrombosis

What the public sensibly calls heart attacks, doctors in the 1950s called coronary thrombosis. This emphasized the importance of intra-arterial clotting, rather than the mural atheroma preceding it. Terminology first reflected, then reinforced, practice, which then depended almost entirely on anticoagulants for a standard 6-week course of treatment, often maintained permanently thereafter. By the 1960s, exaggerated early hopes for anticoagulant treatment had been disappointed, clotting was forgotten, and fashion preferred myocardial infarction. We have now moved full circle, with growing rediscovery of the importance of clot formation and thrombolysis, so I have reverted to the original terminology.

Before the advent of tolerable and effective antihypertensive drugs in the early 1960s, heart failure and stroke were the principal outcomes of high blood pressure seen at necropsy. Now that these are largely preventable, coronary thrombosis has replaced them as the most frequent outcome of treated hypertension. Controlled trials have consistently shown that stroke and heart failure are largely preventable by treatment of high blood pressure in middle age, but that coronary thrombosis is rarely preventable, at least over periods of 5 years or less.

Outcome of Hypertension in Developing Countries

Although coronary thrombosis has a smaller and less reversible association with high blood pressure than stroke, it is a much commoner cause of death in the UK and most industrialized economies, particularly in those under 65 years of age. These countries are rightly preoccupied with control of heart attacks, and tend to see control of high blood pressure as a clinically popular (although relatively ineffective) subset of more general strategies for control of coronary disease.

The situation is entirely different in southern Europe and the less industrialized

65

world, where stroke mortality is still much higher than mortality from coronary disease, and the potential effectiveness of blood pressure control is correspondingly higher.

Despite the low pressures found in a few isolated hunter-gatherer, and some rural, populations, high blood pressure in pre-industrial economies is generally at least as common as in industrialized countries, and, in many cases more so. As mean serum total cholesterol levels (even in cities) are generally low, coronary heart disease remains rare despite both high blood pressure and heavy smoking. Coronary disease is increasingly common in the wealthy in poor countries, but in rich countries is becoming concentrated among the less fortunate.[34, 35] For example, in China, accurate age specific mortality rates for stroke and coronary heart disease, and for the prevalence of risk factors in the general population, are now available for Beijing.[36] Men aged 55 had a stroke mortality of 633 per 100 000 and women 428, compared with coronary mortality rates of 129 and 51 per 100 000 respectively; five times as many fatal strokes as coronary deaths in men, and eight times as many in women. Mean cholesterol levels at age 55 were about 4.6 mmol/l in both sexes, and 67% of men and 16% of women smoked. Similarly, in urban black South Africans hypertension is the main cause of premature non-violent death, mainly from stroke and heart failure rather than coronary disease.[37]

Figures like these are characteristic of most populations in black Africa, South America, Asia, and the Middle East, far more typical than the population in Framingham or others in the industrialized world. Even in Spain in 1979, for example, when well on the road to industrialization, deaths from cerebrovascular disease (37% of all deaths) were commoner than deaths from coronary heart disease (22% of all deaths). In a rural area near Salamanca, deaths from cerebrovascular disease in 1959–84 were five times more common (40% of all deaths) than deaths from coronary heart disease (8% of all deaths).[38]

Effective strategies for health must be both national and local. Progress in primary care depends on the most peripheral health workers gaining confidence in their own ability to solve problems using their own experience from their own research base. This starts from comparison of local with national mortality statistics, which gives at least a crude outline of the local task, and a suggestion of reasonable targets for change.

The world literature still lacks realistic accounts from peripheral health workers of the work they are actually doing or trying to do, and the difficulties and opportunities they encounter, expressed in anecdotal as well as statistical terms. These practical health workers have most to contribute to serious discussion of the most important problem now facing medical science; not how to know more to help a few people, but how to get what we already know implemented for all those in greatest need.

You Have to Die Somehow

The lethal outcomes of high blood pressure are, with few exceptions, relatively quick and easy exits compared with other common causes of death, such as cancer, dementia, or Parkinson's disease. Figure 5.7 shows the course of

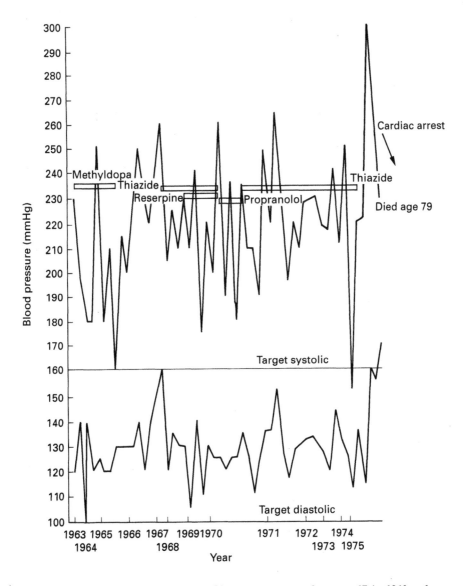

Figure 5.7: Blood pressure record of a Glyncorrwg woman from age 67 in 1963 to her death aged 79.

ineffectively treated high blood pressure in a vigorous old lady who finally died quickly, in 1975, with a massive coronary thrombosis at age 79. Her high blood pressure might have been better controlled by a less tolerant attitude to her systematic non-compliance, mainly caused by side effects from medication then available. It might be easier now.

New (and to me, unexpected) evidence of the effectiveness and tolerability of antihypertensive treatment in the elderly is probably the biggest advance in rational management of high blood pressure during the past decade. However, mortality data which confuse tragedies in youth and middle age with physiological death in the elderly do not contribute to reasoned argument.

References

1. Miall WE and Chinn S (1973) Blood pressure and ageing: Results of a 15–17 year follow-up study in South Wales. *Clin Sci Mol Med* **45**: 23–33s.

2. Austrialian National Blood Pressure Study Management Committee (1980) The Australian therapeutic trial in mild hypertension. *Lancet* **i**: 1261–7.

3. Medical Research Council Working Party (1985) MRC trial of treatment of mild hypertension: Principal results. *Br Med J* **291**: 97–104.

4. Dannenberg AL and Kannel WB (1987) Remission of hypertension. *JAMA* **257**: 1477–83.

5. Parkin DM, Kellett RJ, Maclean DW *et al.* (1979) The management of hypertension: A study of records in general practice. *J R Coll Gen Pract* **29**: 590–4.

6. Miall WE and Chinn S (1974) Screening for hypertension: Some epidemiological observations. *Br Med J* **3**: 595–600.

7. MacMahon S, Peto R, Cutler J *et al.* (1990) Blood pressure, stroke, and coronary heart disease. Part 1: Prolonged differences in blood pressure: Prospective observational studies corrected for the regression dilution bias. *Lancet* **335**: 765–74.

8. Ahmed MEK, Walker JM, Beevers DG *et al.* (1986) Lack of difference between malignant and accelerated hypertension. *Br Med J* **292**: 235–7.

9. Petitti DB and Klatsky AL (1983) Malignant hypertension in women aged

15 to 44 years and its relation to cigarette smoking and oral contraceptives. *Am J Cardiol* **52**: 297–8.

10. Pickering GW (1968) *High blood pressure* (2nd edn, p 414). Churchill, London.

11. MPS Annual Report (1988) *Medical case reports: Blindness from failure to diagnose malignant hypertension*. Medical Protection Society, London.

12. Badran RH, Weir RJ and McGuiness JB (1970) Hypertension and headache. *Scott Med J* **15**: 48.

13. Waters WE (1971) Headache and blood pressure in the community. *Br Med J:* 142–3.

14. Robinson JO (1969) Symptoms and the discovery of high blood pressure. *J Psychosom Res* **13**: 157–61.

15. Sandercock P, Molyneaux A and Warlow C (1985) Value of computerised tomography in patients with stroke: The Oxford Community Stroke Project. *Br Med J* **290**: 193–7.

16. Marmot MG and Poulter NR (1992) Primary prevention of stroke. *Lancet* **339**: 344–7.

17. Shaper AG, Phillips AN, Pocock SJ *et al.* (1991) Risk factors for stroke in middle aged British men. *Br Med J* **302**: 1111–5.

18. Garraway M, Whisnant JP and Drury I (1983) The dichotomy of myocardial and cerebral infarction. *Lancet* **ii**: 1332–5.

19. Garcia MJ, McNamara PM and Gordon T (1974) Morbidity and mortality in diabetics in the Framingham population: Sixteen-year follow-up study. *Diabetes* **23**: 105–11.

20. Yates PO (1964) A change in the pattern of cerebrovascular disease. *Lancet* **i**: 65–9.

21. Charlton JRH and Velez R (1986) Some international comparisons of mortality amenable to medical intervention. *Br Med J* **292**: 295–300.

22. Browner WS, Seeley DG, Vogt TM *et al.* (1991) Non-trauma mortality in elderly women with low mineral bone density. *Lancet* **338**: 355–8.

23. Strachan DP (1991) Ventilatory function as a predictor of fatal stroke. *Br Med J* **302**: 84–7.

24. Beevers DG, Hamilton M, Fairman MJ *et al.* (1973) Antihypertensive treatment and the course of established cerebral vascular disease. *Lancet* i: 1407–9.

25. Dennis M and Warlow C (1991) Strategy for stroke. *Br Med J* **303**: 636–8.

26. Murray FE, Cole AT, Hudson N *et al.* (1992) Possible low-dose aspirin-induced gastropathy. *Lancet* **339**: 1058–9.

27. Pitts JF, Jardine AG, Murray SB *et al.* (1992) Spontaneous subconjunctival haemorrhage: A sign of hypertension? *Br J Ophthalmol* **76**: 297–9.

28. Sutton GC (1990) Epidemiological aspects of heart failure. *Am Heart J* **120**: 1538–40.

29. Smith WM (1985) Epidemiology of congestive heart failure. *Am J Cardiol* **55**: 3A–8A.

30. Kannel WB, Castelli WP, McNamara PM *et al.* (1972) Role of blood pressure in the development of congestive heart failure. *N Engl J Med* **287**: 782.

31. McMurray J and Dargie HJ (1991) Coronary heart disease. *Lancet* **338**: 1546.

32. Fowkes FGR, Macintyre CCA and Buckley CV (1989) Increasing incidence of aortic aneurysms in England and Wales. *Br Med J* **298**: 33–5.

33. Harris PL (1992) Reducing the mortality from abdominal aortic aneurysms: Need for a national screening programme. *Br Med J* **305**: 697–9.

34. Marmot MG (1984) Life style and national and international trends in coronary heart disease mortality. *Postgrad Med J* **60**: 3–8.

35. Marmot MG and McDowall ME (1986) Mortality decline and widening social inequalities. *Lancet* ii: 274–6.

36. Wu Y, Lu C-G Gaao RC *et al.* (1982) Nationwide hypertension screening in China 1979–1980. *Chin Med J* **95**: 101–8.

37. Seftel HC, Johnson S and Muller EA (1980) Distribution and biosocial

correlations of blood pressure levels in Johannesburg blacks. *S Afr Med J* **57**: 313–20.

38. Fernandez Garcia JM (1987) *Apuntes para la lucha contra la hipertension arterial en el medio rural, Ciperez, dos anos de experiencia. II: Jornadas Vitigudinenses sobre hipertension arterial 1986.* Asociacion de Profesionales de la Salud de la zona de Vitigudino, Salamanca.

6

Thresholds for Follow-Up and Medication

Since blood pressure is continuously and positively related to risk throughout its range, and below a diastolic pressure of 130 mmHg symptoms are generally unrelated to blood pressure, diagnosis of high blood pressure cannot depend on presented complaint. It is therefore certainly not an illness, and short of organ damage or the malignant phase, is not a disease in any useful sense. The matter would be clearer if we stopped using the pretentious title hypertension, and spoke only of high blood pressure, 'high' being an obviously relative term.

However, the practice of medicine inescapably depends on sorting people into those who need intervention and those who do not. Intervention must then be justified by a diagnosis; in practice, diagnosis implies treatment, and vice versa.

Criteria for diagnosis of hypertension should therefore be based on current evidence of the point at which therapeutic interventions begin to do more good than harm. This evidence will change as treatments (not necessarily medications) become safer, more tolerable, and more effective, so diagnostic criteria will also change. The WHO definition of hypertension, which starts from a phase–5 diastolic threshold of 90 mmHg, ignores such evidence and is no less arbitrary than the many others which have preceded it.

An American study of factors influencing the decision to treat or not to treat high blood pressure found only 20% of the variance could be accounted for by generally accepted clinical variables such as systolic and diastolic pressure, fundus changes, electrocardiographic and biochemical evidence.[1] This does not mean the other 80% of these decisions were irrational, but that many factors which are ignored in most textbooks do in fact influence clinical decisions. GPs who do not adhere to rigid protocols omitting these other factors should be congratulated rather than condemned.[2]

These other factors include real or presumed patient expectations, work-load, doctors' opinions about the capacity of individual patients to cope with treatment or benefit from it, priority given to other potentially conflicting clinical or social problems patients may have, economic incentives or disincentives for enlarging the scope of care, and the effects of pharmaceutical promotion, which although always denied, are presumably real, since they continue to be well paid for.

A morally defensible basis for decisions on treatment must rest principally on results of controlled clinical trials. These are applicable to our own patients individually only to the extent that they, and the ways we treat them, resemble the patients and treatments in these trials. This means that clinicians must be familiar not only with the main trial results, but with their case material and design.

Evidence from Controlled Trials of Antihypertensive Treatment

Cardiovascular epidemiologists from the MRC, Harvard, Yale, Auckland and other centres reviewed 14 major randomized controlled trials of antihypertensive drugs in middle age, published from 1965 to 1986.[3] These used mainly diuretics and/or beta-blockers, observing 37 000 patients followed for from 1.4 to 7 years, a total of 185 000 patient years. Sexes were almost equally represented, with only a 3% male excess.

Grouped results showed that a mean 5-year reduction of 5–6 mmHg in diastolic or 10–12 mmHg systolic pressure was associated with a 35–40% reduction in stroke events and a 20–25% reduction in coronary events, fatal and non-fatal. Fatal strokes fell by 42%, almost as great as the fall in all strokes, but fatal coronary heart disease fell by only 14%, roughly half the fall in all heart attacks, fatal or non-fatal. Benefit for stroke was much larger, and more quickly attained, than benefit for coronary heart disease. There was no significant effect on non-cardiovascular mortality. The authors concluded that patients compliant with antihypertensive medication, who reduced diastolic pressure by 8–10 mmHg and systolic pressure by 16–20 mmHg, reduced their stroke risks by 50% and their coronary risks by 20% within a few years, and that longer term treatment might reduce coronary risk by about 30%.

Effective antihypertensive drugs first became available in the middle 1950s, and were in wide use by the early 1960s. Except for diuretics, which were for a long time wrongly considered to be only marginally effective, all of them caused serious side effects. Their use in hitherto asymptomatic patients was therefore difficult and generally limited to a small market.

The first evidence that their use could result in a net saving of life came from small controlled studies of subjects referred to hospital specialists with severe and immediately dangerous hypertension, nearly all of them with evidence of organ damage.[4-7] All these studies showed benefit for patients with moderate to severe high blood pressure, sustained over weeks or months in the range 175/105 mmHg or more. There has been an international consensus ever since that treatment is mandatory at this level.

People with mean blood pressures below this threshold but above 140/90 mmHg outnumber these moderate and severe hypertensives by three or four to one, and here there is still no real international consensus.

The MRC Trial

Review of controlled trials of treatment of mild hypertension in the diastolic range 90–104 mmHg prompts a serious question: does medical opinion grow from evidence, or does evidence grow from medical opinion?

The largest controlled trial so far of treatment for mild hypertension in middle age was reported by the MRC.[8] It had more than 17 000 subjects and 85 000 patient years of observation, and was conducted by specially trained nurses in general practice. It had a single blind randomized placebo controlled design, and is likely to be the last trial of this size without actively medicated controls.

Using bendrofluazide and propranolol as its principal drugs for screened men and women aged 35–64, in the diastolic range 90–109 mmHg, it sought to answer two main questions: does treatment for this group reduce strokes or coronary events, and if so, what are the costs of these reductions in terms of iatrogenic impairment and medical, nursing and administrative labour?

Treatment reduced the number of strokes by 45%, agreeing well with all earlier trials. However, strokes in this age group were rare, even in mild to moderate hypertensives, so it took 850 patient years of treatment to prevent each one. An average GP list of about 2000 subjects of all ages will contain around 100 patients in this age and pressure group, so each GP might expect to prevent about one stroke every 8.5 years by finding and treating all of them.

Treatment had no significant effect on coronary events, and worse still, had no effect on all cause mortality for both sexes combined, even if strokes were included. This was because the small reduction in cardiovascular deaths in men was counterbalanced by an increase in non-cardiovascular deaths in women, chiefly from cancer. The principal harm done to patients seemed to be erectile failure in 16% of men taking thiazides, reversible when treatment was stopped and associated with what we now know to be unncessarily high doses.

These results were based only on a 5-year follow-up, and it is probable, although not certain, that additional benefits might have appeared later, if observation had been continued. Figure 6.1 shows that the difference between treated and untreated subjects grew steadily through the 5 years of the Veterans' Administration second trial;[7] it is reasonable to believe that benefits are greater, the longer control is maintained.

Control of mild to moderate hypertension in middle age will probably prevent much heart failure in the elderly, a lot more strokes, and probably much multi-

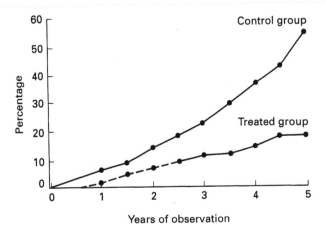

Figure 6.1: Estimated cumulative incidence of all morbid events over a five-year period for treated and control groups in Part II of the Veterans' Administration trial (life table method)[7]. (Reproduced with permission).

infarct dementia.[9] It will prevent some coronary disease, but not a lot; atheroma certainly cannot be reversed quickly, but very prolonged treatment may be more effective.

The Australian Trial

The smaller Australian National Blood Pressure Study (ANBPS)[10] preceded and set the scene for the MRC. With much arm twisting, of which I had personal experience, it was the basis for international guidelines endorsed unanimously by a World Heath Organization conference[11] at Bürgenstock in 1982, before the MRC or Hypertension Detection and Follow-up Program (HDFP) results were available.[12]

The ANBPS followed men and women aged 30–69 with diastolic pressures 95–109 mmHg at entry for 4 years. They were volunteers, so instead of over representing high morbidity, as all the hospital based studies certainly did, this trial was probably selective for well people, with less organ damage and lower risk than the average for the whole population. It allocated subjects randomly to treatment or no treatment; there was no placebo group, so side effects could not be measured. The study was relatively small, and was wound up as soon as differences between treated and control subjects reached lower limits of significance.

An important finding was that the risk of complications in treated subjects was proportionate to achieved pressures rather than entry pressures, and this was subsequently confirmed in other trials, including retrospective analyses of the Veterans' Administration studies. Quality of care was therefore all important in achieving results.

As before, there was a large reduction in strokes, but a barely significant fall in coronary heart disease. The actual number of deaths in the two groups were five in the treated and 11 in the control groups, representing 2000 patient-years of treatment for each life saved.

The Hypertension Detection and Follow-Up Program

Although in 1976 the only available controlled evidence of significant and substantial benefit from treatment of hypertension was based on hospital referred cases and began at a diastolic threshold of 105 mmHg, 78% of doctors in New York State were already prescribing antihypertensive drugs for the general population in the diastolic range 90–100 mmHg. By 1979 (when there was still no controlled evidence of significant benefit) this proportion had risen to 90%.[13]

By the time a large enough American trial could be set up, either to challenge or legitimize this consensus, it was already considered unethical to withhold treatment from anyone with a diastolic pressure over 90 mmHg. So the trial which eventually took place, the Hypertension Detection and Follow-up Program,[12] instead of comparing randomized treated cases with untreated controls, compared the mortality results of a structured system of free treatment and active recall by specially trained nurse practitioners ('stepped care'), with the results of the ordinary American medical market ('usual care'), assuming that purpose built structured care would be more rigorous than marketed care, particularly for mild hypertension.

However, this trial did draw its subjects from random samples of local populations rather than from hospital referred cases. From these it identified 11 000 subjects and observed 55 000 patient-years of treatment, randomized to two groups. The experimental group received 'stepped care' from specially trained nurses, following a protocol which included a variable amount of advice about other problems. Treatment and transport were free and patients were actively recalled to follow-up. The work was done in a variety of ambulant clinic settings, mostly attached to hospitals, as no network of general practice comparable to the UK exists in the USA. The control group received 'usual care' from whatever agency they normally used, whether a family physician, internist, cardiologist, hospital ambulant clinic or emergency room.

After 5 years, cardiovascular mortality fell by 26% and non-cardiovascular mortality by 13% more in the 'stepped care' group than in the 'usual care' group. There were large differences in coronary as well as stroke mortality, which were greater for those in the lower than in the higher ranges of hypertension studied.

The HDFP trial seemed well designed to demonstrate a difference in outcome between the work of a free planned public service, and the consequences of marketed medical care. It is of unique interest in that, so far as I know, this is the only randomized controlled trial ever performed comparing planned public service with unplanned privately marketed care. Needless to say, this aspect has been almost universally ignored. The HDFP was used not to answer the question most appropriate to its design (which of these two kinds of health service works best?), but to reinforce what doctors were already doing.

Differences Between the Trials

How can we account for the difference between the MRC trial, which had little effect on coronary disease, and the ANBPS and HDFP, which had apparently positive results? The ANBPS was a relatively small trial, and was wound up on ethical grounds as soon as marginal levels of significance were reached for all terminations, both strokes and coronary events. Set against the six-fold greater size of the MRC trial, with a better design and equal quality control, the simplest explanation is probably correct; the MRC and the ANBPS results approximate to the same truth, but the MRC comes closer because of its larger scale.

The HDFP was much bigger than the ANBPS and cannot be criticized for insufficient numbers. Interpretation is difficult because of the curious nature of its controls. HDFP results were given for three strata of blood pressure at entry: diastolic ranges 90–104 (Stratum I), 105–114 (Stratum II), and >115 mmHg (Stratum III), with 72% of subjects in Stratum I. In all strata there was a significant reduction in strokes and stroke mortality for patients receiving free stepped care, compared with controls receiving marketed care, a result in line with other studies. Unlike them, however, there was also a 26% reduction in deaths from myocardial infarction, entirely restricted to Stratum I (diastolic 90–104 mmHg). Benefits were greatest in black women, followed by black men, and then by white men; there was no benefit for white women. This suggests that gains from free structured care were greatest for the previously most disadvantaged groups, a theory reinforced by the still unexplained 13% reduction in non–cardiovascular mortality. Finally, 25% of Stratum I subjects were already on antihypertensive medication when they were screened, and their original pressures before treatment were not available; this group was therefore contaminated by an unknown number of more severe hypertensives poorly controlled at entry.

Social Composition of the Trials

An outstanding and somewhat neglected difference between the MRC and ANBPS studies on the one hand, and the HDFP on the other, was their different social composition. The MRC trial recruited volunteer group practices with 10 000 or more patients. Its authors admit, and participating GPs confirm, that these were heavily biased towards comfortable middle class market town and suburban practices, areas with generally low morbidity and certainly not of the same social character as Glasgow, Liverpool, Belfast and the South Wales valleys, the worst areas in Britain for both stroke and coronary mortality.

In contrast, the HDFP drew on generally more sick, more urban, more black, more industrial, and more deprived populations. Tyroler[14] has written interestingly on this. Of male subjects in the HDFP, 30% were black, compared with about 11% for the whole American population. All-causes mortality and stroke mortality in Stratum I of the HDFP stepped care group were each nearly three times higher than in the placebo group of the MRC trial, and coronary mortality was over twice as high. Primary care teams working in high mortality, high morbidity, and high unemployment areas of Britain may well feel greater affinity with the HDFP populations than with those of the MRC trial. Providing it is offered and accepted, perhaps treatment is more effective in neglected populations; if so, the main lesson of the HDFP is once again that treatment should be free, structured and targeted at high risk populations, rather than marketed by entrepreneurs.

None of this helps to define a rational threshold for routine intervention.

Consensus Threshold for Medication

The MRC trial results provide little support for antihypertensive medication in the diastolic range 90–110 mmHg in middle age, except where there is either positive evidence of organ damage, or exceptional risk of such damage, as in diabetics or those with a family history of stroke or early coronary disease. A detailed analysis of the cost effectiveness of treatment in the MRC trial range[15] supports this conclusion. In its consensus guidelines for treatment, the British Hypertension Society[16] concluded that in asymptomatic hypertension without organ damage, medication should start from a diastolic threshold of 110 mmHg, based on three measurements on separate occasions, or from a threshold of 100 mmHg based on repeated measurements over 4 months or more. They also suggested that in every case, three other criteria be taken into account, together with the level and stability over time of blood pressure itself: age, sex, and other cardiovascular risk factors.

The emphasis on repeated measurements, made over months rather than weeks or days, was new. Taken seriously, it implied quite a jolt to customary practice, not only in primary care but also for hospital out-patient departments.

The Working Party report had little to say about systolic thresholds. It appeared 2 years before the report of the SHEP study on isolated systolic hypertension in the elderly,[17] which clearly established the value of controlling systolic hypertension in the systolic range 160–219 mmHg (mean of six readings)*.

Contrary to most expectations, certainly to my own, energetic treatment of hypertension in the elderly has been consistently vindicated, most of all by the most recent Swedish trial showing a 43% reduction in all-causes mortality for treated patients aged 70–84 at entry.[18] In this age group, 66 patient years of treatment prevented one death from all causes. In the light of this recent evidence, further considered in Chapter 21, from age 65 antihypertensive medication should probably be considered routinely from a threshold of 160/90 mmHg sustained through three readings on separate days.

Consensus Target for Medication

There seems to be general agreement that medication should aim at a target diastolic pressure below 90 mmHg, and a systolic pressure below 160 mmHg. Providing pressures fall slowly enough for brain circulation to adapt, the further they fall the better, within reason. How 'reason' is in practice defined will depend on the age of the patient, symptoms, and the personal experience of the clinician in charge.

This is where disagreements begin over the 'J-curve' of mortality in relation to blood pressure. Hypertensives are more likely than other patients to have narrowed arteries causing critically impaired perfusion of some organs, particularly the heart, brain, and kidney. If blood pressure is reduced, particularly if it is reduced rapidly, perfusion may fall enough to compromise organ function, or even to cause infarction. There can be no reasonable disagreement that such a J-curve must exist,[19] even if the numbers involved are too small to be obvious in a generally well population subjected to epidemiological study.

Clinical experience and some trials[20] suggest that there is no such J-curve in hypertensives who feel well and have no evidence of organ damage, and if blood pressure levels well below target threshold can be attained easily and without symptoms, prognosis should be correspondingly improved. Once systolic pressures are consistently below, say, 115 mmHg, most clinicians will rightly reduce medication. If on prolonged follow-up such low pressures are consistently maintained, a trial of withdrawal of medication is the next obvious step, always remembering that, in most of these patients, blood pressure will eventually rise again, and medication will have to be resumed[21]; all such patients should be followed up 3-monthly for at least a year, and annually thereafter.

For patients in early heart failure or with other evidence of organ damage, there are obviously possible risks from reducing blood pressure too far, and even

---

* The BHS Working Party published revised guidelines in 1993 (Sever P, Beevers G, Bulpitt C *et al.* [1993] Management guidelines in essential hypertension: Report of the second Working Party of the British Hypertension Society. *Br Med J* **306**: 983–7).

greater risks from reducing it too fast. The greatest risk of all, however, is not to reduce blood pressure at all.

Is Treatment of Mild Hypertension Worthwhile?

It is difficult, although perhaps not impossible, to justify subjecting over 500 people in the diastolic range 90–109 mmHg to continuous antihypertensive medication and regular monitoring for 5 years, so that three should avoid strokes and one a coronary thrombosis. These are the odds calculable from present evidence on treatment in middle age, and it seems to me they should be put frankly to patients in this category, so they can make their own choice.

Of course, given that choice, most patients still ask, 'But what do *you* advise, doctor?', to which the only justifiable answer must start with 'If I were you . . .', and really mean it. Being myself reluctant to submit to doctors, I am sceptical, and therefore have had few takers on these terms, below a diastolic threshold of 105 mmHg. All terms of this equation change in the elderly, but as antihypertensive medication becomes more effective, alternative modes of death may seem more repellent.

The proportion of middle aged hypertensives for whom medication can now be justified is much smaller (about 10% of most British populations) than most of us once thought and hoped. Can the contribution of personal clinical care therefore be ignored in public health strategy? In a well argued paper, Geoffrey Rose[22] comes close to this conclusion, without quite embracing it. Within the limits of the NHS as it then was, he may have been right. However, 10% of the whole population is not a small number. Judging from the way we deal with diabetes, affecting only 2%, it is a much larger number than we can cope with without substantial redeployment of resources towards primary care.

No one suggests that severe high blood pressure in the range 200/120 mmHg plus should be left untreated, yet this is usually asymptomatic at least until there is organ damage, and often remains so until renal, retinal, or brain damage is irreversible. However high the threshold is set, the only way to identify all those who need antihypertensive medication in youth or middle age is to screen (or case find) everyone between the ages of 30 and 65 at least once every 5 years. Such screening will detect much greater numbers of people below this threshold, although at high relative risk. Are these people to be ignored, or are we going to do something positive to help them?

This is the central paradox of all strategies for blood pressure control; detection and effective treatment for the few at exceptional risk requires organized contact with everyone. Does anyone seriously suggest that such organized mass contact with health workers, potentially motivated for prevention by their own experience of unprevented cardiovascular disease, should not be used to improve personal care?

The answer is to recognize that attempts to reduce blood pressure in isolation from control of other risk factors is futile. The only effective strategy is to accept high blood pressure as one of several risks, and the search for it as only one of several possible entry points to a final common pathway: reduction of premature coronary thrombosis and stroke by control of multiple risk factors, both in the whole population and by concentration of personal care on those at highest risk. As most of the British population is registered with a GP, GPs' responsibility to all of their patients means responsibility to all of the people. Search for high blood pressure is a good entry point to this much larger task, because, for historical reasons, this is what most interested GPs have wanted to do. The same point would eventually be reached by comprehensive search for any other common problem: diabetes, obesity, smoking, airways obstruction, alcohol abuse, hyperlipidaemia, schizophrenia and many others.

Conclusion

For middle age, in the endless discussions about who should or should not be treated with antihypertensive drugs at the broad base of the hypertensive pyramid, we are in danger of losing sight of the apex of severe, imminently dangerous hypertension, in which the need for effective treatment is beyond doubt.

On the best controlled evidence we have in 1993, antihypertensive medication in middle age is mandatory for blood pressure sustained at or over 170/105 mmHg, using either a systolic or diastolic value, whichever is the higher. Below this threshold, decisions to treat with antihypertensive drugs should be based on a family history of stroke for ruptured aorta, rapid progression of pressure, evidence of organ damage, complicating disease (mainly diabetes), onset under the age of 40, or interacting risk factors, which are discussed in Chapter 7. For younger age groups, discussed in Chapter 20, we appear to have no controlled evidence. For older groups, discussed in Chapter 21, the evidence now seems to me to justify a much more aggressive approach, but this will depend very much on what patients want after fully informed discussion.

Decisions to intervene should depend on patients' agreement, which should in turn depend on trust, shared information and understanding. The disappointing results of the MRC trial should not be misused to endorse passivity in tackling necessary and effective work which is still less than half done.

References

1. Gibson ES, Sackett DL, Hayes RB *et al.* (1978) Clinical determinants of the decision to treat primary hypertension. In: Abstracts of the 18th Confer-

ence on Cardiovascular Disease Epidemiology. *CVD Epidemiology Newsletter no. 25*. American Heart Association, Dallas.

2. Smith TDW and Clayton D (1990) Individual variation between general practitioners in labelling of hypertension. *Br Med J* **300**: 74–5.

3. Collins R, Peto R, MacMahon S *et al.* (1990) Blood pressure, stroke, and coronary heart disease. Part 2: Short term reductions in blood pressure: Overview of randomised drug trials in their epidemiological context. *Lancet* **335**: 827–38.

4. Leishman AWD (1963) Merits of reducing high blood pressure. *Lancet* **i**: 1284–8.

5. Hamilton M, Thompson EN and Wisniewski TKM (1964) The role of blood pressure control in preventing complications of hypertension. *Lancet* **i**: 235–8.

6. Veterans' Administration Co-operative Study Group on Antihypertensive Agents (1967) Effects of treatment on morbidity in hypertension. I: Results in patients with diastolic blood pressures averaging 115 through 129 mmHg. *JAMA* **202**: 1028–34.

7. Veterans' Administration Co-operative Study Group on Antihypertensive Agents (1970) Effects of treatment on morbidity in hypertension. II: Results in patients with diastolic pressures averaging 90 through 114 mmHg. *JAMA* **213**: 1143–52.

8. Medical Research Council Working Party (1985) MRC trial of treatment of mild hypertension: Principal results. *Br Med J* **291**: 97–104.

9. Hachinski V (1992) Preventable senility: A call for action against the vascular dementias. *Lancet* **340**: 645–8.

10. Australian National Blood Pressure Study Management Committee (ANBPS) (1980) The Australian therapeutic trial in mild hypertension. *Lancet* **i**: 1261–7.

11. World Health Organization/International Society of Hypertension Conference (1982) *Memorandum on guidelines for the treatment of mild hypertension*. WHO Cardiovascular Diseases Unit, Geneva.

12. Hypertension Detection and Follow-up Program Cooperative Group (1979) Five-year findings of the HDFP, I and II. *JAMA* **242**: 2562–71.

13. Guttmacher S, Teitelman M, Chapin G *et al*. (1981) Ethics and preventive medicine: The case of borderline hypertension. In: Hastings Center Report, February 1981.

14. Tyroler HA (1983) Race, education, and 5-year mortality in HDFP Stratum I referred-care males. In: Gross F and Strasser T (eds) *Mild hypertension: Recent advances*, p 163. Raven, New York.

15. Milner PC and Johnson IS (1985) Treating mild hypertension. *Lancet* ii: 1364.

16. Swales JD, Ramsay LE, Coope JR *et al*. (1989) Treating mild hypertension: Report of the British Hypertension Society Working Party. *Br Med J* 298: 694–8.

17. SHEP Cooperative Research Group (1991) Prevention of stroke by antihypertensive drug treatment in older persons with isolated systolic hypertension. *JAMA* 265: 3255–64.

18. Dahlof B, Lindholm LH, Hansson L *et al*. (1991) Morbidity and mortality in the Swedish Trial in Old Patients with Hypertension (STOP-Hypertension). *Lancet* 338: 1281–4.

19. Cruickshank JM (1992) The J curve lives. *Lancet* 339: 187.

20. Coope J (1990) Hypertension: The cause of the J curve. *J Hum Hypertens* 4: 1–4.

21. Fletcher AE, Franks PJ and Bulpitt CJ (1988) The effect of withdrawing antihypertensive therapy: A review. *J Hypertens* 6: 431–6.

22. Rose GA (1981) Strategies of prevention: Lessons from cardiovascular disease. *Br Med J* 282: 1847–52.

7

High Blood Pressure as a Combination Risk Factor

Risk factors for coronary heart disease and stroke ■ Motivating attributes ■ Smoking ■ Is stopping smoking feasible? ■ Cost benefits for medical services from smoking control ■ How to do it ■ Diet ■ Obesity ■ Energy balance and dietary fat ■ Glucose intolerance and diabetes ■ Plasma cholesterol, cholesterol fractions and triglycerides ■ Measurement of blood cholesterol ■ When should blood cholesterol be measured? ■ Is reduction of blood cholesterol feasible, and does it reduce coronary risk? ■ Familial hypercholesterolaemia ■ Plasma triglyceride ■ Plasma fibrinogen ■ Exercise ■ Social dislocation and isolation ■ Can multiple risk control work? ■ Overstatement ■ Calculating the odds ■ Starting from where we are, with the people we have

Most of the effects, even of severe high blood pressure, overlap with other causes of coronary heart disease, stroke, and other ischaemic organ damage. Like high blood pressure, these causal factors are almost unrelated to symptoms, and the disease model is therefore as inappropriate and misleading for them as it is for high blood pressure. Policies for control of high blood pressure cannot be effective unless they take full account of other risk factors for arterial disease, and accept that people with high blood pressure are rarely ill, at least until subjected to treatment. We are generally dealing, not with disease, but with disordered health.

Figure 7.1 shows the different probabilities of first cardiovascular disease (fatal or non-fatal) during the next 8 years in mildly hypertensive 40-year-old men with an entry systolic pressure of 165 mmHg, according to presence or absence of four other risks: high total cholesterol (335 mg/dl+ = 8.6 mmol/l), glucose intolerance, cigarette smoking, and ECG evidence of left ventricular hypertrophy.[1] There is a 20-fold increase in risk between those with raised blood pressure alone, and those with all five risk factors.

The implications of this are daunting. Instead of measuring, explaining, treating and monitoring blood pressure in the roughly 10% of the total population with blood pressures in the generally accepted hypertensive range (about twice as much work as most practices are doing now), we need measurement, explanation,

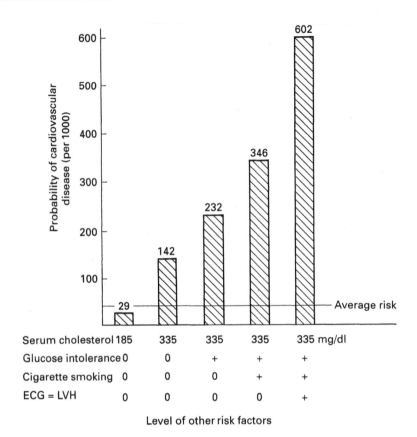

Figure 7.1: Risk of cardiovascular disease (fatal or non-fatal) during the next 8 years in men aged 40 at entry, with an entry systolic pressure of 165 mmHg, according to presence or absence of four other risks: high total cholesterol (335 mg/dl+ = 8.6 mmol/1), glucose intolerance, cigarette smoking, and ECG evidence of left ventricular hypertrophy. (From the Framingham Study 18-year follow-up[2]).

treatment and monitoring of all major risk factors in at least twice that number; we need to know five times as much about twice as many people.

In real life, pursuit of coronary prevention separately from stroke prevention, or of any of their shared risk factors, is always wasteful and sometimes counterproductive. High blood pressure, smoking, obesity, high blood cholesterol, physical inactivity and diabetes do not exist on their own, but are mixed characteristics of real people, distortions of normal physiology usually occurring more than one at a time. It is not possible to take effective action to prevent coronary disease without having some impact on stroke, heart failure, and even airways obstruction and lung cancer; so plans, and measurements of outcome and cost effectiveness should include all these objectives, and all causes mortality.

A joint committee of the Coronary Prevention Group and the British Heart Foundation, on which primary care teams were well represented, has produced a practical 'action plan' adaptable to practices within a wide range of risk burdens and resources, and serving all three subgroups at highest risk (hypertensives, diabetics, and people with established coronary disease), together comprising about 15% of an average practice population aged 35–64.[3] These two and a half pages of good advice are well written, and recommended to all teams as a starting point for discussion.

Risk Factors for Coronary Heart Disease and Stroke

Nihilists suggest that the multitude of alleged coronary risk factors is only a pretentious way of concealing continuing ignorance of *the* cause; but *the* cause does not exist. Why is this concept difficult? We easily understand that there is never a single cause of any fatal road accident. Although there may be one dominant cause in a particular case, for example aggressive driving after a domestic quarrel, many other factors affect the chain of events leading to final outcome. These include vehicle speeds, use of seat belts, vehicle mass, braking systems, road surface, weather, lighting, division of forward from oncoming traffic, availability of off street playspace for children, and countless others. This does not mean we do not know the causes of road accidents or can do nothing about them.

Table 7.1 lists 13 causal risk factors for coronary heart disease and stroke, divisible into three groups: two unchangeable attributes with big effects on risk and therefore useful for motivating both the patient and the team; four changeable behaviours; and seven clinical targets, through which both patients and professionals can measure success in risk reduction.

Each of these factors makes its own contribution to risk, the weight of each varying from patient to patient, just like the causal factors operating in fatal road accidents. Some are commonly more powerful than others, and many are causally linked with one another, so that a shift in one may change others.

Three alterable risk factors emerged ahead of the rest from prospective population studies in the early 1970s and have dominated thought and action ever since: smoking, blood pressure, and plasma cholesterol.

Measuring power by the increase or reduction in risk represented by a shift of one standard deviation in the value of a risk factor, the large USA Pooling Project Research study[4] concluded that smoking was the most powerful risk factor for young men aged 40–44, blood pressure the most important for older men 55–59, and all three were of roughly equal power for men aged 45–54.

Although each makes an independent contribution to risk, risk factors are not independent of each other. Beneficial changes in one variable tend to cause

Table 7.1: Thirteen major causal risk factors for coronary heart disease and stroke

Motivating attributes
Family history
Male sex

Behavioural targets
Smoking
Diet
Exercise
Social dislocation and isolation

Clinical targets
Systolic and diastolic blood pressure
Central obesity
Glucose intolerance and diabetes
Plasma low density lipoprotein (LDL) cholesterol
Plasma high density lipoprotein (HDL) cholesterol
Plasma triglyceride (?)
Plasma fibrinogen

beneficial changes in others, so that a multifactorial approach to treatment is likely to be more effective than simple addition of individual treatment benefits would suggest.

Motivating Attributes

Family history of early coronary disease or stroke is a powerful predictor of individual risk; coronary heart disease before age 50 in a first degree relative probably multiplies risk by two to four times. Patients resemble their siblings more than their parents. Polygenic inheritance of high blood pressure, non-insulin dependent diabetes, and either polygenic or, more rarely, single gene autosomal dominant inheritance of hypercholesterolaemia, account for much of this concentration in families. Some of it is not genetic, but derives from learned behaviour, particularly smoking and eating patterns.

Children learn from their parents both by imitation, and by noting their mistakes and drawing their own conclusions. Early death or disease in a parent or sibling can be a powerful motivator for change, of which care teams should take full advantange, particularly during bereavement counselling. Although inheritance cannot be changed, awareness of higher risk can become either a powerful motivator, or an obstacle to rational thought. From this point of view, early coronary disease or stroke in close friends and colleagues at work is as important as in the family; after such an event, many patients become more receptive to advice. Patients need help and encouragement to choose to learn more about opportunities for reducing their own risks, rather than to ignore them through denial, or discount them through irrational fatalism.

In the USA Framingham study, men aged 35–44 had six times as much coronary disease as women of the same age, and twice as much even at 65–74. Although some of this gender difference was caused by differences in other risks (notably smoking, then, but not now), most of it was independent of other factors. Although elderly women generally have much higher blood cholesterol than men (cholesterol >6.9 mmol/l in 40% of women but only 19% of men aged 65–74), their associated coronary mortality is so much lower that it is difficult to justify either screening or intervention for raised cholesterol in elderly women.[6] Being a premenopausal woman has a powerful protective effect for coronary disease, and as we saw in Chapter 6, oestrogen medication seems to prolong much of this protection after the menopause.

Smoking

Smoking endangers health through not only coronary, aortic and peripheral arterial disease but a wide range of other conditions, including lung cancer, airways obstruction in all its forms, and cancers of the mouth, throat, oesophagus, pancreas and bladder. It is therefore more important to stop smoking than to correct high blood pressure or any other single risk factor, if these sometimes competing priorities conflict. Patients and staff need to understand that the aim of treatment is not just reduction of blood pressure, but reduction of risk.

Stopping smoking does not reduce blood pressure, but it does reduce risk. Cigarettes raise blood pressure a little during the act of smoking, but otherwise smokers generally have slightly lower blood pressures than non–smokers, probably because they eat less and are generally thinner. Patients and many nurses often believe the reason hypertensives should not smoke is that smoking raises blood pressure, and that stopping smoking will made blood pressure fall. This mistaken belief may lead to disappointment and loss of compliance, so it is important to explain the independent effect of smoking on coronary risk, particularly in younger patients in whom this effect is most powerful; nearly all coronary deaths under 45 years of age are associated with smoking.

In the 1950s, before smoking was generally recognized as dangerous, professional people smoked more than unskilled manual workers, because they could afford it (a social pattern still prevalent in the Third World and most of continental Europe except The Netherlands). In the UK, by 1988 only 16% of men and 17% of women in the professional class smoked, compared with 43% and 39% of unskilled manual workers; the proportion of unskilled women who smoked was actually rising. Smoking behaviour correlates strongly with education, and therefore with social class. People with more to live on may also have more to live for, so that attitudes to risk differ between adolescents confident they will get somewhere, and those equally convinced they will get nowhere.

Smoking in treated hypertensives increases their mortality by two or three times,[8, 9] a memorable figure which every hypertensive patient should know. Male doctors who quit smoking halved their mortality after 10 years, and most of this effect was apparent after the first year.[10] Both the added risk from smoking, and the benefit from stopping smoking, seem to be smaller in women, but there is good evidence that smoking may precipitate malignant hypertension in young women on the oral contraceptive pill.[11]

Cigar and pipe smoking seems to be less dangerous than cigarette smoking for all risks except oropharyngeal cancer, apparently because cigar and pipe smokers who have never smoked cigarettes rarely inhale the smoke. However, ex-cigarette smokers who change to cigars or a pipe always inhale, whether consciously or not, and probably do not reduce their risks unless they stop smoking entirely. Change from cigarettes to cigars or cigarillos may actually increase risk.

Is Stopping Smoking Feasible?

In my experience, smoking control through individual counselling is difficult. Personal advice from their own GP results in about 5% of smokers not smoking at follow-up 1 year later[12]; although this seems a meagre health output, it is still better than from any other individual technique applied to unselected populations. More structured approaches to screened patients in an Australian study were ineffective.[13]

In Glyncorrwg,[14] vigorous within-consultation counselling, related wherever possible to personal risks and evidence of lung damage from peak flow rates, may have helped to reduce the proportion of men aged 20–64 who admitted smoking from 61% in 1968 to 36% in 1985. The proportion of women who smoked remained virtually unchanged, at 43% and 42% respectively. These changes followed national trends, and suggest that any effects from individual counselling were small.

We had less disheartening experience with hypertensives, a high risk group with more motivation, better information, and more systematic counselling. At audit of all our 116 treated hypertensives (men and women) in 1989, the proportion who smoked had fallen from 56% before antihypertensive treatment began, to 20%. Our experience with diabetics was similar; the proportion of smokers fell from 44% before treatment to 12% at audit. Systematic advice does work, and works better in these target groups at highest risk, but not simply or easily. Much of the literature available intended to encourage people to give up, and health workers to keep trying, gives the impression that stopping is easy. This is generally far from the truth.

Cost Benefits for Medical Services from Smoking Control

Control of smoking is one of the few preventive measures likely to reduce both work-load and treatment costs for primary care teams and hospitals. Study of a sample of 32 000 people in Exeter[15] showed that male smokers under the age of 45 had 33% more GP consultations, 47% more home visits, 26% more hospital out-patient consultations and 71% more in-patient days than non-smokers.

Over the age of 45, care of smokers seemed to shift towards hospitals, perhaps reflecting the seriousness of the diseases to which they were prone, with below average primary care work-load but a 35% increase in hospital in-patient days. Such data are important in preparing your case for improved staff resources from FHSAs.

How to do it

Serious health workers throughout the world are at war with tobacco, and all who profit from it. No war was ever won on a single front, with only one sort of weapon, or without government support. Governments, by tobacco taxation, control of advertising, and withdrawal of subsidies on tobacco production, have far more power to control this serious health risk than any health worker through personal advice.

The main determinant of smoking habits is cost; consumer spending on cigarettes from 1971 to 1985 rose exactly as the price of tobacco fell.[16] As prices rose, so did tax revenues, showing that finance ministers got it exactly right; they never raised tobacco tax enough to impair revenue. An indication of the seriousness with which governments take their responsibilities for health is the fact that the EEC spends £7.3 million a year on its entire anti-cancer campaign, but £900 million a year subsidizing tobacco production.[17] The UK government has lagged behind even its EEC partners, still opposing legally enforced curbs on tobacco promotion, and ignoring current evidence that advertizing is deliberately and successfully directed at recruitment of women and young people to smoking, including children.[18]

Despite all this, the DoH has now set targets for reduction in the proportion of adults who smoke by the year 2000, from 33% down to 22% for men, and from 30% down to 21% for women, one-third overall.[19] In the run-up to the 1992 general election this target was suddenly revised up to 40%. Primary care teams are expected to help to achieve these targets.

After 30 years of personal counselling against smoking, my impression is that most of us have grossly underestimated the addictive nature of nicotine for many people, including adolescents often assumed to be motivated mainly by a wish to display adult behaviour.

Approaches which recognize this power of nicotine dependence include weaning from inhaled nicotine by substitution by oral or transdermal routes. Although nicotine chewing gum was not significantly effective in unselected patients (because of low acceptability and thus poor compliance)[113], it did help the subset who could put up with the taste, if they were backed up by continued professional advice and support[112]. Nicotine skin patches, which became generally available in 1992, seem much more popular and effective[110, 111]. However, like nicotine chewing gum, skin patches used alone, without organized support, apparently show little effect a year later. Gadgets only work within a shared treatment plan which includes continued advice and support.

Although defiance certainly plays a part in initiating smoking, it soon becomes maintained by addiction in many children, even those who can afford only three or four cigarettes a day. Many of these adolescents will respond to advice from a doctor or nurse, providing motivation to smoke is taken seriously, a personal and confidential relationship is established, enough time is given for full discussion, and evidence from an expired CO meter is used to demonstrate that physiological changes are measurable and real.[20]

Young women are now the main target for advertising, and in the UK, as in most other countries, they now smoke more than young men. When pregnant, few, if any, women are in fact unconcerned about their babies (however they may appear), but only one smoker in 12 gives up in pregnancy, and 65% of these resume smoking after their baby is born.[21] We face similar difficulties in persuading young women to stop smoking when they start taking oral contraception, despite the evidence that this accelerates atheroma.

Apart from continued brain washing by advertisers, our biggest problem is gross underestimation of the size and scope of the task. A simple statement of the facts and a leaflet may be enough to stop smoking in 5% of people a year later, but these are the easiest 5%. The other 95% probably need a more personal and thoughtful approach, integrated with ordinary care and taking advantage of major life events which present opportunities for change.[22, 23] This will not be achieved through the conveyor belt methods favoured by many health promotion clinics.

The following six suggestions are based on experience, confirmed by other workers with similar concerns.

- Update data on smoking at every contact, but act on it selectively: updating reminds patients that this information is regarded seriously by professionals; comment is not always necessary, and must never become routine.

- Use every opportunity to link smoking data with symptoms: in otherwise largely futile consultations about upper and middle respiratory infections, the immediate effects of smoking on acute illness are obvious, and it may be possible to negotiate a stop to smoking for the duration of symptoms; once begun, this may continue.

- Use every opportunity to link smoking data with measured effects, notably peak expiratory flow rate and expired carbon monoxide, compared with expected values in non-smokers of the same age: these are regarded by most patients as objective, non-judgemental data, often more convincing than dire warnings; an expired CO meter now costs less than half as much as an ECG machine, and should be a lot more useful.

■ Use patients' previous experience of stopping smoking, which almost all of them have: their reasons for trying and failing will be personal and therefore important; fears of obesity consequent upon stopping need to be taken seriously, and fully taken into account in any plan for stopping.

■ Use known experience of the effects of smoking in family, friends, and colleagues at work. If you do not know about these, ask; everyone knows Churchill lived to advanced old age despite heavy smoking, but few know any such examples from their own personal experience; bereavement counselling can usefully include discussion of smoking, particularly if the death was smoking related; surviving relatives can accept and even welcome a penance, and may in the midst of death be attracted to constructive action to promote life.

■ At the right moment, try to negotiate an agreed plan for either abrupt or gradual withdrawal from smoking: support this with follow-up visits, and an open telephone line.

Diet

Diet includes all we eat and drink. The main variables affecting coronary and stroke risk are total fat load, the composition of fat (mono- and polyunsaturates, and saturated fats and oils), fibre, potassium, sodium, and alcohol, total energy balance (calories in versus calories out), and the proportion of all calories taken as fat.

There is also mounting evidence that consumption of fresh fruit and vegetables is protective, possibly through increasing intake of ascorbic acid. The volume and composition of diet affects atheromatous plaque formation and the tendency of blood to clot.[24]

There is no evidence that sugar, in any of its forms, as a part of an energy balanced diet (calories in = calories out), promotes high blood pressure, coronary disease, or stroke. Of course, because sugar has a high energy value, balance is easier to achieve with a low sugar diet, but many attempts to demonstrate specific associations between sugar intake and either coronary disease or diabetes have consistently failed. High confectionery containing diets are certainly fattening, but these combine high sugar with high fat intake, above all as chocolate.

Evidence incriminating coffee as a promoter of coronary heart disease is unconvincing. There is some evidence that the Scandinavian habit of boiling coffee promotes coronary mortality by raising low density lipoprotein (LDL) cholesterol, but filtered coffee and coffee powders seem to be free from risk.

It has long been known that blood cholesterol in all its forms is closely related to coronary risk, and the consensus view is that this relationship is both causal and reversible[25], although causality is better established than reversibility.

Cholesterol is not a poison, but an essential body metabolite, an important component of every cell membrane. Patients in the last few years of their lives often have lower blood cholesterol concentrations because their metabolism is impaired, so falling cholesterols are not always a good sign. Cholesterol concentration falls steeply after coronary thrombosis, and may take 6 months or more to return to its pre-infarction value, so measurements during this time cannot be used to assess risk.

Although some cholesterol enters the body ready made in cholesterol rich foods such as egg yolk, liver, and dairy products, most circulating cholesterol is manufactured in the liver from simpler dietary fats, so fat content as well as cholesterol content of foods determines plasma concentration. Dietary fat is the most concentrated form of energy, so its reduction is a prime target in achieving energy balance. It also raises blood pressure, independently of its effect on obesity.

Cholesterol has a special status among the 'big three' coronary risk factors (high blood pressure, smoking, and cholesterol), because coronary heart disease is rare in populations with a low average cholesterol (<4.5 mmol), despite heavy smoking and high blood pressures. Examples of this are Chinese, Japanese and black South Africans, who have high stroke rates but low coronary mortality. Blood total cholesterol levels >4.5 mmol seem to be a necessary (although seldom sufficient) cause of early coronary disease, and are in this sense more important than smoking or high blood pressure. On the other hand, as we shall see later, cholesterol is a difficult target for personal as opposed to population prevention.

National average blood cholesterol levels relate both to the quantity of fat of all kinds in the national diet, and to the proportion of different kinds of fat according to its composition in terms of hydrogen bond saturation. Saturated fats are fats from grain fed or cattle cake fed animals, and some vegetable oils, notably oilseed rape, coconut and soya oils, which still have the largest market share of vegetable cooking oil; the common assumption that animal fats are bad and vegetable fats are good is therefore seriously misleading. Some soft margarines have as high a content of saturated (cholesterogenic) fats as butter; the advantage lies only with those specifically containing polyunsaturated fats. Unsaturated fats include most other vegetable oils, notably sunflower seed and olive oil, fish oils, and fat from animals fed on natural wild pastures.

In 1984 the Department of Health's Committee on Medical Aspects of Food Policy (COMA)[26] recommended a reduction in overall calorie intake, a reduction of the proportion of food energy derived from fat from 42% (as it was in 1981) to 35%, and an increase in the proportion of polyunsaturated fat to shift from a polyunsaturated/saturated fat (P/S) ratio of 0.23 (as it was in 1981), to a P/S ratio of 0.45.

The National Food Survey showed that between 1980 and 1986 average energy intake fell by 7% (from 2230 to 2070 Kcal per person per day). Within this smaller total energy intake, the proportion from fats and oils was unchanged, but the P/S ratio rose from 0.24 to 0.35. There were dramatic changes in demand for milk, butter, and margarine. The average per-person consumption of whole milk fell by 27% from 1980 to 1986, the market share of skimmed milk rose from almost nothing to 19%, the average per-person consumption of butter fell by 44%, and that of soft margarine (not all of it polyunsaturate-rich) rose by 20%.[27]

Fish, particularly fatty fish such as herring, mackerel and salmon, seems to have a protective effect against coronary disease. This was first noticed because of the very low rates of coronary heart disease in unurbanized Eskimos, despite their colossal intake of fat as seal blubber. Interest was sustained because of falling rates in Japan, a high fish consumption country, despite heavy smoking and continued westernization of other aspects of diet.[28] There is some evidence that concentrated fish oils reduce plasma levels of fibrinogen[29] and systolic blood pressure.[30] A 20-year uncontrolled study in The Netherlands showed an inverse relationship between herring consumption and coronary mortality.[31] A randomized controlled trial of two or three extra mackerel meals each week reduced death rates from all causes by 29% over two years, in men who had already had one myocardial infarction.[32]

Fibre, by convention, includes all food residues which cannot be absorbed through a healthy gut. This includes not only vegetable fibres, but also (and more importantly) various gums and mucilages which are not fibrous at all, but have similar cholesterol lowering, and therefore cardioprotective, effects. Good sources include wholemeal bread, potatoes, and beans of all kinds. Vegetables are generally good sources of fibre, but much of their protective effect is lost by cooking, especially prolonged boiling. Addition of soda for vegetable cooking destroys the protective effect of fibre, as well as ascorbic acid. Fresh fruits and salads are excellent sources. Breakfast cereals can be good sources, but sales are often promoted by adding a lot of sugar and salt; for example All Bran contains 15%, muesli 26%, and Sugar Puffs 56% sucrose by weight.[33] Although total bread consumption has fallen since the war by an average 2% per year, sales of brown and wholemeal bread rose throughout the 1980s, and are still rising rapidly, and spreading across a wider social class range.

Fresh fruit consumption in the UK is about the lowest in Europe, and like other 'healthy' foods, particularly fresh vegetables, there are large social class differences in consumption.

Women usually take the practical decisions on what their families eat. Contrary to educated mythology, current national nutritional messages seem to be more or less equally received and understood by rich and poor women.[34, 35] Careful and detailed studies of diet and social class show that the most important constraints are not cultural, but arise from low incomes, and often from control of that income by husbands rather than wives.[36] Evidence shows, perhaps unsurprisingly, that people with low incomes buy food more efficiently than those with high incomes (they search further for best buys, and get better quality and nutritional value per pound spent) but they often cannot afford what they know they need.

As the rich grow richer and the poor become poorer, costs of healthy foods generally rise faster than costs of unhealthy foods.[37]

Dietary potassium load largely depends on intake of vegetables and fruit. There is consistent evidence that high potassium intake lowers blood pressure, particularly if associated with reduced sodium load.

Evidence that sodium intake affects blood pressure was reviewed in the last chapter. Below daily intakes of about 30 mmol (0.69 g sodium or 1.75 g salt) the effect on blood pressure is dramatic, but normal European and North American daily intakes usually lie in the range 150–250 mmol (8.8–14.6 g salt)*. In 1982 the World Health Organization recommended reduction in average daily salt intake to 5 g salt (85 mmol). This is, in my opinion, not feasible with a food culture recognizably similar either to what we eat now, or to what we have ever eaten during the past few hundred years. The choice of 5 g as a threshold is arbitrary, and not justified by any specific evidence. A more feasible, although still ambitious, target would be a reduction to about 110 mmol for an average adult man weighing about 70 kg (big people eat more than little people, and therefore take in more sodium). An important, although generally unheralded, achievement was the 12% reduction in the salt content of bread flour negotiated with British bakers by the Health Education Council in 1986. However, the general trend of food marketing is to promote sales by instant tastiness: more salt, more sugar, and more fat.

Even allowing for benefits discussed later, alcohol has been estimated to cause a net excess mortality from all causes of 28 000 a year at ages 15–74 in England and Wales alone.[38] Relatively few of these deaths are in 'alcoholics' as generally understood. Alcoholic misery short of death, and in families as well as drinkers themselves, remains incalculable.

Intake is now usually measured in 'drinks' or 'units' of alcohol, one drink or unit being equal to the alcohol contained in one glass of wine, half a pint of beer, or one tot of spirits. Obviously this results in substantial error because the strength of wines and beers varies, but it is an easily understood system with the great advantage that it is actually used by most practices which have followed the advice of the Royal College of General Practitioners[39] to ask all adult patients at some time for a detailed account of their normal weekly alcohol intake in units per week.

Even after adjustment for effects from smoking, risk of oral and oesophageal cancer increases fourfold in drinkers taking 56 or more units a week. At only 21 units a week, associated breast cancer risk is increased by about 50% compared with abstainers.[40] As discussed in Chapter 6, chronic high alcohol intake probably raises blood pressure, although not much. It can certainly raise it acutely, which

---

* Sodium, potassium and other blood concentrations are discussed in this book in terms of SI units (millimoles). Conversion from grams is as follows:

1 g NaCl = 17.1 mmol Na
1 g Na = 43.5 mmol Na
1 g KCl = 13.4 mmol K
1 g K = 25.6 mmol K

is probably why strokes so commonly occur during or after bouts of heavy drinking.[41]

The volume of family misery, violence, degradation and exacerbated poverty attributable to alcohol is well known to any experienced GP. This far outweighs any mortality benefits from reductions in coronary disease, and no total abstainer from alcohol should ever be encouraged to start drinking simply in order to reduce coronary risk. However, for the large majority who presently do drink alcohol, especially the heavy drinkers (about 14% of adult men drink heavily enough to cause health or social problems)[42], it is important to tell the truth so far as we know it. This certainly includes heartening and remarkably consistent evidence that moderate alcohol consumption (probably up to about 21 units a week) reduces relative risk of death from coronary disease by about 25%.[43, 44]

A protective effect from moderate alcohol is biologically plausible; alcohol increases concentration of HDL (protective) cholesterol, reduces fibrinogen levels, and reduces platelet adhesiveness.

However, risk of death from all causes, from cerebrovascular disease, from all cancers and from accidents and violence, all increase steadily from a threshold of about 14 units a week. Above 28 units a week, even coronary risk rises, and at very high levels cardiomyopathy becomes a common (and frequently unrecognized) cause of heart failure.

Obesity

Obesity[45, 46] is most easily measured as body mass index (BMI = metric weight/metric height squared, also known as the Ponderal Index or Quetelet's Index). People of different heights can then be ranked on the same scale to assess risk and audit achievement. From a BMI of about 30, death rates increase steeply, mainly from cancer, coronary disease and stroke, but also from breast cancer and airways obstruction.

Note that BMI cannot be measured without the patient's height. The easiest way to do this, and the worst, is to ask people how tall they are; men usually add an inch, and women increasingly do the same. The optimal range of a BMI is usually defined as 20–25, but there is little evidence of excess mortality from 25–29.

Obesity in general has little independent effect on coronary mortality until it is fairly severe, at a BMI of 30 or more. Fat stomachs (central obesity) are much more important for coronary risk than fat arms and legs (peripheral obesity). A convenient way of measuring this is to divide metric stomach circumference by hip circumference; Bjorntorp[47] has shown that coronary risk increases steeply when this coefficient exceeds 1.00. This effect of obesity is not exerted through any association with high blood pressure, because thin hypertensives have a higher mortality than fat hypertensives, when standardized for differences in blood pressure.[48]

Recent work on obesity in animal models suggests that obese people do (as they have always claimed) have a primary metabolic defect ('It's my glands'), although contrary to equally common belief, the second law of thermodynamics still holds: energy in < out you get smaller, energy in = energy out you stay the same, energy in > energy out you get bigger. Obesity, particularly central obesity, is also linked with an unfavourable pattern of blood lipoproteins, with high LDL cholesterol and triglyceride, and low HDL cholesterol. Its secondary effects on sex hormone metabolism lead to polycystic ovaries and infertility, raised cholesterol concentration in bile leading to gallstones, reduced exercise tolerance, impaired breathing, premature crumbling of weight bearing joints, and gross social and psychological disadvantage. The association of obesity with coronary disease is one of the least of its crimes.

Sustained weight loss reverses most of these consequences, including insulin resistance, so the treatment of obesity is potentially one of the largest and most rewarding fields for clinical medicine, although the direct contribution to blood pressure control is generally small, even after considerable sustained effort.[49] In the UK, 6% of adult men and 8% of women have a BMI of 30+, with large social class gradients favouring the better off. In Glyncorrwg, 17% of adults aged 20–79 had a BMI of 30+ at some time during 25 years of practice.[50]

Cade and O'Connell[51] found 98% of GPs thought counselling on obesity was appropriate to their professional role, but most also believed they were relatively ineffective and badly trained for this work. Best experience suggests that results are better with participative group work, using the social skills of patients themselves assisted by dietitians or nutritionists.[46] However, doctors and nurses have much to contribute because of their motivating experience of the ultimate consequences of uncontrolled obesity, and also because the obese are a high risk group requiring skilled clinical observation.

Energy Balance and Dietary Fat

Ideas about the nature of human energy balance have changed dramatically in the last few years, suggesting that one reason our advice did not work was that it was simply wrong.[45] For generations all health workers were taught, and therefore taught their patients, that all that mattered was quantitative energy balance, not the qualitative composition of diet. Energy intake not used as energy expenditure would be stored as fat, whether the surplus originated from fat, carbohydrate or protein; count the calories, and do not eat more than you can use.

There is now persuasive evidence that intake of carbohydrate or protein in excess of requirements is within wide limits balanced by increased oxidation of carbohydrate and raised energy expenditure, even in grossly obese people. Only at extremes of carbohydrate intake is much of it converted to fat.

The reason modern diets lead so easily to obesity is probably not just overeating, but their characteristically high fat content. A main determinant of appetite is glycogen depletion. High fat, low carbohydrate diets lead to more rapid glycogen depletion, and a larger appetite. On this reasoning, energy balance is almost equivalent to fat balance. Slow but steady weight loss has been shown to occur on diets in which only fat is curtailed, not total calorie intake. This approach is particularly important in young obese people, for whom weight control is both easier and more effective in reducing mortality risk.

Hammering on the theme of reduced dietary fat is not enough to help patients who already have a serious weight problem, with a BMI of 30+. A negative energy balance is essential for these patients, and sugar as well as fat remains an important target; a diet sheet for patients is included in Appendix 3. This has been used for the past 10 years in Glyncorrwg, and has been well received by our almost entirely working class patients. Many of these, but most of all the 'giant' obese with a BMI of 40+, have problems of low self-esteem, which may be easily reinforced by doctors or nurses. Sustained weight loss is one of the most difficult, although worthwhile, tasks we or our patients ever undertake, and this needs continually to be recalled when the going gets difficult, as it always does.

Advantages of anorectic drugs over diet alone are marginal, and far outweighed by their considerable disadvantages.

Glucose Intolerance and Diabetes

No team caring for hypertensives can afford not to know and care at least as much about diabetes as it does about high blood pressure. At least 40% of diabetics are hypertensive on WHO criteria,[52] and all of these need assiduous control of blood pressure to prevent or delay renal and retinal damage.

Treated hypertensives are two or three times more likely than other people to develop diabetes, partly because of their treatment (thiazide diuretics are diabetogenic)[53] and partly because non-insulin dependent (NID) diabetics and many hypertensives share a common resistance to insulin.[54] Risk of both coronary disease and stroke is at least doubled in diabetics[55], and largely accounts for the exceptional coronary and stroke risk of South Asians in the UK.[56-58] Much of this added risk arises from higher than average blood cholesterol levels in diabetics.

Prevalence of diabetes in UK adults is roughly 2% of the adult population, of whom about half are diagnosed. About a quarter of known diabetics are insulin dependent (ID). Prevalence of diabetes rises steeply with age, almost entirely because of NID diabetes in the elderly, who account for most of the undiagnosed patients. UK populations of Asian descent have at least a four times higher prevalence than the general population, but those of Afro-Caribbean descent have the same prevalence as whites. Prevalence is also related to social class; as for coronary disease and stroke, it is higher in poorer people.[59]

Impaired glucose tolerance was defined by WHO as fasting glucose below the threshold for diabetes, but with venous blood glucose 7–9.9 mmol/l 2 hours after a 75 g oral glucose load (or 8–10.9 mmol/l for capillary blood or venous plasma). Prevalence in UK adults is about 1%. The concept of impaired glucose tolerance, or glucose intolerance, is of real value because of good evidence that the specific microvascular complications of diabetes (proliferative retinopathy, diabetic nephropathy and neuropathy) do not occur below this diabetic threshold, whereas the risk of macrovascular complications which are not unique to diabetes (accelerated atheroma in coronary and other large and medium arteries, and corresponding mortality from coronary disease and stroke) rises steadily with decreasing glucose tolerance throughout its range.[60]

The importance of diabetes and glucose intolerance to the burdens of coronary disease and stroke continue to be underestimated throughout clinical practice. ID diabetics are generally recognized as a high risk group, but NID diabetics tend to be managed casually, in a way that often reinforces patients' own underestimations of the risk of their disorder if uncontrolled.

The microvascular complications of diabetes seem to depend mainly on the duration and level of raised blood glucose, not on ID or NID status. Most diabetics with good blood glucose control can become physiologically normal people, and whether they achieve this with insulin or oral hypoglycaemic drugs, they must have a serious approach to diet, not only to reduce blood glucose, but to improve generally dangerous cholesterol and fibrinogen patterns. It is particularly important for diabetics to have a low fat, high fibre diet, both to improve glycaemic control and to reduce cardiovascular risk.[61] Best of all is probably a loosely vegetarian diet.

Control of diabetes can now be easily and accurately assessed by measuring blood levels of fructosamine or glycosylated haemoglobin (HbA_1c), both of which vary according to the average level of blood glucose during the previous 3 months or so. Most laboratories do either one test or the other: fructosamine estimation is cheaper. Methods are not yet completely standardized and you should check with your local laboratory about their normal range. The upper limit of normal for HbA_1c is usually taken as 8%.

Plasma Cholesterol, Cholesterol Fractions, and Triglyceride

In the UK, plasma or serum cholesterol is normally reported in SI units, as mmol/l. Traditional units are still used in the USA and some European countries. The conversion formula is 1 mmol/l cholesterol = 38.7 mg/dl.

It is now generally understood and accepted that coronary risk is promoted by low-density lipoprotein (LDL) cholesterol, and reduced by high-density lipoprotein (HDL) cholesterol. Both depend partly on inheritance and partly on diet, and are affected by smoking and exercise. In general terms, LDL cholesterol represents blood fat available to form cholesterol plaque on arterial walls in target organs like the heart and brain, whereas HDL cholesterol represents transport of cholesterol away from these sites, to be stored in the liver, or conjugated with bile and eliminated through the gut. Laboratory measurement of total cholesterol (TC) is still simpler, cheaper, and generally more reliable than separate measurement of the two main lipoprotein cholesterol fractions, LDL and HDL, and TC has long been satisfactorily used to characterize population risk.

Like blood pressure, the coronary risk associated with blood cholesterol is continuously distributed without a threshold. Even in China, with blood TC concentrations ranging from 3.8–4.7 mmol/l and a correspondingly low coronary mortality, at 7% of all deaths, coronary mortality risk is related to individual TC concentration throughout this range.[62]

Measurement of Blood Cholesterol

Individual risk may be predicted more accurately by a lipid profile including measurement of LDL and HDL, but only if these measurements are themselves accurate and reproducible; this can by no means be taken for granted. Many primary care teams now have machines that will measure capillary samples on site, without the delay, cost and inconvenience of taking a venous sample and sending it to the nearest hospital laboratory. Unfortunately, even if practice staff have special training to use this equipment (and many do not), few of them have had sustained training in the general disciplines of laboratory work, and the need for constant vigilance to reduce equipment and observation error. Wherever they are performed, measurements should be monitored by periodic independent sampling to measure laboratory error. This is important, not only to measure risk correctly in the first place, but even more to give accurate feedback information to patients trying seriously to reduce TC by diet.

The news on this front is not good. Using a 'Reflotron', the most commonly used and best validated machine for primary care,[63] in a quality assessment scheme guaranteeing competent and careful use, the correlation coefficient for the dry chemistry machine was only 0.7, with a 10% difference between the correlation coefficient for each of two samples of the same machine. The authors concluded that the 'bedside laboratory' is not yet sufficiently accurate to measure changes in blood cholesterol over time, and therefore to give feedback to patients on their dietary management. With staff working under more ordinary conditions, results are much worse. I have personally seen a shift of 4 mmol/l on the same subject on the same day, because of capillary samples taken from cold hands by a nurse using a demonstration machine, who was employed (and presumably trained) by the manufacturers; cold hands give false low readings.

When Should Blood Cholesterol be Measured?

It was probably always too late to ask this question, because nobody acting as clinical advocate for patients can or should refuse their request to know more about their own personal risk. However, it is another matter entirely to organize community wide detection drives to identify those at high risk from raised blood cholesterol, in the same way that we should undoubtedly do for high blood pressure.

Like blood pressure, LDL cholesterol (or total cholesterol as its proxy) is a continuously distributed risk for coronary heart disease and (although much less so than blood pressure) for stroke. However, there are important differences in principle between them. Screening for high blood pressure defines a relatively small group at very high risk, particularly for stroke and heart failure (severe hypertension, diastolic pressure 120 mmHg+), which can be treated relatively easily and effectively. Measurement of blood pressure is simple, cheap, and with care and suitable training, reproducible. Screening of the whole population for high blood cholesterol, however, defines no such group, at least if we follow current criteria for definition of increased risk (from 6.6 mmol/l).

Coronary morbidity is low under a blood TC of 4.5 mmol/l, but various population surveys have shown that the average TC for the whole population aged 40–59 is over 6 mmol/l.[64] Almost our entire population is therefore at high risk (by world standards) for coronary disease, at least in men. In these circumstances, practice staff who reassure patients that their blood cholesterol is fine, simply because it is less than 6.6 mmol/l or some other arbitrary dividing line related to the UK average, may well increase the population risk of coronary disease by reinforcing people's natural desire to eat what they like. There is good evidence from an Australian study that mass cholesterol screening can, in this way, increase rather than reduce community risk.[65]

Is Reduction of Blood Cholesterol Feasible, and Does it Reduce Coronary Risk?

Claims that cholesterol lowering diets normally used will reduce TC by 10–25%, which are common in popular literature, are not supported by controlled evidence. The Oslo study suggested that reduction in average blood cholesterol concentration by rigorous dieting (a stricter regimen than any of those commonly used in practice) could reduce coronary risk in selected volunteers by a relatively modest 13%.[66] The much bigger and more representative Multiple Risk Factor Intervention Trial in the USA[67] achieved only an average 2% reduction in TC despite intensive patient education and support, using a diet closer to those generally enjoined on patients today, but still relatively rigorous. In Israel, reduction from a group mean 6.3 mmol/l to 5.3 mmol/l was achieved in the special circumstances of a small kibbutz, with centralized catering and exceptional education input time,[68] but no comparable results have been reported from more ordinary circumstances of practice.

There is, therefore, little evidence that individual counselling on diet, as presently performed by non-specialist primary care teams, is effective in lowering blood cholesterol.[69] The current MRC primary prevention trial using low dose warfarin and aspirin screened whole populations to identify about 6000 men aged

45–69 in the top 20% of the risk distribution (taking account of smoking, blood pressure, and blood levels of cholesterol and fibrinogen).[70] Although these men knew they were at high risk, and were sufficiently motivated to enter a trial using low doses of rat poison involving several venepunctures each year, and although they received energetic dietary advice, both at the start and at quarterly follow-up visits, by the end of the first year there was virtually no change in their average blood cholesterol. My own experience in Glyncorrwg, discussed in Chapter 15, was essentially the same; a large (although unskilled) advisory effort yielded only a pitiful outcome.

This may change if cholesterol lowering drugs come to be used in the UK on a similar scale to in the USA, but there is still no convincing evidence that these reduce all-cause mortality except for extreme hypercholesterolaemia.[71] The case for their mass use remains unconvincing. Systematic review of all published controlled trials of blood cholesterol reduction, by diet alone or aided by cholesterol lowering drugs, still shows no net reduction either in coronary deaths, or deaths from all causes. Optimistic assertions to the contrary have depended on selective citation of positive trials.[72]

Skilled dietary counselling can lower cholesterol, and is a new resource badly needed in UK general practice. A study of 90 men with mean initial TC of 7.2 mmol/l at St Thomas's hospital showed that 3 years later, 46% of those randomized to 'ordinary care' had angiographic progression of coronary atheroma, compared with 15% of those given skilled dietary advice and support, and 12% of those also given cholestyramine. There was a significant reduction of cardiovascular events in both intervention groups.[73]

The 'official' recommendations on cholesterol screening remain ambiguous, partly because they have been devised almost entirely by people without experience of primary care, who often seem unsure whether they are talking about what is best or what is feasible, not in terms of work-load, but cost. Health workers at the coal-face are understandably sceptical of strategies better suited to the drawing board than to practical decisions involving patients. Even if we consider only what is most effective, without regard to cost, cholesterol screening on a mass scale still makes little sense.

As for clinical tests, cholesterol measurements should be done only if their outcome will affect clinical decisions. If the whole population needs to reduce its total fat intake below 30% of total calories, increase unsaturated fat intake to 40% more than saturated fat intake, reduce cholesterol intake to less than 200 mg daily, and achieve desirable weight (roughly a BMI of 25) by reducing overall energy intake and increasing energy output, why confuse this message by giving it to some but not others, often in the same family? Eating is a social activity, in which groups and populations may change more easily than individuals, just as periodically certain groups in society insist on wearing hideous fashions, although none would wear them alone.

There are high risk groups which do need initial testing for case finding: first-degree relatives of those who suffer a heart attack under 40 years, diabetics, treated hypertensives, and persistent heavy smokers. Once begun, these tests must be repeated, with accurate feedback from laboratory measurements to reinforce motivation and encourage personal responsibility by patients to produce their own improved outcomes.

Cholesterol lowering diets and drugs are discussed further in Chapters 15 and 16, and in Appendices II and VIII.

Familial Hypercholesterolaemia

Because virtually everyone in the UK has a high fat intake by world standards, differences between individual cholesterol concentrations depend mainly on genetic differences in cholesterol metabolism, rather than on individual differences in fat intake. These genetic differences are clinically important only for people with exceptionally high TC levels, generally 8–10 mmol/l (310–387 mg/dl) or more. These patients should be referred for specialist help if it is available; they usually need cholesterol lowering drugs as well as help from a dietitian. Among these are the estimated 1: 500 people heterozygous for familial hypercholesterolaemia, a specific metabolic error inherited as an autosomal dominant; homozygotes mostly die of coronary disease before they reach 30 years. Heterozygotes have a peak excess coronary mortality at ages 20–39. If they survive to middle age, their coronary mortality thereafter tends to resemble that of the rest of the population.[74]

Plasma Triglyceride

Plasma triglyceride concentration is so closely associated with obesity, and its measurement often so unreliable, that it has always seemed to me more practical to weigh patients rather than send their blood off to a laboratory for the same information in a less useful form. A target weight is more comprehensible to patients than a target triglyceride.

Unexpectedly high triglyceride values in people who are not fat suggest high alcohol intake, but like other laboratory indicators of alcohol (raised mean corpuscular volume and gamma glutamyl transferase), the association is neither specific nor consistent.

Plasma Fibrinogen

Fibrinogen is a principal link in the extremely complex biochemical chain involved in blood coagulation. It has been clear since Stone's work as a research GP in Lancashire[75] and the Northwick Park study[76, 77] that it is at least as powerful a predictor of coronary disease and stroke as blood cholesterol or arterial blood pressure. Recent work shows it is also highly predictive for peripheral arterial disease. Its measurement is not yet standardized for laboratory use, so it is not a part of routine risk calculation, but it soon will be.

Although it has a powerful independent effect, fibrinogen concentration is also positively correlated with nearly all other cardiovascular risk factors: age, blood pressure, LDL cholesterol, smoking, glucose intolerance, obesity, physical inactivity, and the contraceptive pill.[78] Remarkably, it is also associated with lower social class and probably with specific kinds of social and occupational stress, even after allowing for smoking.[79, 80]

Fibrinogen concentration can be reduced by stopping smoking, by moderate intake of alcohol, and by regular exercise. Although several drugs in common use also reduce fibrinogen concentration, none has this as its principal effect, so no specific fibrinogen lowering drug is available. The current MRC GP Research Framework randomized controlled trial of low dose warfarin and aspirin[70] acts on the coagulation pathway represented by fibrinogen. Its results will (probably in about 5 years' time) tell us whether the risks associated with high fibrinogen concentration are reversible by therapeutic reduction on a mass scale. This is certainly a space to watch.

Exercise

Exercise[81, 82] can reduce coronary and stroke risk in many ways. Most obviously, it uses up otherwise surplus calories, and may therefore improve energy balance and assist weight loss directly. The amount of exercise required to do this is large, because most energy consumption occurs at rest, simply keeping the body machine ticking over, so that even if physical exercise is increased by several times, extra energy expenditure remains relatively small. Simple calculations of energy expenditure therefore appear to yield a disappointingly small return for a large investment of effort.

As we shall see, and as everyone who has run a weight reduction group knows, this sad conclusion may be factually correct but is false in practice; people who adopt and sustain serious exercise programmes generally look better, feel better, and lose weight, even though actual weight loss is small because some fat may be replaced by muscle.

There are many reasons for this broad impact on health. Exercise increases metabolic throughput, with apparently beneficial effects on glucose tolerance and insulin resistance; on the other hand, physical inactivity seems to promote NID diabetes.[83] Vigorous and sustained exercise (but not just walking or pottering about in the garden) raises HDL (protective) cholesterol and reduces fibrinogen. It increases bone density and reverses osteoporosis; low bone density in the elderly is actually a better predictor of thrombotic stroke than blood pressure,[84] perhaps because both are promoted by physical inactivity. Exercise has a training effect on heart muscle and stabilizes heart rhythm, reducing mortality of heart attacks even if they occur.

Finally, and perhaps most importantly, exercise tends to restore confidence, self-esteem, and a general feeling that life is worthwhile and can be coped with, so that everything people do is done better. Thus exercise can be an important adjunct to stop smoking programmes, and other apparently unrelated topics.

It is important to understand, and to convey this understanding to patients, that people do not have to be fit already to start an exercise programme. In fact those who benefit most are those with an already substantial impairment, including established angina, claudication, and heart failure. Exercise is an important measure of secondary prevention after recovery from a first coronary thrombosis; controlled trials show a roughly 25% reduction in re-infarction and sudden death.[85]

Obviously, exercise must be graded according to the initial capacity of the patient. It is important for patients to understand that pain or discomfort are not only not necessary, they are positively undesirable and may be dangerous. Static exercises, such as press-ups and weight lifting, raise blood pressure transiently but sometimes dangerously, and are not useful and should be expressly excluded. Patients should do what they enjoy, with preference for non-competitive activities, especially if they involve meeting other people.

Many of the best activities, for example swimming lengths, are inherently boring, but the company of other people doing it can help to sustain compliance. Swimming is a non-competitive form of exercise using all body muscles in a state of virtual weightlessness, so that it remains possible at virtually all ages and despite virtually all other disabilities, notably pain from degenerative arthropathies. More people swim regularly than take part in any other sport, but despite this the UK has only one public swimming pool per 45 000 population. Cycling to work daily over an average return journey of 13 km uses the same energy as 10 minutes' wrestling or 30 minutes of squash, and civil servants who cycle regularly have half the expected number of coronary events.[86] If every primary care team accepted responsibility for mobilizing public pressure for swimming facilities accessible to its whole local population, and for safe routes for cyclists, these might begin to get the political priority they deserve.

Social Dislocation and Isolation

There has long been a large body of diverse evidence suggesting that social dislocation, isolation, and gain or loss of a comprehensive world view such as religion or politics, may affect all-cause mortality.[87–89] Certainly there are aspects of social class other than smoking and obesity which must be invoked to explain the huge and still increasing social differences in coronary and stroke risk, always rewarding those who have most, and penalizing those who have least.[90]

The always substantial placebo effect, so often believed to call into question the basis of all scientific reasoning because it depends on belief, in fact tells us over and over again that belief is always important. By any reckoning, people feel better and generally are better if they can make sense of the world,[91, 92] do not feel completely alone in it, and think they have met someone willing and able to help them. People who think this contradicts science are apparently unable to understand what science is, or at least what it should be.

It is difficult to overestimate the importance to patients, certainly for their compliance, resistance to drop-out from follow-up, and perhaps for their resistance to disease, that they should be able to make sense of what is happening to them, and of the added risks they run, to be able to use information to increase rather than restrict their control over their lives, and to believe that their lives are of real value, not just to themselves but to others too.

Health promotion clinics, and all the other proactive measures which have been developed as medicine moves beyond crude response to end-stage sympto-matic disease toward search for its more simply, cheaply and easily managed asymptomatic precursors, are always in danger of destroying precisely this quality of reactive care: 'My doctor (nurse, midwife, receptionist, etc.) knows and cares about me, and will help me in my trouble'. Clinics follow set protocols in which infinitely complex and variable patients tend to become standardized, personal responsibilities become delegated and fragmented, continuity becomes unimport-ant, patients become passive consumers rather than active participants and pro-ducers, and practice teams become bored and stagnant. These outcomes are not inevitable, but the trend is always there and has to be consciously resisted. All health service bureaucracy, whether imposed from above or generated internally, needs to be seen, not only as a necessary evil, but a serious threat to health.

Can Multiple Risk Control Work?

Age standardized death rates from stroke have been falling in all developed economies for at least the past 50 years. In the USA, age standardized death rates for coronary thrombosis have fallen by 40% in less than 20 years, with bigger and earlier changes in younger age groups. A similar fall is now well under way throughout the UK for all social groups except manual workers and their wives, in whom mortality is still rising.

In a very general way, all these improvements have coincided with reductions in known risk: better control of high blood pressure, some decline in mean blood cholesterol values (in the USA, at least), and above all a substantial fall in smoking. However, it has been surprisingly difficult to demonstrate any convincing effect from medical, pharmaceutical or educational interventions. We have evi-dence on this now both from large trials,[93] and from a few practices which began this work, mostly in the early 1970s, and which are now just beginning to report long term results.

Large scale trials which have used only mass educational methods without personal care, for example the Stanford Heart Disease Prevention Programme,[94] have shown impressive changes in risk factors. Where personal care attempts preventive work on a population scale, such a background of mass education may well be a precondition for success. On the whole, both the BBC and independent television have carried excellent, imaginative educational material on all aspects of coronary disease and smoking risks. Although they have perhaps underplayed stroke prevention, this is largely the fault of the medical profession. Whatever we do in the way of patient education has good public backing from radio, television, and the women's weeklies at least, despite opposition from a mercenary army of tobacco advertisers.

However, where impact of mass education on either all-cause or coronary mortality has been measured, as in the North Karelia Project[95] results have been much less dramatic. Significantly, almost nothing seemed to change in North Karelia during the first 5 years; all falls in both risk and mortality came in the second 5 years. If you want to alter people's behaviour, it takes at least 5 years before they take your intention seriously. The usual 2-year studies, geared to fit funding for doctoral theses and careers, are useless. More worryingly, 5 years after the end of a multifactorial intervention trial including both thiazides and propranolol for high blood pressure, and probucol or clofibrate for hypercholesterolaemia, subjects randomized to intervention had higher death rates than non-intervention controls. This raised mortality was attributed to increased deaths from cardiovascular disease, accidents and violence.[96] There was also a rapid return of mean risk factor levels to their original values in the former intervention groups. One plausible interpretation of this alarming result is that withdrawal from intensive counselling may have rebound effects on behaviour, making it worse than it was in the first place; another is that antihypertensive medication for mild hypertension may have caused a net increase in all-causes mortality.[97]

If educational interventions are made at all, they should be made within a continuing supportive framework, which did not yet exist in the Karelia project; that is, within an evolving personalized primary care system rather than an add-on, knock-off outreach system.[14, 98]

In multi-country studies, for example the WHO European multicentre trial in factory populations,[99] results were good where preventive work was well resourced, with plenty of staff able to give time to patients; where it was badly resourced, in the UK for example, results were poor. Pooled results from Belgium, Italy, Poland, and Britain showed reductions of 6.9% in fatal coronary events, 14.8% in non-fatal events, and 5.3% in deaths from all causes in the intervention factories compared with control factories. However, overall risk in UK intervention factories actually rose by 4%, compared with a 26% reduction in risk for Italian workers, and changes in morbidity and mortality followed the same pattern. In Britain one whole time equivalent (WTE) doctor and one WTE nurse were responsible for 9734 workers, compared with two WTE doctors and one WTE nurse for 3131 workers in Italy, a more than fourfold difference.[100]

The news from pioneering practices is essentially the same; good staffing levels are a precondition for success. This work is impossible unless the reasonable demands of local populations for the care of sick people are already adequately met, and preventive work does not have to compete with this.[14, 101] This is most difficult of all in city populations with a high proportion of South Asians, who not only have exceptionally high rates of diabetes, coronary and cerebrovascular disease, but also high consultation rates, high work-load from many other causes, and both language and cultural barriers to communication.[102] In such areas, even a beginning cannot be made without substantial additional staff time. The Healthy East Enders project[103] is a model of what can be done within NHS general practice even in the most difficult conditions; 60% of young adults had at least one major classic risk factor for coronary disease, and 23% had two or more major risk factors; of this last group, the risk status of 86% were unknown to their family doctors before screening.

The work is difficult and time consuming, and all of us have been poorly prepared for it by our education. Never having been done before, this work lacks experienced teachers, so that teaching derives mostly from the transient and contrived conditions of research trials.

Overstatement

Preventive work must be sustained for many years to get even meagre results, at least in verifiable, audited terms. It is not made easier by exaggerated claims for prevention. Unlike the case for primary prevention of stroke, and for secondary prevention in people who have survived a coronary thrombosis, the case for primary prevention of coronary disease is presently neither overwhelming nor self evident.[104]

A policy of attempting to salvage only those who actually have heart attacks remains arguable, although with diminishing force. The dogmatic certainty with which some advocates of prevention approach this work, which tends to increase as it filters down in simplified form to primary care physicians, nurses, and administrative staff, sits badly with our chastening knowledge that the classic risk factors still account for only about half of all deaths from coronary heart disease.[105]

Figure 7.2 from the Framingham study 18-year follow-up[2] shows relative risks for coronary heart disease, claudication, brain infarction and heart failure for normotensive, borderline and hypertensive subjects, using systolic blood pressure <140, 140–160, and >160 mmHg as thresholds. At first sight the differences are striking: male coronary heart disease is 250% commoner in hypertensives than normotensives (300% in women), claudication is 86% commoner (350% in women), stroke is 800% commoner (750% in women), and heart failure is 650% commoner (450% in women).

However, if you look at absolute rather than relative risks, the picture is very different. What are the chances of individual hypertensives aged 45–74 actually getting one of these complications during the next 5 years? They are: for coronary disease, 12% for men and 6% for women; for claudication, 3% for men and 1%

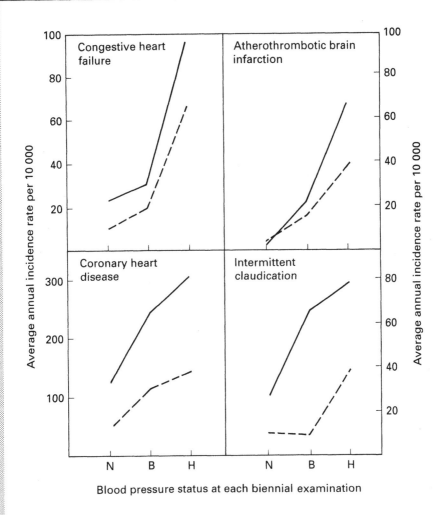

Figure 7.2: Average annual incidence of cardiovascular disease according to blood pressure status at each biennial examination of men (continuous lines) and women (dashed lines) aged 55–64 at entry to the Framingham Study (18-year follow-up). N, B, and H = normal, borderline and high blood pressure at entry (systolic thresholds <140, 140–160, and >160 mmHg)[2].

for women; for brain infarction, 2% for both men and women; and for heart failure, 4% for men and 2% for women.

Calculating the Odds

Life is a gamble, and more so as we descend the social ladder. Calculation of odds can be readily understood by most people at highest risk, if presented truthfully and in practical terms. Primary care teams must either be sufficiently familiar with these figures to be able to give accurate advice, or provide them in written material for patients so they do not have to remember them. Whether verbal or written, this advice should include frank admission that forecasting of mortality risk is still much the same as weather forecasting; it is often wrong, but sensible people still pay some attention to it when planning a journey.

Unlike many of their patients, most health workers are not gamblers. In practice it is difficult to estimate risks involving more than one variable, and almost impossible if there are three or more. Fortunately there is now enough evidence about coronary risks to transfer such calculations to various sorts of slide rule or computer, and several are now available.

The first of these to be widely used in the UK was proposed by Shaper.[25] Its great advantage is that it omits blood cholesterol concentrations from the equation, so a result is calculable immediately at first interview, using data to hand. His justification for this omission, with which I agree, is that virtually everyone in the UK has a raised cholesterol, and therefore needs a change in diet to bring it down.

Shaper's modified score applies only to men, and was derived from study of over 7000 men aged 40–59 randomly sampled from general practices in 24 towns in England, Wales and Scotland. In practice, the top fifth of this distribution identified 53% of men who will have a major coronary event during the next 5 years, and the top 10% identified 35%. The score is made up as follows:

Item	Score
Years of smoking cigarettes	×7
Mean blood pressure mmHg*	×6.5
Diagnosis of ischaemic heart disease recalled	+270
Evidence of angina on chest pain questionnaire	+150
Either parent died of heart trouble	+85
Diabetes	+150
Threshold score for top 10% of 5-year risk	1 091
Threshold score for top 20% of 5-year risk	1 000
Threshold score for bottom 20% of 5-year risk	713
Threshold score for bottom 10% of 5-year risk	647

This was a good system, but like others, for example the Framingham and Minnesota scores, it has been used more for insurance assessment than by primary care clinicians in the field.

More recently, Tunstall-Pedoe[106] has devised the Aberdeen Risk-Disk, its formula derived from 5203 men aged 40–59 in the Whitehall study, and tested against observation of 10 359 men and women participating in the Scottish heart health study. It is a circular slide rule deriving a risk score from data on the three

---

* It is confusing that **mean blood pressure** is not the sum of systolic and diastolic pressure divided by two, but **systolic pressure + (diastolic pressure × 2)/3**. This does fairly accurately average arterial pressure throughout the systolic-diastolic cycle.

classic modifiable risk factors of blood pressure, smoking, and blood cholesterol. Its score is expressed as a risk-rank, rather like a queuing system, on a scale from 1–100 for both men and women. Patients can understand easily where they are in the queue for coronary risk, and whether they are moving forwards or backwards. Unless the Shaper score is included in a computer system, the Risk-Disk is certainly easier to use, its results may also be more comprehensible to patients and staff, and users have reported impressive success in motivating patients by giving them objective feedback on what they achieve.[107]

The Risk-Disk is less than perfect, particularly in that, by concentrating only on coronary risk, it underestimates overall risk from smoking.[108] However, some tool of this kind seems essential now for any team that is serious about coronary prevention, if only as a learning instrument for the primary care team. No such tool is available for stroke, but though the balance of risks is different, good strategies against coronary disease tend to be even better against stroke. The Risk-Disk is available, together with an illustrated instruction manual, from Risk-Disk, CVEU, Ninewells Hospital, Dundee DD1 9SY, Scotland. An educational videocassette and software programme are also available.

Now that about 80% of UK practices have a computer, risk assessment incorporating data on the three classic risk factors plus family history should be incorporated in some of their programmes in the near future. Until this happens none of the available formulae are likely to make much headway.

Starting from Where we Are, with the People we Have

British GPs and primary care teams who have been attracted to organized care of hypertension are generally aware of the preventive nature of this work, and that it must eventually lead to more comprehensive approaches to prevention. Blood pressure is not the only place to make a start, but it is where most of the more progressive teams have chosen to begin.

If we keep looking systematically for severe high blood pressure, which unquestionably needs medication, we shall find two or three times more people with blood pressures high enough to be a high relative risk, but not high enough to justify antihypertensive medication in the light of evidence from randomized trials. These people should be our starting point for the more effective primary care of the future, when we shall have a National Health Service not just a National Disease Service.

The trouble with this strategy is that it may concentrate treatment on single risk factors, within such small population groups that, even if fully operated, it could have little effect on the overall burden of premature cardiovascular disease. Using Framingham data, only 36% of all deaths causally related to systolic pressure >140 mmHg occur in the subgroup >180 mmHg. Even of these, two-thirds are coronary deaths, few of which are preventable by reducing blood pressure alone. In middle age there is no systolic or diastolic threshold below which the level of pressure is unrelated to risk. Even in the diastolic range 80–89 mmHg, risk of cardiovascular death is 39% higher than for people with diastolic pressures <80 mmHg.[109] There is no convincing case for reducing this risk by lowering blood pressure with antihypertensive treatment, but it can and should be reduced by attention to other risks which can be effectively reduced without medication, above all smoking, diet and exercise.

Rhetoric about prevention is cheap, but prevention in practice means sustained and intensely personal work, interfering with other people's lives, and is therefore unsuited to the conveyor belt styles of work generally typical of the private health check industry. Real outputs of prevention are proportional to real inputs, and these inputs are resources of time and labour. On any large scale, the changes in attitude, which we are told are the essential first step towards effective prevention, must follow firm government commitments to resource this vast area of new work, rather than precede them. Where this assurance is absent or not credible, it is hardly surprising that so many GPs hesitate to go down this path, or are unwilling and unbelieving conscripts to it because of the terms of the 1990 GP Contract. Driven by economic incentives alone without large investments in more and better continuing education, staff, information technology and record handling, they will merely comply with the cursory, largely delegated rituals of health checking, and the net health product will not change.

References

1. Gordon T, Sorlie P and Kannel WB (1971) Coronary heart disease, athero-thrombotic brain infarction, intermittent claudication. A multivariate analysis of some factors related to their incidence: Framingham study, 16–year follow-up. In: Kannel WB, Gordon T (eds) *The Framingham study: An epidemiologic investigation of cardiovascular disease, section 27.* US Government Printing Office, Washington DC.

2. Kannel WB (1975) Assessment of hypertension as a predictor of cardiovascular disease in the Framingham study. In: Burley DM, Birdwood GFB, Fryer JH, Taylor SH (eds) *Hypertension: its nature and treatment.* p.69 International Symposium, Malta, 1974. Ciba, Horsham.

3. Working Group of the Coronary Prevention Group and the British Heart Foundation (1991) An action plan for preventing coronary heart disease in primary care. *Br Med J* 303: 748–50.

4. Stamler J and Epstein FH (1982) Coronary heart disease: Risk factors as guides to preventive action. *Prev Med* 1: 27–48.

5. Lerner DJ and Kannel WB (1986) Patterns of coronary heart disease morbidity and mortality in the sexes: A 26-year follow-up of the Framingham population. *Am Heart J* 111: 383–90.

6. Pocock SJ and Seed PT (1992) Cholesterol in elderly women. *Lancet* 339: 1426.

7. Griffin T (ed) (1991) *Social Trends* 21. HMSO, London.

8. Bulpitt CJ, Beevers DG, Butler A *et al.* (1986) The survival of treated hypertensive patients and their causes of death: A report from the DHSS Hypertensive Care Computing Project (DHCCP). *J Hypertens* 4: 93–9.

9. Samuelsson O, Wilhelmsen L, Elmfeldt D *et al.* (1985) Predictors of cardiovascular morbidity in treated hypertension: Results from the primary preventive trial in Göteborg, Sweden. *J Hypertens* 3: 167–76.

10. Doll R and Peto R (1976) Mortality in relation to smoking: 20 years' observations on male British doctors. *Br Med J* ii: 1525–36.

11. Petitti DB and Klatsky AL (1983) Malignant hypertension in women aged 15 to 44 years and its relation to cigarette smoking and oral contraceptives. *Am J Cardiol* 52: 297–8.

12. Russell MAH, Wilson C, Taylor C et al. (1979) Effect of general practitioners' advice against smoking. *Br Med J* ii: 231–5.

13. Slama K, Redman S, Perkins J *et al.* (1990) The effectiveness of two smoking cessation programmes for use in general practice: A randomised controlled trial. *Br Med J* 300: 1707–9.

14. Hart JT, Thomas C, Gibbons B *et al.* (1991) Twenty-five years of audited screening in a socially deprived community. *Br Med J* 302: 1509–13.

15. Ashford J R (1973) Smoking and the use of health services. *Br J Prev Soc Med* 27: 8–17.

16. Townsend J (1987) Economic and health consequences of reduced smoking. In: Williams A (ed) *Health and economics*. Macmillan, London.

17. Townsend J (1991) Tobacco and the European common agricultural policy. *Br Med J* 303: 1008–9.

18. Dean M (1991) Tobacco deaths versus free speech. *Lancet* 338: 1383–4.

19. Secretary of State for Health (1991) *The health of the nation: A consultative document for health in England*. HMSO, London, (Cm1523).

20. Townsend J, Wilkes H, Haines A P *et al*. (1991) Adolescent smokers seen in general practice: Health, lifestyle, physical measurements and response to antismoking advice. *Br Med J* 303: 953–7.

21. Godlee F (1991) No smoking day 1991. *Br Med J* 302: 552.

22. Jamrozik K, Vessey M, Fowler G *et al*. (1984) Controlled trial of three different smoking interventions in general practice. *Br Med J* 288: 1499–503.

23. Sanders D, Fowler G, Mant D *et al*. (1989) Randomized controlled trial of anti-smoking advice by nurses in general practice. *J R Coll Gen Pract* 39: 273–6.

24. Ulbricht T L V and Southgate D A T (1991) Coronary heart disease: Seven dietary factors. *Lancet* 338: 985–92.

25. Shaper A G, Pocock S J, Phillips A N et al. (1986) Identifying men at high risk of heart attacks: Strategy for use in general practice. *Br Med J* 293: 474–9.

26. Department of Health and Social Security (1984) Report of the Committee on medical aspects of food policy: *Diet and cardiovascular disease*. HMSO, London.

27. Editorial Committee of the National Forum for Coronary Heart Disease Prevention (1988) *Coronary heart disease prevention: Action in the UK 1984\1987: A review of progess*. Health Education Authority, London.

28. Lee T H and Arm J P (1988) Benefits from oily fish. *Br Med J* 297: 1421–2.

29. Hostmark AT, Bjerkedal T and Kierulf P (1988) Fish oil and plasma fibrinogen. *Br Med J* 297: 180.

30. Norris PG, Jones CJH and Weston MJ (1986) Effect of dietary supplementation with fish oil on systolic blood pressure in mild essential hypertension. *Br Med J* 293: 104–5.

31. Kromhout D, Bosschieter ED and Coulander C de L (1985) The inverse relation between fish consumption and 20-year mortality from coronary heart disease. *N Engl J Med* 312: 1205–9.

32. Burr ML, Fehily AM, Gilbert JF *et al.* (1989) Effects of changes in fat, fish, and fibre intakes on death and myocardial reinfarction: Diet and Reinfarction Trial (DART). *Lancet* ii: 757–61.

33. Walker CL (1984) The national diet. *Postgrad Med J* **60**: 26–33.

34. Calnan M (1990) Food and health. In: Cunningham S, Burley S and McKeganey N (eds) *Readings in medical sociology.* Tavistock. London,

35. Directorate of the Welsh Heart Programme (1987) Pulse of Wales: Social survey supplement. Heartbeat Report No. 7. Heartbeat Wales, Cardiff.

36. Wilson G (1989) Diet and health. *J Soc Policy* **18**: 167–85.

37. Cole-Hamilton I (1989) Review of food patterns amongst lower income groups in the UK. Health Education Authority, London (unpublished report).

38. Anderson P (1988) Excess mortality associated with alcohol consumption. *Br Med J* **297**: 824–5.

39. Royal College of General Practitioners (1986) *Alcohol: A balanced view.* Report from general practice No. 24. RCGP, London.

40. (1990) Alcohol and cancer (editorial). *Lancet* **335**: 634.

41. Gill JS, Beevers DG and Tsementzis SA (1983) Strokes and alcohol. *Lancet* ii: 1142–3.

42. Wallace PG, Brennan PJ and Haines AP (1987) Drinking patterns in general practice patients. *J R Coll Gen Pract* **37**: 354–7.

43. Lazarus NB, Kaplan GA, Cohen RD *et al.* (1991) Change in alcohol consumption and risk of death from all causes and from ischaemic heart disease. *Br Med J* **303**: 553–6.

44. Marmot M and Brunner E (1991) Alcohol cardiovascular disease: The status of the U-shaped curve. *Br Med J* **303**: 565–8.

45. Ravussin E and Swinburn BA (1992) Pathophysiology of obesity. *Lancet* **340**: 404–8.

46. Garrow J (1992) Treatment of obesity. *Lancet* **340**: 409–13.

47. Bjorntorp P (1985) Obesity and the risk of cardiovascular disease. *Ann Clin Res* **17**: 3–9.

48. Barrett-Connor and Khaw KT (1985) Is hypertension more benign when associated with obesity? *Circulation* **72**: 53.

49. Berglund A, Anderssen OK, Berglund G *et al.* (1989) Antihypertensive effect of diet compared with drug treatment in obese men with mild hypertension. *Br Med J* **299**: 480–5.

50. Hart JT (1992) The Rule of Halves: Implications of underdiagnosis and drop-out for future workload and prescribing costs in primary care. *Brit J Gen Pract* **41**: 116–9.

51. Cade J and O'Connell S (1991) Management of weight problems and obesity: knowledge, attitudes and current practice of general practitioners. *Br J Gen Pract* **41**: 147–50.

52. Turner RC (1985) UK prospective diabetes study. III: Prevalence of hypertension and hypotensive therapy in newly-presenting diabetic patients. *Hypertension* **7** (**supp 12**): 8–13.

53. Salomaa VV, Strandberg TE, Vanhanen H *et al.* (1991) Glucose tolerance and blood pressure: Long term follow-up in middle aged men. *Br Med J* **302**: 493–6.

54. Yudkin JS (1991) Hypertension and non-insulin dependent diabetes. *Br Med J* **303**: 730–2.

55. Rosengren A, Welin L, Tsipogianni A *et al.* (1989) Impact of cardiovascular risk factors on coronary heart disease and mortality among middle aged diabetic men: A general population study. *Br Med J* **299**: 1127–31.

56. McKeigue PM and Marmot MG (1988) Mortality from coronary heart disease in Asian communities in London. *Br Med J* **297**: 903.

57. Simons D, Williams DRR and Powell MJ (1989) Prevalence of diabetes in a predominantly Asian community: Preliminary findings of the Coventry diabetes study. *Br Med J* **298**: 18–21.

58. Balarajan R (1991) Ethnic differences in mortality from ischaemic heart disease and cerebrovascular disease in England and Wales. *Br Med J* **302**: 560–4.

59. Barker DJP, Gardner MJ and Power C (1982) Incidence of diabetes among

people aged 18–50 years in nine British towns: A collaborative study. *Diabetologia* **22**: 421–5.

60. Fuller JH, Shipley MJ, Rose G *et al.* (1983) Mortality from coronary heart disease and stroke in relation to degree of glycaemia: The Whitehall study. *Br Med J* **287**: 867–70.

61. Mann JI (1981) A high carbohydrate leguminous fibre diet improves all aspects of diabetic control. *Lancet* i: 1–5.

62. Chen Z, Peto R and Collins R (1991) Serum cholesterol concentration and coronary heart disease in a population with low cholesterol concentrations. *Br Med J* **303**: 276–82.

63. Curzio JL, Howie C, Kennedy S *et al.* (1991) Measurement of capillary cholesterol level in hyperlipidaemia. *Br J Gen Pract* **41**: 433.

64. Welsh Heart Programme Directorate (1988) *Heart of Wales: Clinical results of the Welsh Heart Health Survey.* Heartbeat Report No. 20. Heartbeat Wales, Cardiff.

65. Kinlay S and Heller RF (1990) Effectiveness and hazards of case finding for a high cholesterol concentration. *Br Med J* **300**: 1545–7.

66. Hjermann I, Velve BK and Holme I (1981) Effect of diet and smoking intervention on the incidence of coronary heart disease: Report from the Oslo study group of a randomized trial in healthy men. *Lancet* ii: 1303–10.

67. Multiple Risk Factor Intervention Trial Research Group (1982) Multiple risk factor intervention trial (MRFIT): Risk factor changes and mortality results. JAMA **248**: 1465–77.

68. Yinnon AM, Blau S and Sardas A (1992) A practical intervention programme aimed at decreasing high serum cholesterol levels in primary care. *Fam Pract* **9**: 167–70.

69. Ramsay LE, Yeo WW and Jackson PR (1991) Dietary reduction of serum cholesterol concentration: Time to think again. *Br Med J* **303**: 953–7, 1551.

70. Meade TW (1990) Low-dose warfarin and low-dose aspirin in the primary prevention of ischemic heart disease. *Am J Cardiol* **65**: 7c–11c.

71. Collins R, Keech A, Peto R *et al.* (1992) Cholesterol and total mortality: Need for larger trials. *Br Med J* **304**: 1689.

72. Ravsnkov U (1992) Cholesterol lowering trials in coronary heart disease: Frequency of citation and outcome. *Br Med J* **305**: 15–19.

73. Watts GF, Lewis B, Brunt JNH *et al.* (1992) Effects on coronary artery disease of lipid-lowering diet, or diet plus cholestyramine, in the St Thomas' Atherosclerosis Regression Study (STARS). *Lancet* **339**: 563–9.

74. Scientific Steering Committee of the Simon Broome Register Group (1991) Risk of fatal coronary heart disease in familial hypercholesterolaemia. *Br Med J* **303**: 893–6.

75. Stone MC and Thorp JM (1985) Plasma fibrinogen, a major cardiovascular risk factor. *J R Coll Gen Pract* **35**: 565–9.

76. Meade TW, Mellows S, Brozovic M *et al.* (1986) Haemostatic function and ischaemic heart disease: Principal results of the Northwick Park Heart Study. *Lancet* ii: 533–7.

77. Meade TW (1987) The epidemiology of haemostatic and other variables in coronary artery disease. In: Verstraete M, Vermylen J, Lijnen R, Amout J (eds) *Thrombosis and haemostasis.* pp. 37–60. Leuven University Press, Leuven.

78. Ernst E (1991) Fibrinogen: An independent risk factor for cardiovascular disease. *Br Med J* **303**: 596–7.

79. Markowe HLJ, Marmot MG, Shipley MJ *et al.* (1985) Fibrinogen: A possible link between social class and coronary heart disease. *Br Med J* **291**: 1312–14.

80. Rosengren A, Wilhelmsen L, Welin L *et al.* (1990) Social influences and cardiovascular risk factors as determinants of plasma fibrinogen concentration in a general population sample of middle aged men. *Br Med J* **300**: 634–8.

81. Dargie HJ and Grant S (1991) The health of the nation: Exercise. *Br Med J* **303**: 910–12.

82. Gloag D (1992) Exercise, fitness, and health. *Br Med J* **305**: 377–8.

83. Helmrich SP, Ragland DR, Leung RW *et al.* (1991) Physical activity and

reduced occurrence of non-insulin-dependent diabetes mellitus. *N Engl J Med* **325**: 147–52.

84. Browner WS, Seeley DG, Vogt TM *et al.* (1991) Non-trauma mortality in elderly women with low mineral bone density. *Lancet* **338**: 355–8.

85. O'Connor GT, Buring JE, Yusuf S *et al.* (1989) An overview of randomized trials of rehabilitation with exercise after myocardial infarction. *Circulation* **80**: 234–44.

86. British Medical Association (1992) *Cycling towards health and safety.* Oxford University Press, Oxford.

87. Borhani NO and Borkman TS (1968) *The Alameda County blood pressure study.* State of California Department of Public Health, Berkeley CA.

88. Cassel J (1976) The contribution of the social environment to host resistance. *Am J Epidemiol* **104**: 107–23.

89. Marmot MG and Syme SL (1976) Acculturation and coronary heart disease. *Am J Epidemiol* **104**: 225–47.

90. Marmot MG, Smith GD, Stansfield S *et al.* (1991) Health inequalities among British civil servants: The Whitehall II study. *Lancet* **337**: 1387–93.

91. Brody H (1987) *Stories of sickness.* Yale University Press, New Haven.

92. Charlton BG (1991) Stories of sickness. *Br J Gen Pract* **41**: 222–3.

93. Borhani NO (1985) Prevention of coronary heart disease in practice: implications of the results of recent clinical trials. *JAMA* **254**: 257–62.

94. Farquhar JW, Maccoby N, Wood PD *et al.* (1977) Community education for cardiovascular health. *Lancet* i: 1192–5.

95. Puska P, Nissinen A, Salonen JT *et al.* (1983) Ten years of the North Karelia Project: Results with community prevention of coronary heart disease. *Scand J Soc Med* **11**: 65–8.

96. Strandberg TE, Salomaa VV, Naukkarinen VA *et al.* (1991) Long term mortality after 5 years multifactorial primary prevention of cardiovascular diseases in middle aged men. *JAMA* **226**: 1255–9.

97. Durrington PN and Bhatnagar D (1992) Wrong lesson from Finnish trial of cardiovascular disease prevention. *Lancet* **339**: 488.

98. Imperial Cancer Research Fund OXCHECK Study Group (1991) Prevalence of risk factors for heart disease in the OXCHECK trial: Implications for screening in primary care. *Br Med J* **302**: 1057–60.

99. World Health Organization European Collaborative Group (1986) European collaborative trial of multifactorial prevention of coronary heart disease: final report of the 6-year results. *Lancet* **i**: 869–72.

100. World Health Organization European Collaborative Group (1982) Multifactorial trial in the prevention of coronary heart disease. 2: Risk factor changes at two and four years. *Eur Heart J* **3**: 184–90.

101. Hart JT (1990) Reactive and proactive care: A crisis. *Br J Gen Pract* **40**: 4–9.

102. Carney T (1989) Ethnic population and general practitioners' workload. *Br Med J* **299**: 930–1.

103. Taylor V, Robson J and Evans S (1992) Risk factors for coronary heart disease: A study in inner London. *Br J Gen Pract* **42**: 377–80.

104. Calnan M (1991) *Preventing coronary heart disease: Prospects, policies, and politics.* p. 32. Routledge, London.

105. Sytkowski PA, Kannel WB and D'Agostino RB (1990) Changes in risk factors and the decline in mortality from cardiovascular disease. *N Engl J Med* **322**: 1635–41.

106. Tunstall-Pedoe H (1991) The Dundee Coronary Risk-Disk for management of change in risk factors. *Br Med J* **303**: 744–7.

107. Tunstall-Pedoe H (1992) Value of the Dundee Coronary Risk-Disk: A defence. *Br Med J* **305**: 231–2.

108. Randall T, Muir J and Mant D (1992) Choosing the preventive workload in general practice: practical application of the Coronary Prevention Group guidelines and Dundee Coronary Risk-Disk. *Br Med J* **305**: 227–31.

109. Kannel WB (1975) Role of blood pressure in cardiovascular disease. *Angiology* **26**: 1–14.

110. Abelin T, Muller P and Buchler A *et al.* (1989) Controlled trial of transdermal nicotine patches in smoking cessation. *Lancet.* i: 7–9.

111. Fowler G (1993) The Indians' revenge. *Br J Gen Pract.* **43**: 78–81.

112. Jarvis MJ, Raw M, Russell MAH *et al.* (1982) Randomized controlled trial of nicotine chewing gum. *Br Med J.* **285**: 537–40.

113. Lam W, Sze PC, Sacks HS *et al.* (1987) Meta-analysis of randomized controlled trials of nicotine chewing gum. *Lancet* ii: 27–30.

Case Finding and Screening

As high blood pressure at any level rarely causes symptoms, it must be looked for. Everyone has a blood pressure, and its value is not known until it has been measured. To achieve this for a whole registered population requires planned organization. In the 1960s everyone would have called this screening, which may be broadly defined as application of any diagnostic procedure to as many as possible of a defined group of the population, regardless of presenting complaints.

Origins of Screening

The screening idea has been with us for centuries, centered initially on problems of military manpower.[1] Since the Second World War, the idea of screening for clinical rather than research purposes began in the early 1960s, as a result of two developments.

The first was the concept of the epidemiology of non-infective disease, which owed much to experience of operations research in the Second World War. This provided a conceptual framework through which strategies for mass diagnosis and intervention could be developed. Although the epidemiological concept was originally a huge step forward, clinical population care now needs to transcend it. Most epidemiological studies gathered their data intensively over short periods, and had an above-down approach, isolated from and ignorant of the street wisdom of primary care teams. Although epidemiologists had to be sensitive to some at least of the feelings and opinions of their target populations, because response rates depended on them, they underestimated the vastly more complex relationships required for the continuing patient care which should result from effective screening.

The second prerequisite for clinical screening was new diagnostic and information technology, which made it logistically possible to generate and handle data on a previously inconceivable scale.

Limitations of Screening

Technical advances have enormously increased our diagnostic power, but this power tends to be used with decreasing precision. Laboratory technology first tempts and then compels us to adopt standardized batteries of tests. These may still answer precisely defined diagnostic questions, but also gather in answers to questions that have never been clearly formulated. The old logical principle that test ordering was a waste of time and money unless it asked a specific question with a clinically useful answer, was generally accepted as long as clinicians did tests themselves, or at least worked close to laboratories. It faltered as work became delegated to pathologists and laboratory workers; with the advent of auto-analysers, which are incapable of offering a simple 'yes' or 'no' to any single question, it collapsed.

These machines produce 10, 12, even 20 biochemical or haematological measurements at a time on a single blood sample. However precise the original question, it leads necessarily to 9, 11, or 19 unrequested and usually irrelevant answers. Information technology has developed even faster, so that all these gratuitous data can, conceivably, be stored and eventually used. Thus clinicians have been prepared for industrialized mass diagnosis, and a general shift from thoughtful testing of specific, individualized hypotheses, to aimless trawling with catch-all diagnostic nets.

The most serious risk of screening, and of all attempts to introduce planned structure, are authoritarianism and bureaucratization of care. These risks are equalled only by those of an abdication from all planned structure, allowing care to be prompted only by presented symptoms. Health workers who cannot learn to understand the creative tension between these two necessary opposites cannot function effectively in a primary care team.

Social Directions of Development of Screening

For all these reasons, all forms of screening are therefore suspect. Beginning in the early 1970s, clinical screening has developed in three different directions.

First in the USA, and to a smaller extent in other fee-paying medical care systems, the idea of earlier diagnosis and earlier treatment by detection of presymptomatic departures from supposed normal values was embraced with enthusiasm, not least because it enormously broadened the market, effectively making the whole population, well or ill, into its customers. Generous investments in staff and multichannel equipment were made, using batteries of tests of the kind just described. The main UK experience of this sort of screening was outside the NHS, mainly staff screening by the British United Provident Association (BUPA) and other entrepreneurs. This sometimes assisted but more often exasperated GPs by sending multiple risk prints and biochemical profiles about many of their NHS patients. Because screening of this kind is based on fees, large proportions of the population at risk but without insurance cover are omitted, and its effectiveness has never been validated against similar controls. As such schemes are self-financing they have attracted little criticism, except for their possible effect in raising expectations of NHS patients which cannot be met.

The second type of screening was developed experimentally, usually with academic and government backing, to evaluate the effectiveness and efficiency of screening procedures before public demand might make them a mandatory and costly addition to the NHS. An early example was the Värmland project in Sweden. Epidemiologists, community physicians, and health economists developed their methodology, generally with little regard for existing systems of primary care (a notable exception was the programme near Glasgow developed by Hawthorne[3]). Generally negative conclusions were quickly accepted for nearly all these non-commercial systems.[1,3]

Typical of these was a large study by the Department of Community Medicine at St Thomas's hospital.[4] This compared ascertainment and control of hypertension in co-operating general practices randomly allocated either to screening assisted by an epidemiological team, or to customary casual case finding, without organization or audit. There were uniformly poor results for follow-up in both groups. Evidently GPs who passively accept screening designed and performed by an outside team, manage and follow-up their hypertensive patients just as badly as GPs whose patients have not been screened. This trial is probably more relevant to the work of health promotion clinics, hastily established to generate practice income under the 1990 GP Contract, than it was to pioneering GP screeners before the contract, who generally reported big improvements in both ascertainment and follow-up.

From this, and other evidence less relevant to general practice, two leading epidemiologists, David Sackett and Walter Holland[5], concluded that there was no case for screening for hypertension. Despite this scepticism, their colleagues in health economics now consider screening of some kind for high blood pressure to be a relatively cost effective exercise, with an estimated cost per quality-adjusted-life-year (QALY) of £5400 (US$9200) for severe and £10 900 (US$18 600) for mild hypertension.[6, 7] This is more costly than GPs' advice to give up smoking at £238 (US$406), but cheaper than a coronary artery bypass graft for severe angina and three-vessel disease at £15 505 (US$26 451) or for single vessel disease at £301 000 (US$515 000) (1987/8 UK prices). Sackett and

Holland conceded only that GPs might usefully continue case finding, which as they described it meant a continuation of presumed standard practice.

Since then screening has become more narrowly defined as an intensive search for cases through active call-up to specialized clinics with protected time, generally separated from other patient demands, and targeting people who feel well. The more integrated alternative is opportunist case finding, actively searching for cases during ordinary contacts prompted by patient demand, usually either by extending ordinary consultations, or by offering measurements to patients while they are waiting.

The advantages of screening as an activity separate from demand-led care are that it makes economical use of staff in protected time, can be used to call up households rather than individuals, and has wide possibilities for group health education. Its disadvantages are that, unless teams acquire sufficient new resources, this protected time may have to compete with the unprotected time of ordinary clinical sessions, leaving less time to help people with problems, that isolation of health maintenance from response to presented problems may lead to staff boredom, and eventually to thoughtless and ineffective conveyor belt care, and that the whole concept of well-man and well-women clinics seems in practice to be much more attractive to middle class than to working class patients.

Social differences in response have been obvious to everyone with real experience of attempts to apply health checks on a mass scale in working class or mixed communities.[8, 13] The difficulty is serious, because poorer and less educated people are generally at much higher risk. It is often assumed that working class people will eventually acquire the consumer preferences of the middle class, so that the well-man/well-woman clinic style will gain more customers and become more effective as time goes on. Both the assumption and the goal are questionable; if health check clinics represent industrialization of medical care, their intuitive rejection by less educated people may be a salutary judgement we should heed.

Case finding, on the other hand, means active search for cases during traditional contacts prompted by patient demand, usually either by extending ordinary consultations, or by offering measurements to patients while they are waiting to see a doctor. It is certainly feasible in the UK NHS, where 65–80% of total registered populations consult at least once a year, 80–95% consult at least once every 5 years, and the social groups at highest risk consult most frequently.[14]

The advantages of case finding are that it starts from where we are, with the people we have. It grows more naturally from traditional patient-prompted contacts, so that active search for modifiable risks can be intelligibly linked to patients' personal problems, and action to change them is more easily incorporated into their own personal stories. This linkage may improve motivation both for patients and for professionals, who may be less likely to slide into thoughtless repetition of diagnostic and instructive ritual.

Its most immediate disadvantage is the illusion that it is already, effortlessly, happening. In the absence of audit, GPs who undertake to implement assiduous case finding as a normal part of their clinical routine do not, in fact, do so. In theory, good clinical care, as taught in medical schools, has always included consideration of every aspect of every case, including social factors and assessment of future risks. Medical students were taught never to question this definition, however impractical it might appear even in centres of excellence, let alone the peripheries in which most would eventually work. They were also taught (usually by example) never to admit their own failures to achieve the impossible. Doctors therefore assumed that if they were seeing most patients every year and nearly all patients every 5 years, and if all these patients came from defined and stable populations, as they generally do in the NHS, the search for need must already be complete. There was therefore no need for any special organization, planning, or division of labour.

Such illusions are now disappearing, under the impact of audits which show again and again that even the best clinical care is normally incomplete against theoretical standards, until subjected to audit and then reorganized to attain defined and measurable objectives. Real advance depends on a continuing cycle of audit, self-criticism, setting of new goals, and then repeated audit to measure their attainment.

Audit of GP recording of cardiovascular risk factors in 24 Scottish practices in 1988 still showed an average of 11% of men aged 35–64 without any recorded blood pressure (range 1–65%), 44% with no information on smoking habit (range 0–89%), and 63% with no record of body weight (range 3–95%)[15]. These relatively good figures followed a series of audits in the same area over the preceding decade, starting from much lower levels of recording. In the Oxford region of England, generally regarded as an area of high quality practice, on the eve of the 1990 contract requiring routine recording of blood pressure every 3 years in adults, only 71% of responding GPs in 1987 aimed to record blood pressure routinely, and only 20% claimed to have some method of identifying patients with no pressure recorded during the preceding 5 years.[16]

Within a care system which permits and depends upon continuity, we need not assume that every patient must be fully assessed at first contact. Traditionally, each consultation has aimed to solve a particular set of presented problems. Clinicians try to do this by selecting economical pathways for testing a limited range of likely hypotheses, excluding information that is not immediately relevant. Extension of ordinary consultations to include not only what patients want (reactive care), but also what professionals think they need (proactive care), requires redefinition of aims. It also requires greater resources, certainly in time and usually in staff. If these resources are not made available, this redefinition will not take place, and necessary work will continue to be assumed in theory but ignored in practice. If payment becomes related to proactive process without regard to audited outcome, as in the 1990 Contract, we are likely to see more of the form but even less of the content of real anticipatory care.

Unit Autonomy

Following considerable investment in postgraduate education for GPs and practice nurses, who shared in developing their own consensus detection and treatment programme, much better results than any yet reported in the UK were found in rural Norway in 1986.[17] Unquestionably, if mass detection of high blood pressure is cost effective and necessary, the most efficient way to do it is through primary care teams, but these need full autonomy to devise their own solutions for the problems of detection and subsequent follow-up on a population scale.

In practice, they are then likely to choose to use both techniques, both formal call-up screening and informal case finding, modifying their choice according to subsequent experience revealed by audit.

This has in fact been the path followed by innovative GPs in the UK, Scandinavia, and The Netherlands, who made constructive use of their autonomy and defined populations in these care systems to set up the first primary care screening programmes.[18-22] Large schemes for organized case finding with planned follow-up were also launched in some countries of the Eastern bloc, notably in East Germany, but virtual elimination of generalist personal responsibility and continuity from these care systems precluded effective innovation on the model of personalized anticipatory care evolving in the West.

Screening by these innovative GPs differed from traditional case findings in aiming to reach whole populations, to audit results over years rather than months, and to build new structures of proactive care on a generous base of reactive care. The few schemes in western Europe were all begun by enthusiasts, a point much stressed by their critics in epidemiology and community medicine, who claimed their techniques were therefore not replicable. A more constructive interpretation might have been that enthusiasim is required for all innovation, and is essential for effective practice, particularly in primary care, and most of all in proactive primary care.

All these early screening or organized case finding programmes initiated by GPs themselves have, as far as I know, prospered, with steadily improving results in terms of high response, sustained reductions in blood pressure in identified hypertensives, and low drop-out rates. I know of only three which have published analyses of their results.[21-24] All performed as well as, or better than, the best specialist hospital clinics, and were tackling a much bigger and more important task, the control of moderate and severe hypertension in entire populations at risk.

Screening and Case Finding: the Sequence

The tasks are to detect high blood pressure throughout the registered population at risk, verify by replication and then offer a full range of treatment to those for whom advantages are likely to outweigh disadvantages. Follow–up must be organized for the entire treated group, and advice on personal risks must be provided for everyone else.

This combination of tasks is much more complex than designers of the GP Contract seem to have imagined. In particular, initial detection is much simpler than organization of consequent investigation, education, and follow–up, which for treated hypertensives will normally be for life.

The old Contract, initiated in 1948 and amended in 1966, assumed that GPs' responsibilities began only when prompted by patients' demands. Inclusion of proactive care in the 1990 Contract in generalized form, that GPs are responsible for organizing prevention of all that is medically preventable, would be an important step forward. What has actually occurred is less a step forward than a step sideways; the Contract undertakes not to resource team reorientation and its progress toward new ends, but to pay individual GPs for specified means. It pays for health promotion clinics as defined in the Act and interpreted by family health service administrators. Some of these administrators had real social imagination, and pushed the Contract towards broad policies of anticipatory care as far as their limited budgets allowed; many more did not. Try as they might to transcend their limited social experience as military, naval, or industrial commanders, they had no experience of actually doing what they were employed to do. So much new screening and case finding went on that more patients must have started on treatment. If, however, the aim was better conservation of health and continued development of general practice teams towards effective anticipatory care, paying for health promotion clinics rather than resourcing a much broader approach will ultimately prove counterproductive. By early 1993, the Department of Health finally began to understand at least some of this message, and revised the Contract to encourage case finding rather than clinics. However, like all development in the NHS, it remains under-resourced.

For optimally efficient, cost effective progress towards any clinical aim, primary care teams must have autonomy, finding their own means to attain national aims. Mistakes will be made, but if they are made at the periphery, by health workers familiar with their particular populations and circumstances, such mistakes will add permanently useful experience on which to build. Mistakes made nationally, regionally, or by area bureaucracies, and then imposed from above without local consultation, will only confirm peripheral cynicism and make the whole task more difficult.

The best teams ignored the terms of the Contract when they could afford it. They found optimal combinations of call-up screening, health check clinics, expanded consultations and follow–up clinics which get the largest response and smallest drop-out from subsequent follow–up, having full regard to local conditions and the particular organizational history of each practice. Having done this, they then saw how much additional staffing and work required could be claimed for under the Contract, bending the rules as far as their FHSA administrators would allow.

Screening the Records

In screening a defined population by either means, call-up or case finding, the first step is to screen not patients, but records, to see what information you already have.

In which age and sex groups will you make this search? You may reasonably assume that little or no blood pressure data will have been recorded for anyone aged under 16. Blood pressures should have been recorded for all women on oral contraceptives, and as it is important for women of child bearing age to have pre-pregnancy blood pressure data to assess the significance of blood pressures recorded later in pregnancy, there is a good case for defining the start of their adult life from age 16. As you will see in Chapter 20, high blood pressure in young adults is much commoner, and eventually more dangerous, than most of us suppose. The Glyncorrwg data set began from age 20, but if I had my life over again it would start at 16 for both sexes. Where should it end? On current evidence, not before age 85. Management in age groups 16–24, 25–64 and 65–85 must be organized differently in each, and your records search should present these data separately.

The best way to start this process is to draw a small random sample of records in the age and sex groups you have chosen, and do a pilot study on these before making any further plans. The whole team can then consider what it is up against.

This record search will yield five different sets of data:

■ Adults with no record of blood pressure at all, or none within the preceding 5 years, either in the text or in hospital letters.
■ Hypertensives currently treated, on initially valid criteria: This may be confirmed by a 3-month search through repeat prescriptions, retrospectively if you have a computer system, prospectively if you do not. Note the date and level of the last blood pressure measurement recorded, and search back through the record and hospital correspondence to identify the average level of the last three pressures recorded before treatment was started.

This procedure will give you the next groups:

■ Hypertensives currently treated, on initially doubtful or unknown criteria: This group will need very careful review. Unjustified treatment may represent a considerable burden on follow-up, but stopping treatment for well controlled hypertensives with initially high levels of pressure can lead to some nasty surprises, sometimes after delays of 6 months or more.
■ Hypertensives previously indentified, who either refused treatment, or started treatment but have been lost to follow-up: This group is likely to be surprisingly large, and may contain some people at very high risk. It is important

to look for initial mean values of pressure, some of which may be alarming and may require urgent and active recall for immediate review. Original refusal of treatment may change on review.

■ People whose status cannot be ascertained from recorded data: These include people apparently on treatment who appear not to be collecting prescriptions, people who appear from hospital correspondence to be on treatment but are known not to be, misfiled data, changed addresses, people not seen for 20 years and of doubtful existence, and so on. Any process entailing contact with all your registered patients will be an important, and usually chastening, experience for the primary care team, at least when done for the first time.

All this is a stern test of the quality of your records. Almost certainly you will find less data than you expected. Perhaps you or your partners have recorded only what you considered abnormal findings, and it may be difficult to understand from the records whether some patients are still on medication, and if so, what. How much information is there about other risk factors, such as smoking, blood cholesterol and obesity? Are weights and heights recorded? When you are looking at patients rather than their records, you can tell easily whether they are fat, but for record review without visible patients, you must have heights to calculate the body mass index (weight in kilograms divided by height in metres squared).

Practices which have never been screened invariably have a lot more hypertensive women than men detected and therefore treated. Keith Hodgkin,[25] for example, reported a male:female ratio of 1:5 in his very thorough analysis of about 30 years' practice, although all epidemiological studies confirm that high blood pressure is both commoner and more dangerous in men than women until middle age, and treatment of men is more effective in preventing organ damage, at least in mild hypertension.[26]

From pilot samples you can estimate roughly how much time and labour will be required, first to screen all your records, then to screen all your patients, and finally to follow up and treat what you discover or rediscover; the number of patients dropped out from treatment is likely to be quite large and will represent an immediate burden on work-load. This is the evidence you will need to assess the additional staff, and possibly the additional space, needed to do the job properly. It is evidence you should include in your practice annual report, which should be your reasoned argument for additional resources from the FHSA, and for support from the community you serve, your patients, who have votes.

Tagging the Records

Having identified the records with missing information, you will need a tagging system to make these omissions obvious next time the people they represent visit your centre, so that whoever is responsible for measuring routine blood pressures or collecting other risk data can know when to do so.

With Lloyd-George* records the simplest way to do this is to get a local do-it-yourself shop to cut up a coloured resin laminate sheet into a number of slats, long enough to stick up out of the record envelope but short enough not to scrape the top of the shelves or drawers, and numerous enough to have one in every record that needs it. As blood pressures are measured, the slats are taken out so that work is not duplicated. When one search is finished you can use the slats for the next. This is the method we used in Glyncorrwg in 1968, when we still used Lloyd-George pocket envelope records.

In 1977 we converted to A4 folders. With these tagging is more difficult; in fact this is the only convincing argument I have ever heard in defence of a record system devised for GPs in 1915, and still used by 95% of English and Welsh practices in 1991. There is no way to attach any removable sign to any part of an A4 folder which will not break loose in the rough and tumble of office consultations and home visits. The simplest method is probably to make one diagonal stroke on the outside of each record with a large felt pen for those with data outstanding, and to cross this out with an opposing stroke when each job has been done. You can use a different colour for the next procedure. As long as A4 folders continue to be made of third-rate cardboard, they will not last more than 10 years, so there should be enough room for lots of marks.

An alternative, which has apparently worked in some practices, is to write (or rubber stamp) an instruction in the text to the next doctor who sees the patient, such as 'BP, SMOKING, WEIGHT AND HEIGHT NEXT TIME PLEASE'. My own capacity to ignore or find excuses for evading such commands has taught me that, for me at least, this does not work. On the whole, nurses and office staff have a more organized approach to their work than doctors, and are less likely to ignore a protocol once it has been agreed and understood, but do not count on it.

* This needs explaining for readers abroad. Lloyd-George introduced the first UK national insurance system in 1912. His medical record was designed in 1915 and first used in 1916. It has a roughly A6-size pocket envelope, originally made of fabric based paper extremely well designed to endure the hard life of a GP medical record, and last the expected lifetime of the patient. The GP's continuing notes are pushed into this envelope, together with all hospital correspondence, laboratory reports and so on, folded up so that eventually they will disintegrate, and thus make room for more notes to go in the envelope. Subsequent governments have downgraded the quality of the paper from which it is made, while at the same time expecting the design to remain immortal. Not one of them has ever understood the clinical importance of good records, or given any material encouragement for their improvement. The Scottish Office has been an honourable exception. Despite these strictures, there are some good features of the UK records system, above all, that records follow patients throughout their lives, moving from one GP to another as patients change their addresses, or choose a different practice.

Boxed Card Indexes

As possible hypertensives are identified, and actual hypertensives are verified by repeated readings, cases found must be listed so that active follow-up and audit are possible. The traditional alternative, simply to tell patients they have high blood pressure and leave it to them to return without any means of recognizing default, will soon return you to chaos. This is particularly true early on in the management of newly discovered cases, because several sessions are usually needed before patients fully understand that they are not ill, but do need lifelong follow-up, and usually lifelong medication.

The answer is simple for computerized practices. Virtually all programs now include facilities for listing and recall of hypertensives. There is an equally simple answer for practices without computers: set up a boxed card index, organized into the months of the year so that, as patients are seen, they move into the next 3-month slot (or whatever interval you have chosen). Having once set up the box, it is important to ensure that subsequent new cases (after the initial excitement of the screening campaign) get into the pipeline. Patients should also be asked to contact someone on the team themselves if they ever find they have been out of contact for more than 3 months, and be informed that practice staff will not issue repeat prescriptions without at least a blood pressure check. This fail-safe device is a useful defence against inevitable organizational failures in even the most sophisticated system.

About 80% of NHS practices now use computers for at least some aspect of patient care. Although these enormously facilitate data retrieval for audit, they are based on the same principles as a card index, and a practice which cannot maintain a good card index is unlikely to use a computer effectively. The whole question of record and information systems is dealt with more thoroughly in Chapter 9.

Contacting the Population

Traditionally, the main way family doctors have tried to reach their patients as a population has been to put up a notice in the waiting room. As we all know, such notices rarely produce an effective response.

If you are planning to contact the whole of your adult population, you will be having a large impact on your local community, and you should think about the public relations aspect of your work in a positive way. Now that government positively encourages self-advertisement and the General Medical Council has virtually abandoned effective opposition, active outreach to your population is much less of a problem. It is still important that any information used to encourage contact should be based on sound evidence. I have seen at least one practice leaflet advertising a well-man clinic which claimed that coronary heart disease was now a wholly preventable condition! In general, however, unrestricted advertising has not been abused by NHS GPs, and there are now many examples of excellent locally produced propaganda material, informing patients of what their primary care teams are doing and plan to do.

In Glyncorrwg we were fortunate in having a stable community despite serious social problems, where people knew and cared about each other. Public meetings on health questions were convened two or three times a year by an elected patients' committee, and were usually well attended, with audiences of 30–60. Explanations of cardiovascular risk factors given to local public meetings are an important way of supplementing individual patient education, and have a lasting effect by recruiting local opinion-formers to your cause and giving them more reliable information than they are likely to pick up by themselves.

A more systematic form of contact is entry to the practice. Many practices now accept responsibility for an initial interview at registration, when patients can give a brief history of major events and a minimum data set can be recorded, normally including at least blood pressure, weight, height, and smoking habit. This first registration contact attracts a fee under the 1990 Contract, which should help to cover the cost. A loophole in the Contract allows new single handed practitioners to claim this one-off fee for their entire practice, so anything short of excellence in their data recording must be hard to justify.

What About Non-Respondents?

A question always brought up at both public and professional meetings is the degree to which we are justified in pushing diagnosis and care at people who have not asked for it and may not want it. In the 1970s this was often raised as a largely imaginary obstacle by doctors trying to find enough difficulties to justify their own inaction, but such evasiveness is now uncommon. The question is important and should be taken seriously; patients who do not want help of this kind must be respected, but they are a dwindling minority, and no excuse for not helping the large majority who welcome proactive concern. This question of patient autonomy seems to worry GPs in Denmark and The Netherlands much more than in the UK.

Another fear commonly expressed is that screening will label well people as diseased, creating feelings of insecurity and increasing work absence. Studies in Canadian steelworkers[27] supported this view. In The Netherlands, van Weel[28] found no evidence that labelling as a hypertensive had any effect on subsequent consulting behaviour other than the direct effects of clinical management.

Providing that both care givers and care receivers fully understand that neither high blood pressure nor any other cardiovascular risk factor is a disease in its own right, and provided that doctors have no economic incentives to create dependence, worries generated by screening are more than offset by the greater confidence engendered by any properly organized health maintenance system. This view is supported by a study of the mostly positive psychological effects of screening in the MRC mild hypertension trial.[29]

There is no doubt that a majority of people would like a more outgoing and more preventively orientated service, but the minority who do not like, or do not think they would like, this style of care, should be recognized and allowed for in all plans for screening. The main reason for not wanting check-ups derives, not from worries about lost independence, but from many people doubting their effectiveness. It seems probable that this may account for 44% of non-respondents to an invitation to a GP health check in Cardiff who said they were not really interested, and another 24% who forgot to attend;[30] only 11% of these non-respondents were opposed to screening in principle. An earlier study[31] showed that 16% of all adult patients were then actively hostile to proactive screening: 5% because they feared discovery of serious illness and preferred not to know, 7% because they actively disliked going to doctors, and 4% for other vague reasons. Acceptance of screening seems to have grown substantially in the last 20 years.

Experience in Glyncorrwg suggests that, when a systematic anticipatory style of care has been developed over a decade or more, it is almost universally accepted. We have about 10 (out of 2000) patients clearly identified as people who reject active medical interest of any kind unless they ask for it, although all but one of these was willing to see a nurse at home about once every 5 years for a blood pressure check.

The Future of Good Proactive Care

Proactive care, with an organized case finding approach, cannot be limited to a search for only one risk, and inevitably leads to a much wider definition of the primary care team's role. As this has narrowed in some other important directions (for example childbirth and most conditions requiring hospital based specialist skills) I see no reason to fear the lurid scenario painted by Ivan Illich[32] and other dystopian prophets, who fear medicalization of the whole world. In public service primary care at least, medical imperialism will be restrained by the time and effort required to do the work. However, if we are made to retreat to fees for service on the French or German models, this safeguard will be lost.

No one who has actually undertaken a serious screening programme in general practice will be anything but sceptical about new suggestions for apparently simple things which should be done for everybody. Unquestionably, the proactive approach will grow, but in our care system I doubt if it will go much further or faster than is endorsed by good evidence.

References

1. Hart JT (1974) A theory of screening in primary care. In: Hart C (ed) *Screening in general practice.* pp 19–29. Churchill Livingstone, Edinburgh.

2. Hawthorne VM, Greaves DA and Beavers DG (1974) Blood pressure in a Scottish town. *Br Med J* iii: 600.

3. Wilson JMG and Jungner G (1968) *Principles and practice of screening for disease.* Public Health Papers no. 34. WHO, Geneva.

4. D'Souza MF, Swan AV and Shannon DJ (1976) A long-term controlled trial of screening for hypertension in general practice. *Lancet* i: 1228–31.

5. Sackett DL and Holland WW (1975) Controversy in detection of disease. *Lancet* ii: 357.

6. Donaldson C and Mooney G (1991) Needs assessment, priority setting, and contracts for health care: An economic view. *Br Med J* 303: 1529–30.

7. Leese B, Hutton J and Maynard A (1991) *The costs and benefits of the use of erythropoietin in the treatment of anaemia arising from chronic renal failure: A European study.* Centre for Health Econmics, York.

8. Amiel S, Bennet J, Dickinson C et al. (1991) Health promotion in general practice. *Br Med J* 302: 257.

9. Pill R, French J, Harding K et al. (1988) Invitation to attend a health check in a general practice setting: comparison of attenders and non-attenders. *J R Coll Gen Pract* 38: 53–6.

10. Pill RM, Jones-Elwyn G and Stott NCH (1989) Opportunistic health promotion: Quantity or quality? *J R Coll Gen Pract* 39: 196–200.

11. Thompson NF (1990) Inviting infrequent attenders to attend for a health check: Costs and benefits. *Br J Gen Pract* 40: 16–18.

12. Waller D, Agass M, Mant D et al. (1990) Health checks in general practice: Another example of inverse care? *Br Med J* 300: 1115–18.

13. Main PGN (1991) Is social mobility enough? *Lancet* 337: 495.

14. Cook DG, Morris JK, Walker M et al. (1990) Consultation rates among

middle aged men in general practice over three years. *Br Med J* **301**: 647–50.

15 Maitland JM, Reid J and Taylor RJ (1991) Two stage audit of cerebrovascular and coronary heart disease risk factor recording: The effect of case-finding and screening programmes. *Br J Gen Pract* **41**: 144–6.

16. Coulter A and Schofield T (1991) Prevention in general practice: The views of doctors in the Oxford region. *Br Med J Gen Pract* **41**: 140–3.

17. Holmen J, Forsen L, Hjort PF *et al.* (1991) Detecting hypertension: Screening versus case-finding in Norway. *Br Med J* **302**: 219–22.

18. Hart JT (1970) Semicontinuous screening of a whole community for hypertension. *Lancet* ii: 223.

19. Coope J (1974) A screening clinic for hypertension in general practice. *J R Coll Gen Pract* **24**: 161–6.

20. Pederson OL and Neilsen EG (1975) Screening for hypertension in general practice. *Dan Med Bull* **22**: 18.

21. Van der Feen JAE (1975) Hypertension and the general practitioner: A challenge. *Huisarts en Wetenschap* **18**: 406.

22. Lindholm L (1984) *Hypertension and its risks: Epidemiological studies in Swedish primary health care.* Department of Community Health Sciences, Dalby, University of Lund, Sweden.

23. Hart JT (1980) Furture strategies of hypertension control by age. In: Coope J (ed) *Hypertension in primary care: An international sypmposium held at Reykjavik, Iceland, April 1978.* pp. 11–12. RCGP, London.

24. Hart JT, Thomas C, Gibbons B *et al.* Twenty-five years of audited screening in a socially deprived community. *Br Med J* **302**: 1509–13.

25. Hodgkin K (1984) *Towards earlier diagnosis: A guide to primary care.* Churchill Livingstone, Edinburgh.

26. Medical Research Council Working Party (1985) MRC trial of treatment of mild hypertension: principal results. *Br Med J* **291**: 97–104.

27. Haynes RB, Sackett DL, Taylor DW *et al.* (1978) Increased absenteeism

from work after detection and labelling of hypertensive patients. *N Engl J Med* **228**: 741–4.

28. Van Weel C (1985) Does labelling and treatment for hypertension increase illness behaviour? *Fam Pract* **2**: 147–50.

29. Medical Research Council Working Party on Mild to Moderate Hypertension (1977) Randomized controlled trial of treatment for mild hypertension: Design and pilot trial. *Br Med J* i: 1437–40.

30. Pill R and Stott N (1988) Invitation to attend a health-check in a general practice setting: The views of a cohort of non-attenders. *J R Coll Gen Pract* **38**: 57–60.

31. Cartwright A (1967) *Patients and their doctors: a study of general practice.* Routledge and Kegan Paul, London.

32. Illich I (1976) *Medical nemesis: Limits to medicine.* Marion Boyars, London.

9

Record Systems

As you collect your new data, you will want to arrange them so that they are readily accessible for future management, without duplicate entry. This is easy with a good computer program, difficult with A4 folders, and impossible with Lloyd–George records.

In England and Wales only 5–15% of records have been converted to A4. Scotland passed 50% about 10 years ago. Most practices are therefore still staggering along with the outdated Lloyd–George system. Although about 80% of practices now use computers, many are still at a stage where they create at least as many problems as they solve. Except for newly registered patients, good computer held data systems are extremely difficult to build without a good foundation of structured written data.

Conversion to Structured Written Records

Practices which undertake screening seriously will begin by screening their records, as outlined in Chapter 8. The search for data should include checking identification data which are essential for efficient practice in general, by updating of addresses, correction of first names and married names, correction of dates of birth, and so on. So much of the work in a manual record search arises simply from getting the records off the shelves, identifying them, and putting them back again, that most practices embarking on this huge undertaking might as well go two steps further, using the opportunity to construct simple major event histories, as well as to update identification data, and to enter these in a computerized database.

Most such practices will already have a computer, with an age/sex register on file, probably downloaded from the FHSA. This will be very inaccurate unless each entry has been verified against local knowledge and an electoral register, and the whole lot has been updated at least once a week.

Practices with A4 records will mostly have information entered in some kind of structure, which will make data retrieval much easier. Few Lloyd-George records are structured, other than continuation cards and hospital correspondence filed in date order. Conversion from Lloyd-George to A4 is probably no longer a reasonable option, except in the growing number of undergraduate teaching practices, where A4 records may provide a good learning area and can help to restore continuity between community based and hospital based care.

It takes about 3 minutes of staff time simply to assemble an A4 folder and enter indentification data: 100 hours of work for a list of 2000. Refiling, date ordering and editing hospital correspondence and investigation reports takes another 3–5 minutes for each folder, making another 150 hours or so, bringing total staff hours to 250.

Making major event summaries and listing repeat prescribing is equally essential for converstion to A4, but so much more time consuming that the idea of doing this for A4 conversion rather than creation of a computerized database seems nonsensical. In my opinion this work cannot safely be delegated, because there will be ambiguities in many records, requiring experience and judgement to sort out. There is probably no escape from each doctor doing all of his or her own personal list. The only possible compromise is to delegate the work to an experienced nurse, with clear remit to set aside any and all records that seem difficult. Hannay and Mitchell[1] found it took 25 minutes to make a summarized history for the average patient, working out at 833 hours for an average list of 2000.

This means most evenings given up for about a year, but the quality of care thereafter has been transformed in every practice I know where this has been done. The work is interesting if you already know the patients; much unexpected material crops up which was either forgotten, or never recorded. Since 1977 all my patients in Glyncorrwg have had fully updated lists of major clinical problems, and I am now amazed that I ever managed without them. The answer is, of course, that I tolerated a much lower standard of practice.

Graphic Flow Charts

Flow charts are a rapid means of scanning changes in selected indicators of clinical progress. I can see nothing in favour of numeric flow charts, which either isolate measurements from other text, or require duplicate entry, and present no obvious story to the patient or professional eye.

Graphic charts are a different matter. I suspect this is the only way to get clinicians to pay as much attention to systolic as they do to diastolic pressures, a long standing and serious problem. Graphic charts have the advantage that, through them, patients and professionals can see and understand what is going on, relating changes in pressure to patterns of medication and to compliance, and to the original pressures which prompted the decision to treat in the first place. All Glyncorrwg patients had a simple fine-graded graph sheet in the record, but before we got a computer these were only updated about once in 2 years, and therefore served no useful purpose in management.

As all blood pressure records become fully computerized and graphics are designed as an educational tool, this problem will vanish.

Patient-held Co-operation Cards

These again were something I always advocated but seldom practiced. Like graphic flow charts, they will not really happen until computers make it easy to reproduce data quickly and easily in a variety of forms. Judging from experience with antenatal records, about 5% may be lost, about the same as the proportion of medical records missing in an average general practice at any one time, and about half the proportion missing in most hospitals. Once there is a computer-held record, these losses hardly matter, because backed-up data can always be duplicated.

Again, from antenatal experience, we know that patients read records if they hold them, and begin to consider more carefully what the various figures mean. They are therefore an important potential aid to patient education, and could reduce confusion over medication.

A Records System Crisis

All GP medical records in the NHS are either currently in crisis, or soon will be, for four reasons.

The first and most obvious is that the 1990 Contract requires clinical audit and annual reports as conditions of service, which will ultimately be enforced. This means that data must not only be recorded, but easily and rapidly retrieved and analysed.

Secondly, since the 1970s there have been dramatic increases in the quality, but therefore also in the volume of GP clinical records. Really bad records, with virtually no clinical or social information in them except correspondence from specialists, have become almost as uncommon today as good ones were 20 years ago. This means that in high morbidity areas at least, Lloyd-George envelopes are bursting at the seams. When these are released to the space of A4, recording is no longer cramped, but then explodes faster than ever. Many of my own A4 records accumulated 10 or more double sided sheets over the 11 years 1977–87, compared with only five or six Lloyd-George double sided A6 cards over the 15 years 1961–76. This huge volume of potentially useful information is almost wholly wasted in written records, because it cannot be retrieved without hours of work which will never be available.

Thirdly, as innovative practices have either acquired computers, or at least begun serious planning for them, no ground rules have yet emerged about how computer-held information should relate to written records, nor has any common format or language emerged so that computer systems in different practices can be networked, or connected with area hospitals, FHSAs or health authorities. Almost all this development has occurred agaist a political and economic background of deregulation, in which government and health authorities have assumed that responsibility for public service information systems can safely be left to market forces, with minimal academic guidance or tax-funded support. Many different computer systems now compete for ascendancy in this overcrowded market. The ultimate victor will be bigger and richer than those which fail, but will almost certainly not be better. This is a field in which above all we need relatively unprofitable long term policies for software development, requiring substantial change from traditional ways of thinking and recording. Competitive advantage, however, will lie with user friendly software which perpetuates obsolete modes of thought and recording, creating huge logistic obstacles to rational future growth.

Fourthly and finally, the legal right of patients to see their own medical records has opened up entirely new areas for sharing information, and ultimately for sharing responsibility for clinical decisions. This will accelerate division of record systems into separate functional compartments, one for information (evidence), the other for interpretation (judgement). All these developments are becoming practically feasible for the first time, because of the ease with which computer held data can be duplicated and then modified to multiple uses.

This crisis cannot be solved simply by computerizing all data and leaving written records to wither away. We have got to look more seriously at the various functions of all forms of recording, allocating some to continued written records, and others to computers, with the least possible overlap between the two. A principle which no bureaucrat will ever understand, but all staff in every practice understand only too well, is that no person ever consistently and reliably records the same information twice; we are lucky if we have time to record it at all, particularly if data are regarded as normal or negative. Staff who are asked to write blood pressures in the paper record, and also to key it into the 'prevention' screen of a networked computer, will either give priority to one medium or the other, but not both. Alternatively they will record sometimes in one, sometimes the other, or they will get so exasperated that they look for another practice.

Written records will certainly continue in most practices, despite some experiments with wholly electronic records, but there is general agreement that the more structured and accountable style of primary care introduced by the Contract will be permanent, even if its entrepreneurial features are eventually discarded.

141

We need a division of labour between written and computerized records, but none has yet been suggested. Even the legal status of computer held data remains uncertain.

This crisis can be solved only by a most rigorous reappraisal of the real rather than rhetorical aims of medical care, translated into new ways of conceptualizing and structuring recorded data. The whole issue was first perceived by Weed[2], whose thoughts on the matter are still worth considering:

'There is no practical way for literally millions of patients to benefit from application of the highest standards except through use of structured information to acquire, and adequate communication techniques to transmit rapidly, the appropriate information. Whether this necessary reminding of the physician involves books, cartoons, an abacus or a computer is not important. What is important is that the proper care gets to all the people. We should continually remind ourselves that not to think quantitatively about the needs of all of the people has qualitative implications for most of the people; and in our efforts we should neither worship nor fear the computer and technology, but rather we should simply use them as long as the benefits outweigh the losses in an honest accounting that does not leave, as many present methods do, thousands of people without care and without even being taken into account and weighed in the balance.'

All this is peculiarly relevant to the management of high blood pressure. Of all possible clinical models, high blood pressure is the commonest, simplest, and most easily understood in quantified terms. Record systems that perform well for detection, management, and audit of high blood pressure may, with minor modifications, serve well for all other chronic or recurrent health problems that can be expressed as quantified risks of qualitative outcomes, in other words for all the most problematic areas for personal and continuing primary care of populations.

Some such systems, for example ELIAS in The Netherlands, are now developing rapidly and are in widespread use (ELIAS has replaced paper records for about 10% of all Dutch GPs).[3] Experience with these systems shows that they do not, and never will, replace the best human judgement. It will never be either possible or desirable to enter into a computer all the biological, social and historical variables that should influence even the simplest clinical decisions. However, computer software development compels human judgement to improve, to look more openly and accurately at itself, to set quantified objectives and measure their attainment, to value scientific honesty more and to deflate mere technical competence.

Data Entry in Computerized Records

Possession of a practice computer is no guarantee that it will be used to improve clinical care. By 1988 Scotland was well ahead of England, with over 25% of practices, 32% of GPs, and 30% of the Scottish population using a single Home and Health Department sponsored software system given free to all GPs willing to buy compatible hardware (GPASS). However, when these computers 'in use' were interrogated through an 'electronic questionnaire' designed to evaluate the data they held,[4] only 20% had any clinical or morbidity data entered, and only about 10% contained any blood pressure data. Only 60% of practices had their whole registered population entered on the computer.

More complete data entry has been achieved in practices which accepted heavily subsidized low cost computers from VAMP and AAH Meditel, on condition that they maintained entry for prescription linked clinical data at a rate of not less than 80%. These data were then anonymized and sold to marketing departments in the pharmaceutical industry. One study covering 2491 patients in 58 practices showed that 87% of consultants' clinical diagnoses were entered in the VAMP low cost scheme.[5] Both these schemes were eventually non-viable commercially in their original form, and wobbled on the brink of bankruptcy in 1991. Although the information they contained was clearly vital to public service and included about one-third of all computerized practices, the English Department of Health (DoH) and the Welsh Office washed their hands of responsibility, apparently accepting that if a section of the computer market collapsed, the public information it contained would go with it.

GPASS failed because the Scottish Home and Health Department slowed funding of software development to a virtual halt. VAMP and AAH Meditel almost failed because their first duty was not to public service but to shareholders. However, if government ever again accepts responsibility for providing the best currently feasible means for family doctors to keep good (i.e. computerized) records, there is no reason why it should not negotiate similar contracts for high information input in return for free data systems, enforced with the same excellent results, more dependable funding, and aimed at improved public service rather than higher pharmaceutical profits.

Once the hard initial work has been done, first of record scanning and transfer of data to computer, then of case-finding supplemented by call-up screening, microcomputers permit a sustained continuous screening rate of 90–95%. Within 2 years, Difford and colleagues[6] had recorded blood pressures for 92% of adults on their list, within the previous 5 years. About 73% of new screening measurements were obtained through opportunistic case finding without a computer prompt, 34% followed prompts from the computer indicating that measurement was due at the next consultation, 21% came from patients who responded to a computer generated letter inviting them to attend, and 8% were missed. Monthly computer generated worksheets were produced for the whole practice staff, which could be modified according to other pressures of work.

Depreciation and running costs for this computer system amounted to about 1.6% of total practice expenses (£1000 a year at 1986 prices), and mailing costs came to 0.1% of practice expenses (£0.15 per patient at 1986 prices). However, the authors did not specify the computer program they used, nor whether they had skills required to develop some of it themselves. Most off the shelf systems cost more than this, and were at that time much less flexible and efficient.

My only working experience is with the VAMP system, one of the most widely used in the UK. It is well adapted to initial screening, less well to follow-up. The same seems to be true of most systems now in use in the UK, few if any of which have developed critical prompt systems to assist clinical judgement, as in the Dutch ELIAS system, or really good graphic representation of control over time in relation to treatment.

Choosing a Computer System

Most computer systems installed by GPs in the next 10 years will be selected by second-time buyers, who already have experience at least of a word processor. However, few UK medical or nursing schools as yet offer any hands-on experience of using a computer for any purpose,[7] and training practices still exist without any computer in use. Any inexperienced first-time buyers reading this book would be well advised to buy a PC now, so that before taking any larger decisions they are at least familiar with a word processor.

The main factor influencing choice of first system is nearly always its short term cost. Readers who already have experience of any system attempting to cover all aspects of care will already know how wrong this is. The far more serious question which should determine choice of system is its capacity for sustained growth and development in an era which is already upon us, and is rapidly making obsolete most of the clinical categories we now use. Above all, we need systems that can handle the quantified evidence that first justifies intervention and then monitors its effect, rather than arbitrary disease labels. The only one I know of with capacities in this direction is EMIS.

Probably the most effective way to choose between existing systems is to get a list of two or three accessible practices for each, ask them nicely (*very* nicely; you will not be the first) and then arrange for at least two of your team, preferably including a nurse and someone from office staff, to visit and observe the system in operation. You will learn almost nothing from any demonstration by a salesman, who will be using a small artificial population containing no real data. If the system you observe works really well for all aspects of blood pressure control, it will probably have a good future for management of other chronic or recurrent clinical problems which involve quantitive measurements as well as qualitative decisions. It may not matter too much whether this system has been adapted to handle these other problems; if the model is right, it is at least potentially available for other purposes.

It is extremely important that whatever system you choose should be based on a standard language such as MS-DOS, able to run on a wide range of hardware, and easily integrated with the very wide range of business programs available for IBM-compatible PCs. The single most popular system, VAMP, as yet still fails this specification. Primary medical care is a very small market in commercial terms, with correspondingly little specific software development, available only at high cost. It is essential that you are able to use ordinary business software developed for less specific purposes, much of which can be readily adapted by a competent programmer at low cost.

Installing a Computer

However convinced you may be that your practice must computerize, the rest of your team is unlikely to share your enthusiasim, at least until they have seen how the computer behaves in practice. Given that doctors, particularly those reputed to be computer literate, have all the power, office staff and nurses naturally fear that the new machinery will be used to shift work previously performed by doctors to other 'less costly' (and therefore 'less valuable') workers in the team, and that most of the new work the computer requires will fall on them also.

It is first of all necessary not to tell lies. The immediate effect of the computer will not be to make anyone's life any easier. Computers can perform an extraordinary range of valuable tasks which were previously unimaginable, mainly those requiring data recall, but they can do very few tasks traditionally undertaken manually. You should straightaway admit that, although the computer can enormously improve patient care, it will generally speaking expand rather than contract the work of supporting staff. This means that you will almost certainly need more labour.

You will not carry your team with you unless you make it clear from the outset that any additional hours for existing staff will be paid for, and that you accept the alternative of taking on more staff, because many part-time health centre staff really do not want more hours.

Secondly, the few previously manual tasks which computers can do well should be developed as your first priority, to reduce the load of monotonous work for your staff. Repeat prescriptions are obvious, less obvious is generation of two or three sheets of sticky name and address labels for insertion in every A4 record, which can then be stuck on to investigation request forms or letters to patients. Modem connnections to fax hospital reports and correspondence are also obvious, and already more economic than postage.

Development of your computer system should proceed in consultation with your whole team, preferably overseen by a practice manager as chairperson, rather than one of the doctors. If this procedure is followed, even elderly and experienced staff can be won over surprisingly quickly to confident use of the computer. The whole team then for the first time begins to be able to see an overall picture of what they are doing. Far from depersonalizing and industrializing its work, the team can begin to use all of its brains in a co-ordinated but uncoerced way. If, on the other hand, the computer is imposed on the team without consultation, the capacity of entrenched staff to sabotage any system may be fully expressed.

Long-term Requirements for Computer Programs in Primary Care

The great advantage of computer held over written data is the ease, speed, and low cost with which data can be recalled, duplicated, and expressed in graphic form. The advantage is much greater for continuing primary care, in which lifetimes of data accumulate and move with the patient, than for episodic hospital care.

All consultations are constrained by time. The time required to extract data even from a structured written record ensures that this can rarely be done completely within even a generous consultation time of 10 minutes. Clinical habits, and the same time pressures, ensure that personal medical records are seldom reviewed thoroughly at other times. If they are, it takes several hours to produce (for example) graphic charts of blood pressures, set against time and changing treatment, over periods of 20 or 30 years, like those in this book. Yet data of exactly this kind are needed to make best possible judgements and learn from experience, using not only the general information available in medical literature, but all the information specific to particular patients, which together compose the human experiments we are privileged to undertake.

Data of this sort are needed so that patients also learn from experience to become not passive consumers, but active and thoughtful producers of their own health. Even the most structured written records trap information which cannot be released quickly or easily, unless they include graphic flow charts, which are logistically impossible to maintain manually as a routine procedure.

The answers any computerized data system can give will never go beyond the questions its programmers have anticipated, but if only some answers are paid for, inhibited growth in other directions is guaranteed. In a commercial system in which GPs get cheap computers in return for providing useful information on prescribing, software development gives first priority to questions asked by the marketing departments of pharmaceutical companies, and second priority to whatever minimum data set a generally unimaginative government requires from GPs, leaving minimal scope for the imagination of users. A distant and vulnerable third priority may go to questions now classified as 'research', which have only become feasible with the advent of computerized data systems, but experience shows that this is more rhetoric than reality. We are only at the beginning of even formulating the questions we need for better patient care.

Future Requirements

The most difficult and important clinical responsibilities of primary care teams concern qualitative either/or decisions (treat or not treat, refer or not refer) based upon quantified evidence. This evidence comes from one or more (usually several) different measurements (for example, systolic and diastolic pressure, blood cholesterol, weight for height, peak expiratory flow rate, number of epileptic fits or migraine attacks diary-recorded in the past month, or severity of menstrual pain marked on a linear analogue scale). Most of these measurements are continuously distributed throughout the general population, without abrupt breaks to signify a clear difference between sickness and well being.

Decisions about sickness or well-being do, however, have to be made. They are now made intuitively, drawing partly on a wide variety of knowledge, or at least informed supposition, about our patients, partly on vaguely remembered values previously recorded which we have no time to verify, and partly on crude rules of thumb which have acquired authority through consensus use (diastolic 90 mmHg in the USA, diastolic 100 mmHg in the UK, wheezing regardless of flow rates, and so on).

For health problems in which best clinical practice is still primitive, for example most cancers, diagnosis still concentrates almost exclusively on qualitative, either/ or evidence, but even this is beginning to change. The origins of cancers are ceasing to be seen as one-off and irreversible, and are becoming recognized as probably quite common events, encountering variable host resistance. Even for risk factor distributions, not all significant variables are continuously distributed. For example, there is a qualitative difference between smokers and non-smokers, although smokers can be ranked quantitively. In general, however, as we turn from single minded concentration on end-stage disease toward concern for its beginnings, we shift from relatively simple qualitative (either/or) evidence, to difficult quantitative (how much?) evidence.

On the other hand, as we approach irreversible organ damage and end-stage disease, the landmarks we learned in our hospital based medical schools become more easily recognizable. We become more comfortable with and confident in our disease labelling, and although decisions may be difficult, there is at least no doubt that they have to be made. Perhaps because computer development has been led by the expectations of hospital specialists, it has so far seemed to help more at this sharp, easy end of clinical decision making, than at its complex, ambiguous and uneasy beginnings. This will continue as long as we accept systems that depend on qualitative disease labelling rather than quantified deviations from health, and fail to formulate questions more appropriate to our work.

For health problems in which best clinical practice is already fairly advanced, for example high blood pressure, asthma, diabetes, or epilepsy, we already have quantified indicators of present severity and future risk, which permit more than either/or labelling. We can already tell patients the truth: that all these conditions have graded severity which we can usually control, and evoke host resistance which we can assist, so that minor asthma no longer has to be emphasized to wheezy bronchitis, and first (and commonly last) epileptic fits need no longer be described as something else. We already perceive multifactorial causes and therefore can accept multifactorial decisions, using quantified data extending back as far as patients' records allow, normally to their birth, sometimes to the lives of their parents and grandparents.

Our present intuitive decisions are dominated by the immediate evidence to hand, plus a caricature of the patient, which is normally all we are able to keep in our heads; better than nothing, but inadequate. Computer software prompting qualitative decisions derived from quantified cumulative measurements could at last make it possible for us to think and act not just intuitively, but using all data we have recorded but cannot in practice recall.

The next generation of computer systems needs to concentrate, not upon labelling, but on more imaginative, graphic representation of patients' lives, along multiple quantified tracks relevant to probable health outcomes, helping to clarify the options open to them and to us to assist change. Programs for detection and management of high blood pressure provide an excellent model for this, as the ELIAS system has shown.

References

1. Hannay DR and Mitchell S (1985) Storing summary patient data as a microcomputer file. *J R Coll Gen Pract* **35**: 525.

2. Weed LL (1971) *Medical records, medical education and patient care.* Case Western Reserve University Press, Cleveland, Ohio.

3. van der Lei J, Musen MA, van der Does E *et al.* (1991) Comparison of computer-aided and human review of general practitioners' management of hypertension. *Lancet* **338**: 1504–8.

4. Taylor MW, Ritchie LD, Taylor RJ *et al.* (1990) General practice computing in Scotland. *Br Med J* **300**: 170–2.

5. Jick H, Jick SS and Derby LE (1991) Validation of information recorded on general practitioner based computerized data resource in the United Kingdom. *Br Med J* **302**: 766–8.

6. Difford F, Telling JP, Davies KR *et al.* (1987) Continuous opportunistic and systematic screening for hypertension with computer help: Analysis of non-responders. *Br Med J* **294**: 1130–2.

7. Jones RB, Navin LM, Barrie J *et al.* (1991) Computer literacy among medical, nursing, dental and veterinary undergraduates. *Med Educ* **25**: 191–5.

Measurements

10

Sources of error: the patient ■ Home readings ■ Anxiety and fear ■
Cold ■ Full bladders ■ Circadian rhythm? ■ Sources of error: the
observer ■ Measurement technique ■ Digit preference ■ Bias ■
Attitudes to measurement ■ Sources of error: the instrument ■ Cuffs
■ A cautionary tale ■ Aneroid sphygmomanometers ■ Mercury
sphygmomanometers ■ Research sphygmomanometers ■ Electronic
sphygmomanometers ■ Diastolic phases 4 and 5 ■ Systolic and
diastolic pressures

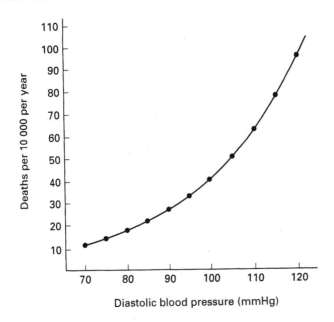

Figure 10.1: Risk function for mortality against diastolic pressure in men aged 35–44
years (mean of three readings, phase 5), free from organ damage at entry[1].

Figure 10.1 shows the association between the mean of three readings of phase
5 diastolic pressure and subsequent annual mortality, for men aged 35–44, free
from organ damage at entry.[1] Case finding and follow-up measurements aim to

149

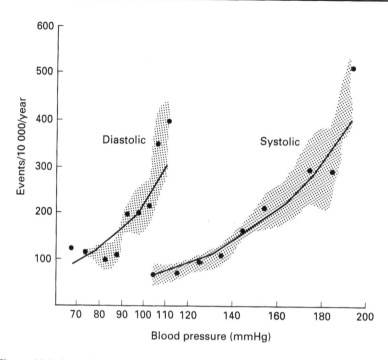

Figure 10.2: Annual incidence of cardiovascular events in both sexes at Framingham over 18 years of follow-up, by level of blood pressure at entry. This is derived from the same data on which Figure 10.1 was based. Shaded areas indicate 95% confidence limits[2].

place individual patients accurately on this predictive curve, so that we can be sure that treatment is worthwhile.

As this graph transforms the raw data actually observed into a smoothed curve illustrating the association between diastolic pressure and mortality, it eliminates both observer bias and digit preference, particularly in the diastolic readings. These can be seen easily for diastolic, but not for systolic pressure, in Figure 10.2, which shows the raw data on which Figure 10.1 was based.[2] Bias is caused by the practical need for observers to allocate patients unambiguously to treatment or non-treatment categories. There is no bias apparent for systolic pressures, presumably because the clinicians recording the pressures were, probably unconsciously, using only a diastolic classification of risk. Where consensus decision points are recognized, for example diastolic 90 mmHg in North America, 95 mmHg in Australia, or 100 mmHg in the UK, a visible step appears in all large groups of data. This is exaggerated still more by digit preference, the tendency of observers to record blood pressures ending in 0, because the gauge on a mercury manometer is most clearly graded at 10 mm intervals.

Some idea of the potential error from the variability of arterial pressure can be seen in Figure 10.3, showing pressures recorded at 5 minute intervals from an intra-arterial catheter worn by a hypertensive patient over a 24-hour period.[3] The fall during early sleep is remarkable, and occurs even in malignant hypertension.

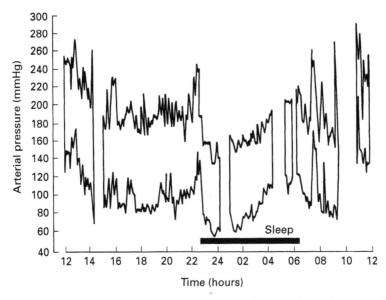

Figure 10.3: Ambulant arterial pressure plotted at 5-minute intervals over a 24-hour period, in a patient with primary high blood pressure. A period of sleep is indicated by the horizontal bar, preceded by a peak during coitus[3].

Your hypertension control programme can be no better than the measurements on which it is based. Good quality data for personal care of individual patients are not less but more important than for epidemiological research on groups, because they lead to clinical decisions; but you would hardly think so from the way these measurements are usually made, either in general practice or hospitals.

Sources of Error: the Patient

Measurement errors mean inaccurate decisions to put people on expensive, potentially uncomfortable, and occasionally dangerous medication which they do not need, or to ignore blood pressures that should be more actively treated. There are three main sources of error: the patient, the observer, and the instrument.

However carefully conditions are standardized and patients put at their ease, attempts to characterize any patient's average pressure throughout the year by a single reading will obviously fail. It is true that, in a group of patients, group average casual seated arterial pressure closely approximates to mean pressure as measured throughout the waking day by portable semi-continuous recorders for subjects not doing any heavy manual work or taking strenuous exercise.[4] It is also true that, in the Framingham study, a single initial casual pressure reading was

151

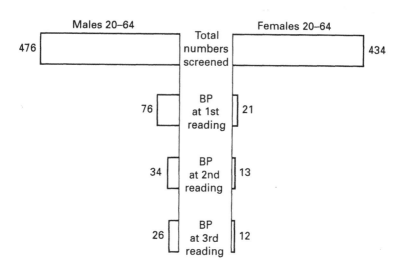

Figure 10.4: Persistence through three readings of diastolic pressures classed as hypertensive: Glyncorrwg, 1968 screen[6].

found to be almost as good a predictor of risk as the mean of several readings.[5] These are conclusions from grouped rather than individual data; the fact that the average male takes a size 8 shoe is no reason for not making other sizes.

Figure 10.4 shows what happened in Glyncorrwg[6] when we repeated readings on patients aged 20–64, found initially to have diastolic pressures high enough to require treatment on the criteria we then used (men<40 years: diastolic 100+ mmHg; men 40–64, diastolic 105+ mmHg; women <40, diastolic 115+ mmHg; women 40–64, diastolic 110+ mmHg). The 97 found in the first wave of case finding fell to 47 after two readings, and 38 after three readings. A study of a large sample of practices in northwest London in 1982[7] showed that 46% of all anti-hypertensive treatment was initiated after a single reading. Had I followed that course in Glyncorrwg, nearly three times as many people would have been started on treatment.

No patient should ever be started on antihypertensive drugs on the evidence of one reading. Even in a true hypertensive emergency, it should be possible to record three replicate pressures; even these often show a substantial fall as the alerting reflex subsides. Of course the patient will need treatment, but at least you have some measure of the severity and stability of the condition you are treating, which may otherwise never be known. Cases picked up by case finding are not emergencies, even with very high pressures, providing retinal haemorrhage and oedema have been excluded. With these there is always time to repeat measurements at least three times on separate days, which also allows more time for all-round assessment, patient education, and the beginnings of a good contractual relationship.

When our nurses find a high pressure, they now arrange for the patient to return twice for repeat readings, without any prompting from the GP. Even so, in many borderline cases we are uncertain whether to begin treatment. The alternatives are either to arrange for weekly readings by the practice nurse over a couple of months, or to teach patients to measure their own pressures and bring back the results.

Home Readings

With about 5 minutes of teaching from a practice nurse and using an electronic sphygmomanometer, almost any patient or relative can learn to measure blood pressure as accurately as most doctors do now. Asked to measure pressure twice a day for 2 weeks, virtually all patients will do so, usually to a high standard.

Home readings by patients have been shown to agree well with hospital out-patient readings by doctors.[8] Mean pressures at home (measured by continuous intra-arterial readings by ambulatory monitoring) have been higher in some studies (by about 14 mmHg systolic pressure) than in the same patients admitted to a hospital ward, even when rest and activity in the two situations are taken into account.[9] Conditions of hospital out-patients seem to resemble those of patients in a family doctor's office more closely than those of hospital in-patients.

Home readings are stable and have been shown to be a reliable technique for initial assessment.[10] From 28 home readings it is a simple matter to work out the mean with a pocket calculator and take a decision based on it, easily shared with patients because they gathered the evidence.

Home readings are of great help in identifying those who hyper-react to office measurements, however carefully these are made. These hyper-reactors are a small minority, but the gap between mean office and home measurements can be remarkable. An example is shown in Figure 10.5. They may still have an important problem, and need prolonged follow-up before any final decision whether or not to medicate. The Framingham data suggest that people with hyper-reactive pressures are at higher risk, of the same order as people whose high pressures are more stable, and that, in any case, variability of blood pressure is not a sustained characteristic.[11] It is difficult to interpret this evidence in a practical way. Probably the best policy is simply to keep an eye on these people by annual blood pressure checks without treatment, a policy which patients seem to find intelligible and acceptable. Most of them eventually develop higher pressures needing treatment, often after many years of observation.

There is a valuable hidden agenda in this exercise. Patients are usually astonished at their own discovery of the variability of untreated pressure under reasonably constant home conditions. They can then begin to understand the

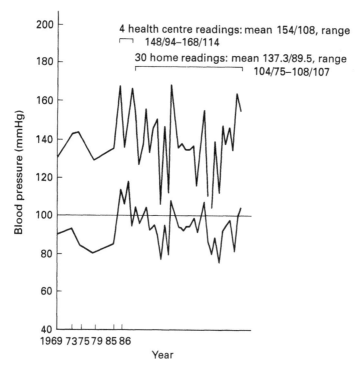

Figure 10.5: Blood pressures recorded at Glyncorrwg health centre, and then at home, in a woman aged 33 in 1969.

probabilistic nature of human biology and rational medical care, the dangers of blind faith and the value of constructive scepticism. However, this assumes that home readings are supported by scientifically informed interpretation.

Judging from the behaviour of Russian emigrants to Israel, home measurements of blood pressure seem to have been common in the USSR, and used there by patients to decide whether or not to treat themselves with antihypertensive drugs on a day to day basis. Consumerism of this sort is indefensible.

Anxiety and Fear

Obviously it is a waste of time to record pressures in frightened or angry patients, but these moods may not be apparent. Untreated patients with normal or slow pulse rates are unlikely to be stressed in this way, and routine recording of pulse rates provides useful additional evidence for interpreting pressure values in individual cases. It would be much more useful if observers could be induced to write their own comments when they observe anger or distress, but in my experience they rarely do so (just as nurses seem hardly ever to record their observations of half-hearted blowing into peak flow meters).

In may often be helpful to ask patients whether they do feel anxiety, fear or anger when they visit a doctor (sometimes, any doctor). Many admit to these feelings when asked directly, and once this has been done, it may be the first step towards overcoming them.

The effect of anxiety or even mere curiosity has been beautifully shown by studies in Milan, plotting continuous intra-arterial readings in 48 hypertensive and normotensive subjects lying in hospital beds.[12] In nearly all cases pressures rose as doctors arrived at the bedside to measure blood pressure in the usual way, by a mean 27 mmHg systolic and 15 mmHg diastolic pressure above the previous resting intra-arterial value. There were big individual differences in the extent of this rise, with a range of 4–75 mmHg systolic and 1–36 mmHg diastolic pressure.

Although it is essential to bear this sort of evidence in mind, it is difficult to use it intelligently in practice.[13] One way to avoid it, routine use of ambulatory monitoring, is now enthusiastically endorsed by some very experienced family doctors.[14] However, the evidence on which rational management policies have hitherto been based comes not from intra-arterial readings and ambulatory monitoring, but from casual seated blood pressures measured in much the same way as in ordinary general practice. I doubt whether a general turn from traditional casual readings to ambulatory readings can be justified until we have good prospective data comparing the outcomes, first of detection, and second of management, using the old and new methods.[15] Better diagnosis needs to include the patient as well as the doctor, and home readings achieve this more simply and cheaply than ambulatory monitoring. The search for 'true' blood pressures, uncontaminated by response to the real world our patients live in, which so occupied the minds of pioneers like Smirk in New Zealand, was probably futile. It has now been shown that basal pressures are no better correlated with organ damage than casual pressures.[16]

Cold

Chilling of the body raises blood pressure substantially, and this seems to account for systematic differences between pressures recorded in summer and winter, which are well known to epidemiologists,[17] and obvious to most thoughtful clinicians; summer audits, therefore, give more optimistic results than winter audits! Obviously, waiting rooms should be warm, but with an efficient appointments system this may not be much help on a cold winter evening. We have found that the only thing we can do about it is to remain aware of the problem. In a really cold winter, the proportion of clinic patients with poor control always rises substantially.

Full Bladders

Stretched bladders are potent and often forgotten elevators of blood pressure. The minority of junior surgical staff who measure blood pressure routinely in emergency admissions frequently send for their physician colleagues to pronounce an opinion on old men with acute retention. These patients then return home after prostatectomy with their original normal blood pressures, plus an expensive and redundant array of antihypertensive drugs. This ancient observation has recently been rediscovered.[18]

Full bladders also happen in full waiting rooms, with the same misleading effect. The man who stopped off for a quick pint on the way to the doctor suddenly realizes that if he goes to the toilet he may lose his place in the queue. He grits his teeth, clenches his sphincters, and raises his diastolic pressure by 20 or 30 mmHg. As Charcot said, listen to the patient and he will tell you the diagnosis.

Circadian Rhythm?

There have been bitter arguments about whether there is, or is not, a systematic difference between morning and evening blood pressures. Blood pressure falls dramatically during sleep, usually even in malignant hypertension. There is good evidence of a substantial rise just before waking and for an hour or two after, but a huge American study of 10 000 men and women aged 30–64 showed no significant difference between systolic or diastolic pressures measured in the morning and the afternoon,[19] the relevant times for primary care clinics.

Sources of Error: the Observer

As the Milan study of 'white coat' effects on blood pressure showed, observers may influence pressure by inspiring fear, love, loathing, and doubtless other passions in patients, perhaps most often just irritation. All these may modify pressure, and probably account for the systematic differences between pressures recorded by nurses and by doctors, discussed in Chapter 11. A study in New York showed only 'white coat hypertension' in 22% of patients diagnosed as borderline hypertensives by ordinary clinical readings.[20]

Observers influence measurements in four other important ways: measurement technique, digit preference, bias, and their attitude to the results.

Measurement Technique

Detailed instructions on how to measure blood pressure with a standard mercury sphygmomanometer are given in Appendix 4 (use and care of sphygmomanometers). Most medical and nursing students learn to measure blood pressures in antenatal clinics, the majority of which have frankly appalling traditions of measurement.[21] Even if you think you know all about how to measure blood pressures, you will be wise to read Appendix 4 before going further in this chapter; there will almost certainly be something you have forgotten.

Digit Preference

An example of this has been given already in Figure 10.1. Digit preference is the name applied to a clinical fact, that when asked to mark a descending target against a vertical scale of measurement marked at 2 mm intervals with unnumbered lines, and at 5 mm intervals with terminal 5s and 0s, observers prefer 0s to 5s, and 5s to even numbers. Those who consistently read 0s are clearly reading to the nearest 10 mmHg. We are seldom told whether they choose the nearest 10 up or the nearest 10 down, so the potential error is huge. This seems a casual way to get evidence for important clinical decisions.

Is this kind of approximation common in otherwise good clinicians? Table 10.1 shows some evidence from hospital correspondence containing a total of 39 readings concerning five randomly sampled patients from the Glyncorrwg practice. For comparison, I give 110 readings by our practice nurses for the same patients over the same period. If the true measures were randomly distributed, obviously 10% of the readings would end in 0s, another 10% in 5s, and the rest in other digits.

Table 10.1: Percentages of various terminal digits in blood pressure at hospital and a primary care clinic, 1985.

| | Hospital letters | | GPs and practice nurses | |
	No.	%	No.	%
Systolic				
Terminal 0	37	95	27	24
Terminal 5	2	5	2	2
Other	0	0	81	74
Diastolic				
Terminal 0	33	85	20	18
Terminal 5	6	15	4	4
Other	0	0	86	78
Total	39	100	110	100

These data include correspondence from a university department of cardiology. If you have a look at your own records you will probably find much the same monotonous preference for zeros, but, as you see, you are in good company.

Bias

This also was illustrated in Figure 10.2. Bias is the unconscious tendency of observers to 'make sense' of measurements by allocating them unambiguously to one side or the other of a cutting point habitually used for clinical decision. If you return to Figure 10.2 you will see a relatively even distribution of systolic pressure values over the range 105–175 mmHg, with an unexpected dip at 185 and a rise at 195 which could be partly explained by smaller numbers and therefore greater sampling error. There is little evidence of bias, because in the early 1960s, when these data were collected, systolic pressures were virtually ignored in clinical decision making in English speaking countries. If you look at the diastolic pressures, on the other hand, there is a clear break exactly where you would expect to find it, if the population were neatly divided into normotensives up to and including 90 mmHg, and hypertensives over 90 mmHg. Indeed, the values are distributed as a three-step staircase rather than a curve; normotensives, mild hypertensives, and severe hypertensives.

Is this a slander on the honest and conscientious group of experienced observers who pioneered the Framingham study? Not at all; this is how all clinicians behaved, until they became aware of this universal tendency.

Figure 10.6 shows a study[22] comparing readings by Norwegian cardiovascular epidemiologists using conventional sphygmomanometers (as used in the entry phase of the Framingham study), with readings by the same observers using a random zero sphygmomanometer.[23] This instrument allows observers to record a reading before they can know its value, and is therefore bias free. The illustration shows systolic values rather than diastolic, but as continental European doctors pay a lot more attention to systolic pressures than Anglo-Americans, the effect is obvious; a cleavage at systolic 140 mmHg, apparent with conventional sphygmomanometers, disappears when a random zero machine is used, to give unbiased readings.

Bias is important in two situations: initial categorization of a screened population, and follow-up of treated cases. Publications comparing different antihypertensive treatments or auditing clinical managements are of questionable value if they are based on measurements with conventional sphygmomanometers. The best, but expensive, solution to this problem is to use a Hawksley random zero sphygmomanometer for all measurements. This has been our policy in Glyncorrwg; since 1974 all office and most home readings were made in this way. A cheaper and more practical solution is to use electronic sphygmomanometers, which also exclude digit preference (which the random zero machine obviously cannot). These have some serious limitations, discussed later in this chapter, but

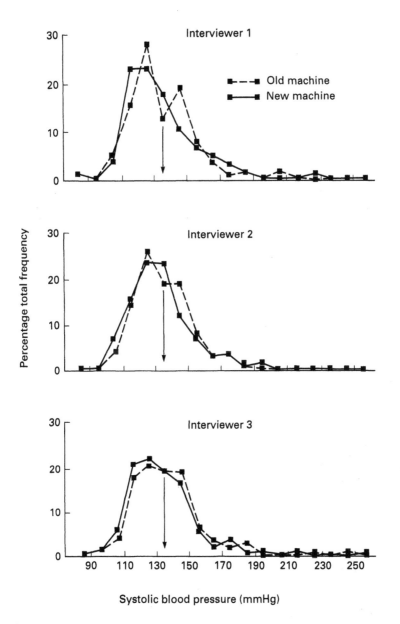

Figure 10.6: Frequency distribution of readings of systolic pressure in a large Norwegian population, by the same observers using conventional sphygmomanometers (as used in the entry phase of the Framingham study), and random zero sphygmomanometers[22].

they are wonderful for teaching unbiased measurement technique, which can be learned. Fully retrained observers, who have become conscious of both bias and digit preference, can use conventional sphygmomanometers accurately.

Attitudes to Measurement

This pedantry may be all very well for epidemiological research, but does it really matter for day to day clinical medicine? Do the statements 'BP 120/70' or 'BP 170/100' reveal an experienced clinician, aware of the fallibility of these measurements and careful to avoid the spurious precision implied by the statements 'BP 124/68' or '166/102'? The answer is 'no' because control of high blood pressure in a general practice population is not a one–off onslaught, but a sustained search for precise targets, with many opportunities for collecting the evidence necessary for accurate decisions.

This evidence, on which a decision whether or not to intervene must at some point be made, should be of the highest possible quality. We need the best measurements we can get, repeated many times before reaching a conclusion.

Sources of Error: the Instrument

There are basically four types of sphygmomanometer available: aneroid, conventional mercury, research, and electronic. All of them have one thing in common, an inflatable cuff. This is the commonest serious source of error arising from the instrument itself.

Cuffs

Cuffs which are too small may grossly exaggerate both systolic and diastolic pressures. World experts disagree about whether cuff length[24, 25] or width[26] is critical, but there is no doubt at all if you try to measure all adult blood pressures with the same cuff, you will get grossly incorrect values for both very fat and very thin people. Eighty-two per cent of adult British arms are too big for the 23 cm standard UK cuff, and 50% of American arms are too big for the 26 cm standard US cuff.[27] The effect is purely artefactual, and has nothing to do with the true association of hypertension with obesity.

Cuff sizes recommended by an expert committee of the American Heart Association[28] are shown in Table 10.2.

Adults with giant obesity (BMI 40+) often have arms which are too short to accommodate a sufficiently wide cuff. Their blood pressure must then be measured either at the forearm or thigh.

Table 10.2: Cuff bladder sizes recommended by an expert committee of the American Heart Association.

Arm circumference (cm)	Cuff name	Width (cm)	Length (cm)
5–7.5	Newborn	3	5
7.5–13	Infant	5	8
13–20	Child	8	13
17–26	Small adult	11	17
24–32	Adult	13	24
32–42	Large Adult	17	32
42–50	Thigh	20	42

A Cautionary Tale

In 1983 a woman of 47 years moved into my practice. She had been taking various anti-hypertensive drugs continuously for the previous 18 years, having been started on treatment at age 29 after a single reading of 145/100 mmHg, presumably using a standard cuff. In 1983 she was 5ft 1in (1.51 m) tall and weighed 14 st 2 lb (89.9 kg), giving a body mass index of 39.4. Her previous GP record showed the readings given in Table 10.3.

Table 10.3: Blood pressure readings of a 47-year-old woman as noted in her GP record.

Age	BP(mmHg)	Events
29	145/100	Started antihypertensive medication
	130/80	
	130/80	
37	160/90	
43	190/100	
45	170/105	
	170/105	
	160/96	
	170/96	
47	162/100 (standard cuff)	
	142/80 (outsize cuff)	
		Treatment stopped: 'hypertension' cured

The answer is, of course, to get outsize cuffs and use them. This is no longer as difficult as it was. Both Accoson and Baumanometer, the chief suppliers, now make a full range of cuff sizes, although you may have to be very persistent to obtain them. Both brands use a system of transverse lines (easier to use than to describe) which give an immediately obvious indication of whether you are using the right cuff. As most arms are 'outsize' our team normally used 'large adult' as standard, occasionally replacing it with 'normal adult' or 'very large adult' when we needed to.

Nearly all cuffs now use Velcro binding, which tends to make the bag rather rigid; tuck-in cloth cuffs are better, if you can get them. After a few years the nylon hooklets on Velcro lose their grip and begin to slip; they will usually recover if cleaned by vigorous scrubbing with a nylon toothbrush.

Aneroid Sphygmomanometers

Aneroid sphygmomanometers are compact; otherwise they have no advantages, and many serious disadvantages. Fisher[29] compared over 3000 aneroid machines in use with a standard mercury manometer and found an error of more than 7 mmHg in 10% of them. The dial is small so that precise readings are difficult over the very compressed scale available.

If anything begins to go wrong, measurements drift up or down imperceptibly, producing a systematic error over all readings, which may go on for months or years before it is suspected. Aneroid machines require adjustment above sea level, which they rarely receive, and errors increase at higher levels of blood pressure.

Mercury Sphygmomanometers

Mercury machines are cumbersome, particularly for home visits, and need annual maintenance, which they rarely receive, but they have the great advantage of simplicity. When they break down the fault is usually easy to find. Leaks at male/female tube joins, and valve filters blocked with fluff, are two very common faults which can be easily put right. Details of routine maintenance are given in Appendix 4, which should be photocopied for use by practice staff responsible.

Spot checks of hospital sphygmomanometers in regular use generally show about half of them to be seriously faulty[27, 30], because of a long medical and nursing tradition that all instruments endure without care, testing, or maintenance until they can no longer be made to work at all. One of the pharmaceutical companies (Riker Laboratories) offers a free sphygmomanometer maintenance service for GPs, but a good primary care team should make someone who can use a screwdriver responsible for this task.

Research Sphygmomanometers

The greatest research need is for a non-invasive, portable sphygmomanometer which will give semi-continuous readings over about 24 hours, and permit the subject under study to lead a normal home and working life, ideally an instrument with much the same qualities as a portable ECG monitor. Despite some claims to the contrary, at the time of writing no such instrument yet exists; none of the ambulatory machines can be used to measure during exercise. It seems likely that one will eventually be developed, perhaps using measurement of pulse wave velocity as a surrogate.

The standard research instrument for indirect measurement of blood pressure remains the cumbersome, expensive, but reliable and easily maintained random zero machine[23] marketed by Hawksley, and familiar in many British practices because of its use in the MRC trial. Direct measurements using brachial artery catheters have been used for many years in Oxford and other research centres. Really difficult diagnostic problems should be referred to such centres for 24–hour ambulatory monitoring.

Electronic Sphygmomanometers

The potential advantages of electronic sphygmomanometers are so great that they are bound eventually to replace mercury machines in most circumstances. They eliminate digit preference and bias, and with an adjustable deflation rate can eliminate rapid descent as a major source of error, providing staff do not use this adjustment to speed up their work, as is usually the case on hospital wards. These qualities taken together virtually eliminate differences between observers (including patients as their own observers), except for patient personality related emotional effects. They are generally easy to use, and are therefore particularly suitable for home readings.

Despite these potential advantages, their general use cannot yet be recommended. Thorough evaluation of the electronic machines available in the 1970s at the start of the HDFP trial revealed none that were better or more reliable than the random zero machine, and the designers of the later MRC trial seem to have reached the same conclusion. There are still problems about reliability and cuff size.

One problem with electronic machines is that if they begin to go wrong this may not be apparent to the user, and a systematic error may be introduced which may continue uncorrected for years. If a mercury machine goes wrong this is usually obvious, and the machine can be cleaned and repaired on the spot. If an electronic machine goes wrong, the error will probably be silent and certainly incomprehensible. Makers' literature is always inadequate, often transliterated from Japanese, and rarely contains anything about possible faults, not even so simple or frequent a matter as the effects to expect from a dying battery. Both salesmen and many purchasers seem to have such faith in all things electronic that any differences between readings obtained with a mercury and an electronic machine are automatically attributed to the traditional equipment, although nearly always the reverse is the case.

The cheaper machines rely on a microphone in the cuff which picks up an

163

acoustic signal from the brachial artery, just as the ear does through the stetho-scope. Accurate placing of the centre of the cuff over the artery is even more important than with a mercury machine. The more expensive ones operate from a very sensitive pressure transducer, programmed to distinguish a pulse wave from other extraneous signals, a big step forward which may eliminate many possible sources of error.

Unfortunately, both types complicate the cuff problem. I know of only one make, the Phillips machine, that is able to supply an outsize cuff on request. This is not big enough for really large arms, but will cope with most if used as standard. This is the one we have used for our home readings, but we have had a lot of trouble with it, particularly with diastolic pressures, and have now reverted to a standard mercury machine.

We must hope that one day the British Standards Institution or the Consumers' Association will test these various electronic machines, telling us how many of them have meaningfully different concealed insides, as opposed to visibly different (and therefore saleable) outsides, encouraging the more responsible suppliers to improve their products and assisting the early demise of most of the rubbish now on the market.

Diastolic Phases 4 and 5

Until the early 1970s, most British doctors were taught to use phase 4 (muffling of the Korotkoff sounds) as a diastolic end-point, and American doctors were taught to use phase 5 (disappearance of sound). There followed a period of uncertainty, after which doctors on both sides of the Atlantic seem finally to have agreed on phase 5.

Two sets of arguments have been deployed for and against these alternatives. First, there are arguments about which most nearly approximates to intra-arterial diastolic pressure. The evidence from various studies is conflicting, but phase 4 seems to average about 8 mmHg and phase 5 about 2 mmHg above intra-arterial diastolic pressure. Secondly, and I think more importantly, phase 5 is much easier to recognize and therefore easier for nurses (who will actually do most of the measurements) to use. Doctors have been found to show twice as much variability in recording diastolic as systolic pressures, and nurses three times as much.[31]

Although phase 5 should now be standard practice, there are patients in whom sounds never completely disappear down to 0 mmHg, even with all clothing removed from the upper arm. There is then no alternative to using phase 4. When this happens, the fact should be noted. The conventional correction is to subtract 5 mmHg to give equivalent phase 5 diastolic pressure, but the gap between phases 4 and 5 varies from almost nothing to about 10 mmHg, and the average difference is probably around 8 mmHg.[32]

Systolic and Diastolic Pressures

A simple way of avoiding all the ambiguities of diastolic pressure is to pay more attention to systolic pressure, and all the evidence favours this course from middle age onwards.

Enlargement of the heart,[33] heart failure,[34] ischaemic heart disease, stroke[35] and ECG response to antihypertensive treatment[36, 37] are all more closely related to attained systolic than diastolic pressures. In both men and women over the age of 40, systolic pressures are better predictors of subsequent cardiovascular disease than diastolic pressures at all ages and all levels of pressure,[38] although at lower ages diastolic pressure remains a better predictor.[39]

Unfortunately, in the English-speaking world we have all learned to speak diastolic language, and in practice, doctors avoid taking clinical decisions along two scales rather than one. Although all innovating clinicians have known the superiority of systolic over diastolic measurements for many years, we continue to speak and write 'diastolese' for fear of being ignored or misunderstood. Diastolic pressures therefore continue to be used as thresholds both for entry to treatment and for assessment of control at all ages. This may have serious consequences for older patients. Very high systolic pressures, say over 200 mmHg, have been frequently ignored in both initial assessment and follow-up, if the diastolic pressure is reassuringly low, as it frequently is. This is legitimized by the persistent myth of systolic hypertension as a normal accompaniment of old age, which 'only reflects the state of the peripheral arteries'. As the state of peripheral arteries, including those supplying the heart and brain, is our principal concern in treating high blood pressure, the logic of this argument escapes me.

References

1. Kannel WB and Gordon T (1970) *The Framingham study: An epidemiological investigation of cardiovascular disease, section 26.* US Goverment Printing Office, Washington DC.

2. Anderson TW (1978) Re-examination of some of the Framingham blood pressure data. *Lancet* ii: 1139–41.

3. Bevan AT, Honour AJ, Stott FH *et al.* (1969) Direct arterial pressure recording in unrestricted man. *Clin Sci* 36: 329–44.

4. Sokolow M, Werdegar D, Kain HK *et al.* (1966) Relationship between level of blood pressure measured casually and by portable recorders and severity of complications in essential hypertension. *Circulation* 34: 279–98.

5. Kannel WB and Sorlie P (1975) Hypertension in Framingham. In: Paul O (ed) *Epidemiology and control of hypertension*. pp. 553. Stratton Intercontinental Medical Books, New York.

6. Hart JT (1974) The marriage of primary care and epidemiology. *J R Coll Physicians Lond* 8: 299–314.

7. Kurji KH and Haines AP (1984) Detection and management of hypertension in general practices in north-west London. *Br Med J* 288: 903–6.

8. Wilkinson PR and Raftery EB (1978) Patient attitudes to measuring their own blood pressure. *Br Med J* ii: 824.

9. Young MA, Rowlands DB, Stallard TJ *et al.* (1983) Effect of environment on blood pressure: Home versus hospital. *Br Med J* 286: 1235–6.

10. Jyothinagaram SG, Rae L, Campbell A *et al.* (1987) Stability of home blood pressure over time. *J Hum Hypertens* 1: 269–71.

11. Kannel WB, Sorlie T and Gordon T (1980) Labile hypertension: A faulty concept? *Circulation* 61: 1183–7.

12. Mancia G, Bertinieri G, Grassi G *et al.* (1983) Effects of blood pressure measurement by the doctor on patients' blood pressure and heart rate. *Lancet* ii: 695–7.

13. Webb DJ, Stewart MJ and Padfield PL (1992) Monitoring ambulatory blood pressure in general practice. *Br Med J* 304: 1442.

14. Coope J and Coope G (1992) Monitoring ambulatory blood pressure in general practice. *Br Med J* 305: 53.

15. Webb DJ, Stewart MJ and Padfield PL (1992) Monitoring ambulatory blood pressure in general practice. *Br Med J* 305: 716–17.

16. Caldwell JR, Schork MA and Aiken RD (1978) Is near basal blood pressure a more accurate predictor of cardiorenal manifestations of hypertension than casual blood pressure? *J Chron Dis* 31: 507–12.

17. Hawthorne VM and Smalls M (1980) Blood pressure and ambient temperature. *Br Med J* 280: 567–8.

18. Ghose RR and Harindar V (1989) Unrecognized high pressure retention of urine presenting with systemic arterial hypertension. *Br Med J* 298: 1626–8.

19. Mayer K, Stamler J, Dyer AR *et al.* (1978) Epidemiologic findings on the relationship of time of day and time since last meal to five clinical variables: Serum cholesterol, hematocrit, systolic and diastolic pressure, and heart rate. *Prev Med* **7**: 22–7.

20. Pickering TG, James GD, Boddie C *et al.* (1988) How common is white coat hypertension? *JAMA* **259**: 225–8.

21. (1991) Practice imperfect [editorial]. *Lancet* **337**: 1195–6.

22. Humerfelt S (1966) Methodology of blood pressure recording. In: Gross F (ed) *Antihypertensive therapy.* Springer Verlag, Berlin.

23. Wright BM and Dore CF (1970) A random–zero sphygmomanometer. *Lancet* i: 337–8.

24. Croft PR (1982) Sphygmomanometer cuff sizes. *Lancet*, ii: 323–4.

25. King GE (1982) Selection of blood pressure cuff design. *Lancet* ii: 492.

26. Geddes LA (1991) *Handbook of blood pressure measurement.* Humana press, Clifton NJ.

27. Conceiçao S, Ward MK and Kerr DNS (1976) Defects in sphygmomanometers: An important source of error in blood pressure recording. *Br Med J* i: 886–8.

28. Kirkendall W, Feinleib M, Fries E *et al.* (1984) Recommendations for human blood pressure determination by sphygmomanometers: American Heart Association, Dallas TX 1981. *Circulation* **54**: 1145A–55A.

29. Fisher HW (1978) *Cardiovasc Med* **3**: 769. Quoted Paul O (1979) Clinical aspects of the natural history of mild hypertension. In: Gross F, Strasser T (eds) (1979) *Mild hypertension: Natural history and Management*, p. 15. Pitman Medical, London.

30. Burke MJ, Towers HM, O'Malley K *et al.* (1982) Sphygmomanometers in hospital and family practice: Problems and recommendations. *Br Med J* **285**: 469–71.

31. Richardson JF and Robinson D (1971) Variations in the measurement of blood pressure between doctors and nurses. *J R Coll Gen Pract* **21**: 698–704.

32. D'Souza MF and Irwig LM (1976) Measurement of blood pressure. *Br Med J* iv: 814–15.

33. Kannel WB, Gordon T and Offutt D (1969) Left ventricular hypertrophy by electrocardiogram: Prevalence, incidence, and mortality in the Framingham study. *Ann Intern Med* 71: 89–105.

34. Kannel WB, Castelli WP, McNamara PM *et al.* (1972) Role of blood pressure in the development of heart failure. *N Eng J Med* 287: 781–7.

35. Kannel WB, Verter J *et al.* (1970) Epidemiologic assessment of the role of blood pressure in stroke. *JAMA* 214: 301–10.

36. George CF, Breckenridge AM and Dollery CT (1972) Value of routine electrocardiography in hypertensive patients. *Br Heart J* 34: 618–22.

37. Ibrahim MM, Tarazi RC, Dustan HP *et al.* (1971) Electrocardiogram in evaluation of resistance to antihypertensive therapy. *Arch Intern Med* 137: 1125–30.

38. Kannel WB, Gordon T and Schwartz MJ (1971) Systolic versus diastolic blood pressure and risk of coronary heart disease: The Framingham study. *Am J Cardiol* 27: 335–46.

39. Lichtenstein MJ, and Rose G (1985) Systolic and diastolic blood pressure as predictors of coronary heart disease mortality in the Whitehall study. *Br Med J* 291: 243–5.

11

Divisions of Labour

Anticipatory, proactive primary care for whole populations, not only responding to wants but seeking for needs, is frankly not feasible for family doctors working alone. Simply to detect and manage all moderate or severe high blood pressure and all diabetes in a total population of 2000 before the 1990 Contract, we found in Glyncorrwg that we needed the following additional annual staff time, over and above what we required before screening[1]:

■ doctors
69 hours consulting time
3 hours administration time

■ nurses
159 hours consulting time
3 hours administration time

■ receptionists
70 hours consulting time
15 hours administration time

■ manager
11 hours administration time

■ total new staff time = 330 hours.

In a large, multi-ethnic, high turnover inner city practice in the East End of London, Robson and his colleagues[2] showed not only that multi-risk factor control for arterial disease was possible in such a population, but also mounted a randomized controlled trial to show that nurses prompted by a computer program obtained much better results than doctors working in a traditional way. The team is here to stay, but must be resourced: like myself, Robson had to get research funding to support innovation which should have been resourced by the health authority.

It is usually taken for granted that work should be delegated downwards as far as possible. Doctors who automatically regard themselves as more skilled and more valuable than anyone else in the team eventually discover they never had one. A more effective approach is for the whole team to consider thoroughly and in detail what has to be done, who are or can be made available to do it, who are most interested, and what further learning may be necessary.

Discussion will be greatly improved if some sort of audit material is obtained before the meeting, even if this is just an analysis of some randomly sampled adult records. Discussion based on evidence becomes less subjective and personal. Responsibility may then be agreed on a trial basis subject to revision at later meetings, when new decisions can be taken in the light of further audit and experience.

Who Should Do What?

One of the first questions is 'who will do routine blood pressure readings?'. Granted a short period of appropriate retraining, nurses measure pressures more accurately, with fewer preconceptions, and alarm patients less than doctors. Figures 11.1 and 11.2 show the distributions of systolic and diastolic pressures measured by nurses and doctors on the same group of patients.[3] Nurse-measured pressures are consistently lower than doctor-measured pressures, particularly in the high systolic range.

Other tasks undertaken by nurses in Glyncorrwg were:

- checking medication (patients were asked always to bring their medication with them)
- organizing repeat blood pressure measurements, measuring weights and heights, measuring pulse rates (always recorded routinely with BP measurements as indicators of alarm) and entering results both in the written record and the computer
- updating smoking histories: smoking status was confirmed whenever BP was measured, although not usually commented upon
- measuring haemoglobin when indicated, drawing venous blood for all investigations, centrifuging and preparing blood slides, urine testing (tapes and dip-cultures), measuring peak expiratory flow rates, and recording ECGs.

These tasks were not taken on all at once but developed over several years. Our nurses did not initiate, modify, or change medication, but, with suitable

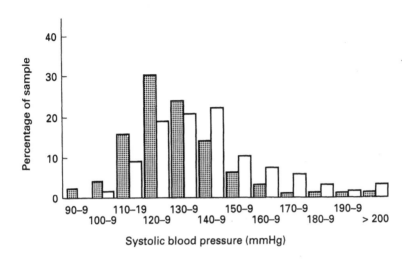

Figure 11.1: Frequency distribution of systolic blood pressures measured by nurses (black squares) and doctors (white squares) on the same group of patients[3].

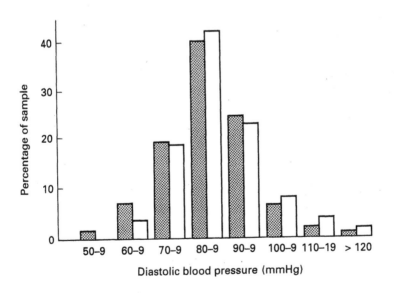

Figure 11.2: Frequency distribution of diastolic blood pressures measured by nurses (black squares) and doctors (white squares) on the same group of patients[3].

additional training (not then available), I see no reason in principle why they should not do so. Once the nature of a task has been clearly defined, limits of competence have been agreed, and adequate time has been made available to perform it, nurse-practitioners work as well as doctors with appropriate training, and better than those without it.[4]

In Glyncorrwg, tasks undertaken by doctors but not nurses were:

- integrating blood pressure management with management of other problems and risk factors
- searching for specific side-effects such as lethargy, depression, diminished libido and impotence
- updating alcohol histories
- examining fundi through dilated pupils in patients whose pressures were badly out of control (diastolic pressure 120 mmHg or more); otherwise fundi were not checked routinely
- asking about breathlessness and fatigue, then examining neck veins for raised venous pressure, lungs for crackles, and hearts for evidence of valvular disease, triple rhythm and arrhythmias, and legs for oedema
- asking about chest and leg pain on exercise, and if present, requesting ECG and examining feet for dorsalis pedis and posterior tibial pulses
- taking all decisions about starting, stopping, or changing anti-hypertensive medication, and initiating all requests for laboratory and imaging investigations.

Every one of these tasks could, in my opinion, be done reliably by an experienced nurse with appropriate training, but this was our division of labour in 1987 when I retired from directing the unit. Laboratory and imaging request forms were completed by doctors, not delegated, because our nurses already had more than enough unskilled, boring and repetitive work to do, and interest and morale needed to be actively sustained. Computer generated name and address labels are now a great help. We kept a full sheet of these inside each record folder, and printed new sheets as these were used up.

Tasks shared by both doctors and nurses were:

- friendly chat and open-ended questions about health and worries, updating smoking histories
- discussion of and responsibility for chasing up defaulters; these were discussed at the end of each clinic.

These divisions of labour evolved over many years, and will continue to change. They partly depended on the aptitude, interests, and often the family responsibilities and other pressures on time of nurses and doctors. The idea that divisions of labour can be set for all time by higher administration or professional bodies obstructs progress and ignores the huge, still largely unrealized potential of continuing in-service education.

Obstacles to Team Development

British family doctors in public service are more fortunate than their southern European colleagues in that they retain full clinical autonomy. They have to tolerate much less professional hierarchy, and have had some responsibility for patient care even as undergraduates.[5] British GPs expect to have considerable autonomous responsibility for patient care even as trainees, and certainly when they become GP principals.

Nurses still have much less autonomy than doctors. Traditionally they were handmaidens, trained rather than educated, to do rather than to think, to obey rather than to lead. New ideas of independent professionalism are now supposed to have swept through the nursing profession, and blind obedience to doctors is on the way out. I wish the same might be said about blind obedience to nursing officers. Much of the military tradition in nursing persists, although the officers have changed sex and uniform. Despite the exciting blueprint of 'Nursing 2000', there is a long way to go before nurses are generally valued intellectually, or value themselves intellectually, as a rule rather than an exception.[6]

Obstacles to team development were obvious in the UK before the NHS (for example, the bitter rivalry between GPs and midwives, and between GPs and health visitors). They remain obvious wherever medical trade is still important, and doctors therefore see nurses as potential competitors. The nurse-practitioner idea, born in rural USA when doctors wanted to work only in cities, was quickly discarded as soon as they rediscovered the security of the countryside.[7] Even in the UK, only about one third of family doctors accept nurse-practitioners even as a future objective.[8]

Despite our long tradition of general practice as a free public service, three big changes are necessary in the UK if we are to achieve real teamwork in primary care: doctors must drop assumptions that they are automatically more competent and valuable than anyone else, nurses must drop assumptions that their responsibilities can begin and end with the practical task in hand, and both must become more interested in understanding and expanding the limits of their personal competence, and less interested in defending professional skills assumed to exist only because of qualifications, unsupported by recent experience.

In practice, it is impossible to lay down impersonal ground rules for who should do what, except in terms so general as to be meaningless. In every case, it depends on the actually existing attitudes, interests, abilities, and experience of staff, the time and space for their work, the further training locally available, and what the local population is willing to try. As insulin dependent diabetics have known for more than 60 years, there is virtually no limit to what anyone, nurses, office staff, patients, or their families, can do, if they only have literacy, motivation, and opportunities to learn. These are the three keys to team development.

Responsibilities for Management and Leadership

Doctors have a long period of training in which they are stuffed with technical knowledge produced by science, but are seldom trained in scientific thought. Once they have tenure, and no longer face examiners, only a minority of doctors (a large minority, it's true), either in hospital or general practice, continue to follow serious medical literature or to innovate, applying the generalities of the literature to the specific local circumstances of their own populations.

All good GPs are specialists, not in a part of the body but in a part of the world. From 1961 to 1987 I occupied a unique chair in 'Glyncorrwgology'. If GPs accept such responsibility, they are usually better placed to adapt the medical literature to local circumstances than anyone else in the team.

Once movement begins, almost anyone, doctors, nurses, office staff, and patients, may develop a leading role for at least some aspect of care. In any case, with time, a team working correctly becomes a collective within which all can work autonomously to extend the limits of their competence in a common effort to improve patient care.

The key to this process is agreement on measurable objectives, with regular audit of the extent to which they are being achieved. Authority must be based on evidence rather than status, and, despite continued retreat in society as a whole down the path of command managerialism, in primary care we can and should retain respect for consensus.

Some senior doctors still refuse responsibility for leading this work, and the question then arises of whether anyone else can. Junior doctors may have sufficient diplomatic skill to manoeuvre their seniors into a position of only apparent power, and nurses or practice managers may wangle grudging agreement to pursue their own schemes, as long as they do not disturb anyone else. Changing to another practice is an ultimate solution, but not helpful for patients.

Uses of Audit

The most effective method for securing real change in any practice is to present a problem in quantified clinical terms which compel respect from doctors, nurses, office staff and patients alike, to set modest objectives by consensus agreement, and then to measure attainment of these objectives.

The person pushing a new idea can draw out a random sample of 25 records for people aged between 40 and 64 and spend three evenings evaluating the recording of information about blood pressure, smoking, and weight for height (or three minutes, if this information is computerized); or take out the records of 25 randomly sampled known hypertensives, to see how many have been seen and checked within the last 4 months, how many have a clear account of current

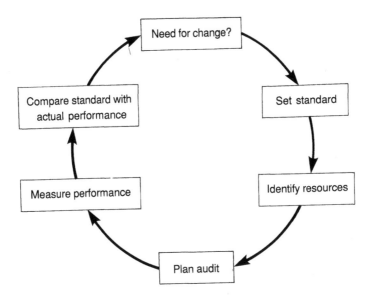

Figure 11.3: The audit cycle[9].

medication, and how many were started on medication on reasonable criteria; or take out the records of 25 randomly sampled known diabetics to see how many have been reviewed in the past year, how many have had their fundi examined with pupils dilated, how may have blood pressures recorded and controlled, and how many have smoking status recorded. Other audit suggestions are listed in Chapter 13.

Discussion of how these results could be improved should involve the whole team, and should lead to discussion of divisions of labour. Once targets are agreed (and if they are realistically modest, they will be difficult for the most conservative doctor, nurse or office staff, or patients to resist), the rest follows. Once begun, the audit cycle[9] (Figure 11.3) is usually unstoppable.

However note that like other cycles, it falls down if it does not keep moving. Providing targets are realistic and take full account of the capacities and interests of the staff available, the cycle will roll.

Employed and Attached Teams

The 1990 Contract has rapidly expanded employed practice staff, and encouraged at least the outward forms of innovation. Nearly three quarters of practices now have a practice manager, and 88% employ one or more practice nurses.

Excellent work has been done for many years in some prevention orientated practices by facilitators attached on an area basis, with a specific remit to assist the birth of community blood pressure control in a number of practices, not to do the work themselves, but to demonstrate possibilities and initiate training of existing or newly recruited staff. One of the first of these, and the best known, was led by Elaine Fullard in Oxford, with imaginative leadership from community physicians and nursing officers willing to commit real resources.[10]

Facilitators with similar job definitions have now been appointed in most regions throughout the UK. It is too early to assess their impact, but I have no doubt at all that it will be large and positive, although the impact on cardiovascular morbidity is likely to be much less than unrealistic early forecasts suggested.

Compared with many other countries, the UK has been slow to develop clinical policies at area level. This negative aspect of our generally useful tradition of clinical autonomy remains unappreciated by most of our family doctors, although obvious to visitors from other countries which actually try to practice community medicine, Spain being the most obvious example. Until the late 1980s progress in the UK depended almost entirely on personal initiatives by individual family doctors, without interest, encouragement, or practical support from regional or area health authorities. The FHSAs (formerly Family Practitioner Committees) were totally ignorant of, and indifferent to, clinical standards and policies in the practices for which they were nominally responsible, acting only as paymasters and guardians against extreme fraud or neglect.

The upheaval throughout the NHS accompanying the introduction of managerialism, industrialization, and internal markets in 1991 has profoundly changed this relationship, in contradictory ways which are incompletely evolved. Only the most tentative judgements are therefore possible.

Even before this upheaval, some FHSA managers were looking for active roles in promoting clinical policies at area level.[11] Although most of the new FHSA managers have industrial or military, rather than NHS, experience of administration, they do at least transcend the paymaster role to which the old FHSAS were constrained. They accept and understand the language of planned development and verifiable production, even if few of them have as yet the haziest notion of what they need to produce. Most are unable to distinguish between the social advances made possible by recognizing medical care as a form of production, and the social retreat inherent in the assumption that medical care must therefore converge with managed industrialism.[12] Because any activity must be better than none, FHSAs have therefore become relatively open to planned innovation at an area level, despite generally savage constraints on all other forms of public spending and investment, a paradoxical growth area surrounded by increasingly arid desert.

Appointment of facilitators, a generally permissive attitude to funding for employed practice nurses and an increasingly imaginative range of other primary care staff, mostly working in the 'health promotion' field, therefore continued despite retreat in most other areas of the NHS*. Of course, this has not been universal, but in general FHSAs seem to have interpreted their role progressively, for 'health promotion' at least. Predictably this advance has generally halted as FHSAs have run up against the buffers of local budgets.

Although most facilitators have had previous experience as health visitors and few have been practice nurses themselves, my impression is that an increasing proportion of them favour recruitment of more GP-employed practice nurses rather than attachment of community nurses employed by health authorities (HAs). Certainly such policies are favoured by many GPs who, given the chance, prefer to control primary care teams themselves, rather than participate as equals. However, it has to be said that many attached community nurses have faced real difficulties of divided loyalty, to local medical and nursing colleagues on the one hand, and their nursing hierarchy on thé other. It is probably this perception which has led so many facilitators to prefer the practice nurse option. Because HA-employed community nurses have generally not been given authority to take autonomous policy decisions, they have been unable to share fully in team decision-making.

Typical questions in my personal experience have included whether an attached nurse can take venous blood, visit patients' homes, scan records for audit, or be assured continuity once she has some experience in a unit.

Such problems should be settled informally and locally; they should depend, not on formal policies (which cannot and should not cover all contingencies), but on what people want, are able or can get in-service training to do, with a generous but realistic assumption that all on the team are normally doing the best they can, both to improve patient care and to respect each others' responsibilities.

GP-employed nurses have rich experience of the disadvantages of their position. Although (pressed by a seller's market) they are improving, family doctors generally have been bad employers. They have paid less than Whitley scale or union rates where they could get away with it, have been slow to adopt pension schemes, have delegated monotonous work thoughtlessly, and have delegated responsible work without organizing paid leave for training. Despite all these failings (which have dwindled rapidly in the last couple of years), to most nurses they seem to be less unattractive employers than HAs. This is probably because GP-employment offers more flexible hours, shorter travel to work, greater variety, and, most importantly (and paradoxically), far more clinical autonomy. GP-employed practice nurses are increasingly able to make their own clinical decisions, with

* This should not be taken to imply that FHSA managers with commercial backgrounds present no threat to the integrity of the NHS, or of those who still work in it as a vocation. For example, appointment of specialized stoma care nurses was one of the great advances of the past decade, but it cost money. About a quarter of all NHS stoma care nurses are now sponsored by stoma product manufacturers, at a cost of £20–30,000 a year each. There are about 70 000 stoma patients in the UK with 17 000 new cases a year. Each patient may be worth £4–8000 a year to a stoma company. This conflict of interest having been acceptable to government, is there any reason in principle why cardiovascular health promotion facilitators should not be sponsored by manufacturers of antihypertensive drugs?

informal relationships with their colleagues, and autonomous and continuing relationships with individual patients, for whom they become personally responsible for widening aspects of care. These relationships often become deeper, at least in some directions, than those formed between the patient and the doctor. All this results in high job satisfaction and high motivation, which must in the long run mean greater efficiency and cost effectiveness.

Delegation Without Responsibility

Doctors who try to do everything themselves are certainly dangerous, but equally dangerous are doctors who delegate work without responsibility.

Table 11.1 shows a real example of blood pressure readings recorded by HA-employed attached community nurses. This man first presented to his GP in 1977, at a teaching practice in another town, with a left hemiplegia; he was then 66. They started him on antihypertensive treatment with methyldopa 250 mg three times a day, and asked their attached community nurses to follow him up monthly, while the practice continued to provide repeat prescriptions. Three years later he and his wife moved to Glyncorrwg temporarily, while their home underwent extensive repairs. They came to me to arrange for our local nurses to continue supervision. He had obviously recovered well from his hemiplegia.

I asked him if he knew what his original blood pressure was, before his stroke. He didn't, but instead he offered the following list of blood pressure values recorded by community nurses at monthly intervals throughout those three years, during which his treatment remained wholly unchanged.

Table 11.1: Blood pressures recorded 1977–80 in a hemiplegic man (mmHg).

1977–8	1978–9	1979–80
162/98	250/150	200/130
180/90	198/134	220/130
190/210	190/130	200/130
220/120	190/110	180/110
220/120	200/130	190/110
230/120	190/130	170/100
180/120	180/100	180/120
220/150	180/90	180/120
220/140	200/130	180/110
230/140	200/130	170/100
180/140	180/120	
120/100	240/110	
190/100	250/120	

His blood pressure when he was first seen in our clinic was 210/110 mmHg.

We added 2.5 mg bendrofluazide to his medication and thereafter saw him once a month, with the following readings: 182/88, 154/80, 146/78, 150/69 and 118/64 mmHg. He then went back to his reconstructed home, and was still alive and well at 79 years when I last heard from him.

How can such things happen? The handwriting showed that at least three different community nurses saw him during the 3 years while he was observed but not cared for. Doctors have no right to assume that nurses have been taught to interpret the data they record. If they want nurses to take clinical decisions, they should specify what these are, with clear criteria for referral back for revision of treatment. It is easy to say that nurses should not accept work without asking what it is for, or what they should do with the results; the negative answers they got when they asked such questions in the past ensure that, all too often when critical thought is needed, it is no longer available. This can happen easily if attachment is so loose that community nurses are not really a part of the team, so that their work is never evaluated or discussed.

Although there has been some discussion of a possible role for health visitors in preventive work among the middle aged, this is hopelessly unrealistic unless there is a huge expansion of the health visitor work force, as well as a radical redefinition of their responsibilities. Health visitors seconded to work in this specific field, without responsibilities for children or the elderly, would be a different matter.

The Expanded Team

Even in a blood pressure clinic with a family doctor and a nurse, it is difficult to do justice to control of other risk factors, particularly smoking, obesity, reduced fat diet, and development of exercise programmes. Everything depends on patient education, but that takes a lot of time, and needs reinforcement with specific literature which is often better if it is locally produced.

There is a great unmet need for mature, intelligent, honest, friendly, but not over-professionalized women and men who might be employed to take responsibility for individual and group health education, for developing and making readily available short leaflets covering the specific things patients need to know and remember, in terms that link up with common local experience. Large numbers of these people are now being wasted in unemployment, who would certainly apply for such jobs if they were offered.

The Oxford randomized controlled trial of anti-smoking education produced disturbing evidence that structured advice from nurses is less effective than advice from family doctors.[13] Some have assumed that this difference is attributable to the greater authority of doctors compared with nurses, but that begs the question where such authority comes from. Some of it probably derives from the different relationship between patient and professional in an expanded, informal consultation prompted by the patient, than in the teacher-pupil relationship in a structured episode of teaching prompted by professionals. As anti-smoking advisers within ordinary consultation, doctors are able to draw on a rich variety of experience, which in a patient-prompted encounter may be applied with more sensitivity and imagination, than in a more formal and isolated educational contact, whoever the teacher may be.

We need much more imaginative, local research into the possibilities of developing use of lay counsellors for lateral referral within the practice, because there is no way that all this can be done by doctors.

Training

Training programmes are now an urgent need, for nurses and practice managers who are moving into this field, for attached community nurses, and hopefully for the lay counsellors described in the last paragraph. National metings for these groups, notably the biennial Anticipatory Care Teams (ACT) conferences, have been well supported, and even now there is a large unsatisfied demand, particularly for local courses adapted to the needs of part time workers with family responsibilities. Pharmaceutical companies which, in the absence of DoH initiative, remain responsible for meeting most of the cost of postgraduate education other than vocational training, are beginning to include nurses and other practice staff in their invitations and on their platforms. This is a disgraceful, and ultimately costly solution (the companies pay because they rightly assume greater sales in consequence), which no responsible government should tolerate.

There remains a serious shortage of locally organized courses, which could not only provide training, but also serve as forums for discussion between professionals tackling the same job in different places, and devising their own solutions. This should be a top priority for district health authorities, or better still primary care authorities, if these eventually replace FHSAs, as the Royal College of Nursing and of General Practitioners have both proposed.

There is also a shortage of teachers. Practical preventive work cannot be taught effectively by people without experience of doing what they teach, so this shortage will continue until we have a first generation of doctors, nurses and practice managers, who have already achieved enough to give them the confidence and credibility to teach others. It is particularly important that whatever training courses are set up should not be weighed down with academic experts, but be conducted in a participative, small group style, discussing real and representative data, brought by participants from their own practices.

References

1. Hart JT (1991) Background reading: An agenda for the next hundred years. In: Roberts G. (ed) *Prevention in practice: A team approach*, pp 6–11. Radcliffe Medical Press, Oxford.

2. Robson J, Boomla K, Fitzpatrick S *et al.* (1989) Using nurses for preventive activities with computer assisted follow-up: A randomized controlled trial. *Br Med J* 298: 433–6.

3. Richardson JF and Robinson D (1971) Variations in the measurement of blood pressure between doctors and nurses. *J R Coll Gen Pract* 21: 698–704.

4. Spitzer WO, Sackett DL, Sibley JC *et al.* (1974) The Burlington randomized trial of the nurse practitioner. *N Engl J Med* 290: 251–6.

5. Brearley S (1992) Medicine in Europe: Medical education. *Br Med J* 304: 41–4.

6. Clark J (1991) Nursing: An intellectual activity. *Br Med J* 303: 376–7.

7. Spitzer W (1984) The nurse-practitioner revisited: Slow death of a good idea. *N Engl J Med* 310: 1049–51.

8. Georgian Research Society (1991) The attitude of general practitioners towards practice nurses: A pilot study. *Br J Gen pract* 41: 19–22.

9. Koppel I and Schofield T (1991) Evaluation in practice. In: Roberts G (ed) *Prevention in practice: A team approach*, pp 53–8. Radcliffe Medical Press, Oxford.

10. Fullard E, Fowler G and Gray M (1984) Facilitating prevention in primary care. *Br Med J* 289: 1585.

11. Allsop J and May A (1986) *The emperor's new clothes: Family Practitioner Committees in the 1980s*. King's Fund, London.

12. Hart JT (1992) Two paths for medical practice. *Lancet* 340: 772–5.

13. Sanders D, Fowler G, Mant D *et al.* (1989) Randomized controlled trial of anti-smoking advice by nurses in general practice. *J R Coll Gen Pract* 39: 273–6.

Verification ■ What about other risk factors? ■ Family history ■
History, examination and baseline measurements ■ Laboratory tests
■ Are there other complicating medical problems?■ Is there a common
cause of secondary hypertension? ■ Is there a rare cause of
secondary hypertension? ■ What resources and limitations does the
patient have? ■ Suggested sequence for early data collection

Your hypertensive patients are identified chiefly by organized search and occasionally by presenting symptoms, but always through measurement of a single variable,
blood pressure itself.

According to classic teaching methods, which for all I know may still continue
in some medical schools, the next diagnostic steps are first to verify that the high
pressure is real and sustained, secondly to search for causes, thirdly to assess
organ damage, and finally to assess social context.

For a referred out-patient, the first of these is likely to be completed by
replicate readings at the first interview, and the others will usually be completed
at one or two subsequent interviews, at the end of which the patient will probably
embark on a lifetime of treatment. 20–30 minutes will normally be available for
these initial encounters, with nursing assistance for measurements, blood sampling, and form filling.

In general practice, the time available for each interview still averages about
7–8 minutes' face to face time with the doctor. In Glyncorrwg we eventually
managed to extend this to an average of 10 minutes, plus about 5–10 minutes of
nurse time. There is no way we could do all that needed to be done at the first
encounter, or often even at the first three encounters. We therefore extended both
verification and the collection of data over anything from three to seven encounters, doing a little each time, and using each opportunity to convey information
to the patient in small and hopefully memorable amounts. A suggested sequence
for this data collection is given at the end of this chapter.

Verification

There can be few more reckless gambles in clinical medicine than to start a patient on a lifetime of antihypertensive drugs on the evidence of a single reading, but on records from 71 GPs who permitted audit of their records in 1976, this is what then happened in about one-third of cases[1]. The proportion of subjects with high pressure (using any theshold) falls by about half on second readings (on separate days), and by about 20% on the third reading. After this it is fairly stable, but there is still a large minority of patients whose blood pressures fall substantially over 3 or 4 months on observation alone.

In a well organized practice few patients are seen for whom antihypertensive treatment is so urgent that they could not benefit from a delay of a few weeks or even months, during which a full assessment can be made, uncontaminated by the effects of drugs. Even for the tiny minority who have neuroretinopathy or heart failure when first seen, it should still be possible to record at least three replicate readings spaced over 20 minutes or so. The fact that these often differ by 20 mmHg or more may be important evidence later in assessing the apparent effects of antihypertensive drugs.

The routine in Glyncorrwg was that, when any pressure at or over a threshold of 170/100 mmHg was recorded, another two visits to our nurse were organized, to give us three readings to consider at the next doctor consultation. About half our newly discovered hypertensives (mostly those with erratic or borderline readings) borrowed an electronic machine to record 14 days of morning and evening readings, so that the decisions to treat or not could be taken on the mean of 28 readings.

What about other Risk Factors?

Two other principal cardiovascular risk factors, smoking and blood cholesterol, should be checked in everyone found to have a high pressure, whether or not you decide to start antihypertensive treatment.

Smoking status should always be checked at the same time as blood pressure, as a normal part of the same standard procedure. This helps to link the two risks in the minds of both patients and staff, and to emphasize the futility of treating hypertension while continuing to ignore smoking.

Many authorities deny the value of routine measurement of blood lipids in hypertensive patients, mostly on grounds of cost. This is trivial compared with the cost of much antihypertensive medication. Although there is a positive association between total blood cholesterol and obesity, and weight reduction is the first target in all cholesterol lowering diets, there are plenty of skinny people with prodigiously high cholesterols; obesity is not a reliable indicator of cholesterol status. After many years of avoiding it (because it entails even more work for an already overworked team), I was driven by the weight of evidence to the conclusion that action should be taken to reduce not only unusually high cholesterol values (say 7.5 mmol/l), but all values over 5 mmol/l (about 200 mg/dl) in patients with one other major risk factor.

If such action is to be effective it requires measurement, not guesswork. If we take trouble, so may our patients. Where subsequent measurements show that cholesterol is not falling, it is probably not worth wasting any more feedback, but if a useful fall is obtained, it probably should be verified annually thereafter.

Family History

Every patient should be asked about stroke, heart attacks and diabetes in parents and siblings, and also their smoking habits, and anything known about their blood pressure, although such information is seldom reliable. This is important partly to assess risk, but chiefly to develop motivation. Illness in the family is potentially the most valuable experience patients have to help them to make rational decisions about their own lives. We put this information at the top of the summary sheet, so it was always readily available.

History, Examination and Baseline Measurements

Starting antihypertensive drug treatment without taking a directed history and without a physical examination of any kind is still common, although shortage of time is not much of a problem if data collection is spread over several visits. At the stage when most cases of high blood pressure are picked up in a well-organized general practice, few hypertensive patients have gross evidence of organ damage. Routine physical examination therefore may seem a pointless exercise, except to impress the patient.

In fact, the main aim of both history and physical examination is not to make a diagnosis, but to record baselines against which to evaluate future events. Except for coarctation, rare causes of secondary hypertension are most often detected by careful re-evaluation of cases with anomalous response to treatment, and are seldom obvious enough to be discovered through any initial routine.

Patients should be asked routinely about sternal pain on exercise and 'indigestion' pains, about calf pain on walking or running, and about breathlessness. Paroxysmal nocturnal dyspnoea rarely has to be asked for – it presents readily enough because it is so frightening – but a history of angina and claudication often have to be actively elicited.

Patients should also be asked whether they have any symptoms which they themselves attribute to high blood pressure. This attribution is rarely correct, but it is important, particularly at this early stage, to know how patients themselves conceive of their 'disease', and to discuss this with them before matters are complicated by the effects of antihypertensive drugs.

There is little point in recording standing and lying pressures, unless there are positive reasons for suspecting autonomic neuropathy, as in diabetics or elderly patients, or in patients complaining of faint spells.

Heart rhythm should be noted. A large heart is obvious in a few patients, and can be confirmed by chest radiograph. Unless there are symptoms of heart failure, or there is some other indication, routine chest radiography for all hypertensive patients is not helpful or necessary, nor is routine pyelography.

We do an initial routine electrocardiogram (ECG), chiefly in order to have a previous tracing available in the event of later chest pain. It is particularly useful always to know whether bundle branch block is old or recent; in the absence of baseline evidence it may be impossible to interpret later ECG evidence of infarction, which may exactly resemble left bundle branch block. We try to avoid overstatement of the prognostic value of ECGs to patients, who tend to have exaggerated faith in machinery of all kinds.

Lungs should be checked for crackles, and whether these clear on coughing. Peak expiratory flow rate should be recorded for all patients and matched against predicted values for sex, age and height, because all hypertensive patients are likely at some stage to be treated with beta-blocking drugs. All asthmatics, overt or latent, should be identified before rather than after prescriptions of beta-blocking drugs, which can be lethal even in previously unsuspected chronic asthmatics.

The abdomen should be felt and murmurs listened for, bearing in mind the possibilities of renal artery stenosis or aortic aneurysm. Posterior tibial and dorsalis pedis pulses should be noted, again mainly as baselines for future events.

Fundi should be examined once at an early stage, with pupils fully dilated with a mydriatic. This will almost always be normal[2], but an early note of, for example, white spots from toxoplasmosis in infancy, may save a lot of worries later on. A fleeting glance through an undilated pupil is a futile gesture.

Laboratory Tests

Urine should be tested for glucose and protein, and one dip-culture should be set up to screen for renal tract infection. In obese older patients with a BMI at or over 30 or a family history of diabetes, we take blood for glycosylated haemoglobin (HbA$_1$C) as a further screening test for diabetes; fructosamine serves as well, and is cheaper.

We also ask for routine baseline measurements of blood electrolytes, urea, creatinine, urate, and gamma glutamyl transferase (gamma GT), and a full blood count for mean corpuscular volume (as another indicator of alcohol problems) and packed cell volume, an important risk factor for stroke.

Are there other Complicating Medical Problems?

Most of our patients over the age of 50 have some other major medical problem complicating management of high blood pressure. Consequent problems are discussed in Chapter 18.

Is there a Common Cause of Secondary Hypertension?

Undergraduate teaching tends to leave the impression that the known causes of hypertension are rare, and since essential hypertension is by definition of unknown cause, there is no point in searching for common causes. However, patients always wonder why their blood pressure is raised, and some effort to answer this question is worthwhile, apart from the most obvious of all, an evaluation of family history.

The contraceptive pill is a fairly common cause of secondary hypertension, which may be severe. It should be excluded in every hypertensive woman of reproductive age. She may be getting the pill from another source, such as the Family Planning Association. Pressure usually falls within a month or two of withdrawal. Other iatrogenic causes are carbenoxolone and large doses of sympathomimetic amines, often bought across the counter from a chemist.

Although obesity on average makes only a small causal contribution to hypertension in middle age, and weight reduction has a correspondingly small effect in controlling it, this is not necessarily true of individual cases, and is certainly not true for patients under 40 years. Careful sequential measurements of blood pressure and weight may suggest that this is an important cause, and feedback to the patient (in terms of reduced pressure) may be an important incentive to maintain weight control.

Alcohol is a common, important and reversible cause of hypertension which should be considered in every case, by taking a full alcohol history and checking mean corpuscular volume (MCV) and gamma GT. A full alcohol history means asking how much beer, wine and spirits is habitually taken on each day of a typical week.

Depression (but not other psychiatric disorders) seems to be a common cause of hypertension. Blood pressure falls as mood improves. Unless pressure is sustained over a threshold of above 200/120 mmHg, or there is evidence of organ damage, antihypertensive drugs should not be started until depression resolves or is controlled. All antihypertensive drugs cause depression in some people, and this is rarely a risk worth taking.

Whether or not chronic anxiety causes sustained hypertension, acute anxiety and overwhelming personal problems can certainly raise pressure transiently, and sufficiently to cause alarm to doctors, whose fears may then be transmitted back to the patient, setting up a vicious circle perpetuated by hasty inception of antihypertensive drug treatment.

Asking patients in a general way whether they have worries is rarely effective. Patients worried out of their minds by failing marriage, a child in trouble or bills that cannot be met, will not complicate their troubles by discussing them with you, unless they believe you can help. They are more likely to simplify matters by denying any problems whatever, just as most of us answer the question 'How are you?' by answering 'Fine, thanks', even if we feel at death's door. The approach should be more circumspect, with an eye for the patient who seems ill at ease or on the brink of tears. Often the best question is to ask patients why they think their blood presure might be raised. Material of this kind often comes out when the spouse is seen, an essential step at some point in the induction phase. As with depression, patients with acute anxieties rarely benefit from immediate treatment, and it is often best to agree to follow them up without treatment until they are coping better with their other problems and then reconsider medication.

Patients who, from evidence of previous contacts, are likely to complain of minor non-specific side effects such as headache, tiredness or loss of libido may benefit from a couple of weeks on placebo before active medication begins, followed by open discussion of the results. Our experience has been that patients afterwards accept this as a reasonable way of separating the effects of apprehension from real drug induced side effects.

Is there a Rare Cause of Secondary Hypertension?

Some of the rarities are covered by initial routine baseline measurements. Three-quarters of all cases of primary aldosteronism (Conn's syndrome) should turn up with an unexpectedly low serum potassium. Do not forget that for accurate potassium estimations, red cells must be separated from plasma less than 30 minutes after venepuncture. Even if your centre is near a hospital or you have a good collection system, your blood samples may lie around for hours before they are attended to; there is really no alternative to possession of a centrifuge. About a quarter of all cases of primary aldosteronism have serum potassium within the normal range. If diagnosis is a guide to action rather than a puzzle for professional entertainment, this rarely matters, since impairment is caused either by hypokalaemia (which they have not got) or the hypertension itself, which can nearly always be readily controlled with antihypertensive medication[3].

Coarctation of the aorta mostly presents in the first year of life, but those who survive this long rarely have symptoms thereafter until they get a stroke, suffer heart failure, get subacute bacterial endocarditis, or rupture their aortas. They should be detected by routine search for foot and ankle pulses.

Polycystic kidneys should turn up on the family history, and most renal hypertension on a history of renal disease plus the results of your baseline measurements of blood urea, creatinine, and urate, and your search for proteinuria and bacteriuria. Chronic nephritis should be sought if you find chronic microhaematuria, which is present in about 10% of treated hypertensive patients in general practice[4], although few of these actually have a nephropathy. Routine pyelography in the absence of a history of renal disease is not justified. Of 952 routine pyelograms performed at the Glasgow MRC Hypertension Research Unit, 18% showed renal tract abnormalities, but these influenced management in less than 1%[5].

Renal artery stenosis is a rare cause of hypertension. It is reversible by surgery in about 50% of cases; the rest still have to be controlled medically. Renal artery stenosis rarely causes symptoms unless it presents with the malignant phase, a renal infarct, or hyponatraemic hypertensive syndrome, with thirst, polyuria, no glycosuria, and salt craving. About half of all cases have an abdominal systolic murmur over the renal arteries, but most such sounds are caused by atheroma rather than primary stenosis, and are a result rather than a cause of hypertension. So even this classic sign is fairly useless, and there is really no satisfactory screening test for this disorder[6]. The Glasgow MRC Hypertension Research Unit suggests two groups commonly seen by the GP in whom investigation could be reasonably cost-effective. The first group comprises patients under 45 years with moderate or severe high blood pressure. To this I would add 'and a negative family history of hypertension and with no alcohol problems'. This narrows the field very considerably, as high blood pressure in young men is fairly common, but nearly all cases have one or usually both parents hypertensive, or are heavy drinkers. The second group is of compliant patients with treated high blood pressure whose control deteriorates rapidly and unexpectedly. This may signal thrombotic or embolic occlusion of a renal artery.

Phaeachromocytoma is said to have a prevalence of between 0.1 and 1% in the general population[8]. About 10% are familial and 5% are associated with neurofibromatosis; these latter patients get diagnosed sooner, otherwise most are diagnosed over the age of 40. The tumour releases a variable mixture of adrenaline (epinephrine) and noradrenaline (norepinephrine), sometimes continuously, sometimes intermittently. Classically there is unstable high blood pressure with paroxysmal symptoms of anxiety, sweating, tachycardia, palpitations, nausea, flushing, vomiting, and tremor. High blood pressure is frequently sustained and stable, or if adrenaline release predominates, may not be present at all. The diagnosis may be suspected when high pressure is first recorded because of some or all of these paroxysmal symptoms or wide variations in pressure, or when response to treatment is erratic and incomprehensible. Diagnosis is usually by measurement of degradation products of adrenaline and noradrenaline in 24-hour samples of urine. If amine release is intermittent, so are the raised concentrations of their metabolites in urine, so collection should begin when the patient feels characteristic symptoms. The most widely available test is for vanillylmandelic acid (VMA), although this seems to be less sensitive and specific than measurment of free catecholamines and normetanephrine. Bananas, coffee, tea, chocolate, vanilla, phenolic drugs like aspirin, and citrus fruits should all be excluded from the time urine collection is proposed, as all can give false high values for VMA. Several tests may be necessary before you pick up the tumour, and if you really suspect it, persistence is essential. Routine screening is ineffective, and nearly all suspected cases turn out to be anxious people with panic attacks. Treatment is surgical. In patients awaiting surgery, blood pressure is usually controlled with the tyrosine hydroxylase inhibitor metirosine, sometimes combined with the alpha-receptor blocker phenoxybenzamine.

Cushing's syndrome (glucocorticoid excess) is equally rare, and causes hypertension in about three-quarters of all cases[9]. Its appearance is familiar because of the hypercortical facies of steroid treatment. The diagnosis is confirmed by the dexamethasone suppression test, measurement of plasma cortisol the day following a bedtime dose of 1 mg dexamethasone.

What Resources and Limitations does the Patient have?

At some point close to the inception of treatment, patient and spouse should be seen together to discuss a long term plan for management. This should include not only antihypertensive medication, with discussion of possible side effects, but also plans for changes in smoking, eating and drinking. Social and occupational difficulties should be discussed, and an informal contract for treatment agreed upon, which takes into account both the resources available to patients and their families, and the limitations they perceive.

Plans must be realistic. Doctors are poor judges of what patients can or cannot do; they are unable to predict who will succeed and who will fail in adhering to treatment plans. Contrary to medical folklore, no sociodemographic variables except extremes of age show any consistent association with compliance[10]. We do know, however, that GPs can do rather better than hospital specialists in securing compliance[11], and that patients do best if they share in devising treatment plans themselves.

Suggested Sequence for Early Data Collection

■ First (identification) visit.
   Explain that one raised pressure has been found, which needs to be

verified; check smoking status, and weight for height as BMI; arrange for repeat blood pressure measurements on at least two more separate days, then if mean pressure warrants it, arrange second visit.

■ Second visit.

Explain the likely significance of the mean value of three readings; obtain family history of stroke, coronary disease, diabetes, and causes of death in parents and siblings.

Obtain current symptoms, especially those attributed by the patient to high blood pressure.

Verify current medication, especially oral contraception and antidepressants.

Obtain baseline ECG, peak expirary flow rate, ankle and foot pulses, fundoscopy, urine for glucose and protein, examination of heart and lungs, blood for FBC, urea, creatinine, urate, total cholesterol and gamma GT; request glycosylated haemoglobin (HbA$_1$c) or fructosamine if BMI = 30+ or there is a family history of diabetes.

Invite spouse to third and fourth visits.

■ Third visit.

Review results of baseline measurements with the patient; if MCV = 95+, or triglyceride or gamma GT are raised, search again for high alcohol intake.

Take a diet history concentrating on fat and alcohol.

Record current exercise at home and at work, past and potential future interests in excercise, and local availability of pools, tracks, etc.

Are there any major problems at home or at work? Ask both partners specifically about sex function.

■ Fourth visit.

Discuss investigation results; agree a plan for control of other coronary and stroke risk factors.

Take decisions to: Review blood pressure annually; or teach patient or spouse to do home recordings and return in 2 weeks with 28 readings; or initiate antihypertensive medication and return to follow-up clinic in 4 weeks.

References

1. Parkin DM, Kellett RJ, Maclean DW *et al.* (1979) The management of hypertension: A study of records in general practice. *J R Coll Gen Pract* **22**: 590–4.

2. Dimmitt SB, West JNW, Eames SM *et al.* (1989) Usefulness of ophthalmoscopy in mild to moderate hypertension. *Lancet* **i**: 1103–6.

3. Swales JD (1983) Primary aldosteronism: How hard should we look? *Br Med J* **287**: 702–3.

4. Ryan WA (1981) Microscopic haematuria in hypertension. *Lancet* **ii**: 994.

5. Atkinson AB and Kellet RJ (1974) Value of intravenous urography in investigating hypertension. *J R Coll Physicians Lond* **8**: 175–81.

6. Choudhri AH, Cleland JGF, Rowlands PC *et al.* (1990) Unsuspected renal artery stenosis in peripheral vascular disease. *Br Med J* **301**: 1197.

7. Mackay A, Brown JJ, Lever AF *et al.* (1983) Unilateral renal disease in hypertension. In: Robertson JIS (ed) *Handbook of hypertension. Vol 2: Clinical aspects of secondary hypertension*, pp 33–79. Elsevier, Oxford.

8. Ball SG (1983) Phaeochromocytoma. In: Robertson JIS (ed) *Handbook of hypertension. Vol 2: Clinical aspects of secondary hypertension*, pp 238–75. Elsevier, Oxford.

9. Kaplan NM (1983) Cushing's syndrome and hypertension. In: Robertson JIS (ed) *Handbook of hypertension. Vol 2: Clinical aspects of secondary hypertension*, pp 208–21. Elsevier, Oxford.

10. Haynes RB, Sackett DL, Taylor DW *et al.* (1977) Manipulation of the therapeutic regimen to improve compliance: Conceptions and misconceptions. *Clin Pharmacol Ther* **22**: 125–30.

11. Drury VWM, Wade OL and Woolf E (1976) Following advice in general practice. *J R Coll Gen Pract* **26**: 712–18.

13

Organization of Follow-up and Compliance

Clinical medicine as traditional puzzle solving is important and great fun, but has hardly anything to do with successful control of high blood pressure and its associated risk factors in large numbers of people. Organized detection of high blood pressure is relatively easy. Because 60–70% of adults consult their GP at least once a year, and about 85% consult at least once in 5 years, case finding is an efficient method of mass detection. This can be supplemented by call-up.

The real problem is not detection but continued follow-up, without which detection is a wasted effort. Even in practices conscientious enough to participate in audit, published evidence suggests that this remains a serious problem[1], despite some progress from the frankly disgraceful standards prevailing in the 1970s[2].

Starting with a complete population screen in 1968–1970, and using a treatment threshold of diastolic 105 mmHg (plus hypertensive patients below this threshold with organ damage or diabetes), in Glyncorrwg we usually manage about 130 patients from a population of about 2000 (all ages). These patients are seen once every 3 months if they are well controlled, more often if not; this results in the organization of at least 600 visits a year.

Clinic or Regular Surgery Session?

Many GPs are opposed in principle to special clinics in general practice, and I still have some sympathy with their view. They believe that any and all clinics eventually degenerate into impersonal, over-structured conveyor belts, on which a fixed set of delegated standard procedures are performed by nurses, while doctors sign forms. I have known many clinics like this, and refused to segregate care of the hypertensive patients in my own practice for as long as possible because of the same fears.

About 3 years after our screening was completed we did our first team audit. The results were appalling. Many patients were rediscovered who had either lapsed from treatment altogether, or were collecting repeat prescriptions without any medical supervision. We set up first a monthly and later a fortnightly clinic, with a check on defaulters at the end of each session and a full audit once a year. Since then our compliance and control figures have been as good as or better than any figures reported from teaching hospitals, although unlike theirs, our results were based on a whole population, and on an intention to treat basis, including all drop-outs.

If those who oppose clinics in general practice can achieve 80% control (blood pressure <160/90 mmHg) and 80% attendance (treated patients seen within a 4-month span and untreated patients seen at least once a year) by seeing patients only in ordinary demand-led sessions, they deserve every success; our team was unable to operate at this level using that system.

The position is analogous to antenatal care, which until the 1950s was often scattered through the jumble of patient demand, and presented the same problems of ensuring that a minimum data set be obtained, and regular contact maintained, without degeneration into ritual. Many antenatal clinics, especially fully industrialized ones in hospitals, are insensitive and inhuman, but the answer to this is not abolition but reform, making them smaller, more flexible, more personal, and closer to the communities they serve. The best GP antenatal clinics are a good and familiar model for what is needed in GP blood pressure clinics.

Just as pregnant women need to discuss whatever worries they wish at a patient-orientated antenatal clinic, but may also need to discuss their pregnancies when consulting at other times, it is impossible to push all blood pressure related consultations into an appropriate clinic, or to confine clinic consultations to high blood presure and its related risks. If hypertensive patients consult for some other reason a week or so before their clinic day, it is mean, petty, and counterproductive to insist they return another time for a blood pressure check. If, during a blood pressure clinic, patients have other problems they want to discuss, reasonable flexibility should be shown in accepting them. If you do not do this, compliance will fall. We found that about 25% of our hypertension consultations, including all the induction phase, occurred outside our clinic structure.

How Often?

We operated on a 3-monthly cycle, not only for treated blood pressure follow-up, but also for oral contraception monitoring and follow-up of most chronic disease and long term certification. We found this simple to remember for both staff and patients and it fitted in with reasonable quantitites for repeat medication. Although the DoH rule is that prescriptions should cover a maximum of one month's supply, in reality this has not been enforced in practices with a good record for prescribing costs.

Roughly 20% of patients booked for a clinic do not come, about half of them because they have already been seen in a normal surgery session, the other half because they have forgotten, work impossible hours, or are persistent defaulters. This means that with a 3-month cycle, about 10% of the patients are actually seen on a 4-month or even 5-month cycle.

Some practices operate a 6-month cycle, and thus reduce work-load. Even on a 3-month cycle, at least 20% of patients will have pressures above target level, and I do not beleive we could have extended our cycle without impairing quality of care.

How many Patients?

We booked about 20 patients for each follow-up session, of whom 15–18 turned up. About two-thirds of these were dealt with entirely by a nurse, and of the other third, who wanted to see the doctor for another reason, about half had blood pressure related problems (usually poor control). The rest had some other problem. The blood pressure clinic was run concurrently with an ordinary office session, so that from the doctor's point of view, the feared monotony of special clinics could not arise.

Which Staff?

The bare essentials are a nurse and a doctor. Undoubtedly, a nurse who follows a logical plan for continuing care is safer and better than a doctor who does not, and there are cases where individual nurses have more of the qualities needed for innovation than any doctor available in a group. However, these are exceptional, and generally there are as many 'job-and-finish' nurses as there are 'job-and-finish' doctors.

It is important to remember that divisions of labour within the team should change over time, as members of staff gain confidence and experience, and develop new skills and interests. All members of the team should be encouraged both to read and to contribute to the professional literature at an appropriate level, starting with the Local Medical Committee, FHSA, or RCGP Faculty newsletter. None should continue in post longer than 2 years without going away for some kind of further training, even just a one-day conference.

For educational work, particularly on associated risk factors, more people are needed, preferably less professionalized. This point is discussed in Chapter 11.

Preconditions for Compliance

Studies in the USA have shown that up to 50% of people who are identified as hypertensive fail even to enter the treatment and follow-up pipeline, another 50% drop out of care within the first year, and over 30% of those who remain fail to take enough medication to control pressure[3]. In the USA at least, it seems that compliance and drop-out are worst in the patients at highest risk; they are worse in blacks than in whites, and worse in men than in women[4]. Anecdotal experience strongly suggests that we have similar associations with male sex and low status in the UK. There are six preconditions ('six C's') for compliance.

- Credulity.
- Continuity.
- Concern.
- Comprehension.
- Contract.
- eConomy.

Credulity

Doctors who think they can predict who will or will not be a 'good patient' overestimate their powers. Apart from old age[5], no sociodemographic variables are consistently predictive of compliance, control or drop-out[6,7], and doctors are poor predictors of patient behaviour[8].

The first condition for maximal compliance is therefore an open mind; all patients who really need antihypertensive treatment should be offered it, with an initial presumption of innocence.

Continuity and Concern

Finnerty[9] studied drop-outs from a USA inner city out-patient hypertension clinic. He reduced the annual drop-out rate from 42% to less than 4% in 2 years. He also got 85% of his patients at or below target blood pressure, so his conclusions are worth listening to.

'We rapidly learned that patients dropped out not because they were uneducated or did not care about their health, and not because they could not afford the medication.

Rather, they abandoned the clinic because they were treated like cattle, herded from one room to another, left waiting for hours, then examined by a different doctor on each visit, leaving no opportunity to develop any kind of relationship . . . The average waiting time for the doctor was 2.5 hours, and the average waiting time for drugs at the pharmacy was another 1.8 hours . . . the average time actually spent with the physician was only 7.5 minutes.'

His solution was to develop an effective appointments system (average time spent by patients in the clinic fell from 4 hours to 20 minutes), and ensure continuity of staff-patient relationships. Continuity turned out to be more important than staff qualification.

'Most important was the assignment of every patient to his or her own paramedic, seen at every visit. The paramedics frequently came from the same neighbourhood as the patient . . . chosen not so much because of prior experience or education but because of friendly and sympathetic personality and ability to identify with the patients.'

Perfunctory care has perfunctory results. Antihypertensive drugs vary in many ways, but they have one feature in common; none of them work when dropped into the toilet, or if the patient stops coming for prescriptions. If we want patients to show effective concern for their health, we must show effective concern ourselves, by ensuring both continuity of care and a flow rate that allows time to listen and to explain. Continuing personal responsibility by a known professional greatly improves compliance with medication in general[10], and evidence is accumulating to support what experienced family doctors have long known, that health outputs from consultation relate closely, not only to the technical quality of input, but much more to development of close and caring human relationships between professionals and patients[11].

Comprehension

In contrast to non-insulin dependent diabetics with poor initial control, in whom it has been hard to demonstrate significant outcome changes from formal patient education, courses of education for poorly controlled hypertensives do improve blood pressure control compared with uneducated controls[12]. Doctors given 2 hours' instruction to become educators get better results in terms of blood pressure control than doctors without such training[13].

Whether and how people take their medication, and whether they continue follow-up, depends on their own system of beliefs about health and disease in general, and about high blood pressure in particular, with whatever modifications professionals can teach. All patients have minds of their own, and these minds already contain thoughts, of which teachers must take account if they want to be effective. For commonly presented symptoms, agreement between professionals and patients about the nature of problems seems to be more relevant to good outcomes than history taking, examination, investigation, or prescription[14]; for patient satisfaction at least, this is likely to be even more true of a normally asymptomatic condition like high blood pressure. Diabetic patients allowed substantial input into initial consultations attain better control of blood glucose 18 months later than patients who had less initial input[15].

Lassen in Copenhagen showed that compliance was correlated strongly with attention to six specific features in all consultations:

- patients' expectations for the consultation
- patients' ideas about health problems
- information
- explanation
- patients' opinions of the quality of information and explanation
- discussion of patients' perceived obstacles to compliance with advice.

Most patients start with an initial conceptual model for high blood pressure which is both grossly misleading, and tenaciously held, not least because some doctors and many nurses still reinforce it. Studies of hypertensive patients attending clinics in Baltimore showed that 92% were unaware that even very high blood pressure rarely caused symptoms, 81% were unaware of any possible side effects from their medication[17], and 97% thought that the word 'hypertension' meant 'worry, tension, or nerves'[18]. Of 42 patients seen in a Detroit hospital with a hypertensive emergency, 39% had been on antihypertensive treatment which they had stopped because they felt well[19]. Although these studies were done 20 years or so ago, these ideas remain the point of departure for most patients until they are informed and persuaded otherwise.

Patients fear the diagnosis of high blood pressure, but except in the few cases of malignant hypertension or impending stroke for whom immediate fear is justified, fear is a bad motive for compliance. Patients quickly discover that whatever fortuitous symptoms first brought them to the doctor have disappeared, and from then on they soon find they feel better without either medication or supervision. The word 'hypertension' should first be explained, and thereafter never be used. The most suitable term is 'high blood presure', with an initial explanation of exactly what this does and does not mean.

The educational leaflet for patients suggested in Appendix 1 has been carefully written, revised and simplified after many years of experience running the Glyncorrwg clinic and I strongly recommend that this be copied and used by other practices, revised according to local circumstances and changes in available medication.

Similar leaflets devised by pharmaceutical companies, even when not directly promotional, have not been written by people with experience of primary care or vernacular language, nor have they been tested in the field.

Patients rightly question hasty or dogmatic disease labelling. If they are helped to consider their own personal data (including family history), preferably using their own home measurements, ranked in an approximate distribution of population risk, they can understand quickly the nature of high blood pressure and its clinical management. The stage is then set for intelligent and critical compliance with advice.

Contract

The informed patient is in a position to negotiate an unwritten, but nevertheless real, contract. The primary care team has rules which patients must respect if they want to receive care efficiently. These rules cannot command respect unless we acknowledge the right of patients to explanations of what we do and why we do it, what consequences there may be, and share in choosing alternatives where these exist.

For example, we have no right to start a man on thiazide diuretics without explaining that this entails a roughly one in five risk of causing erectile failure, that if this occurs it will stop when the drug is withdrawn, and that several alternative drugs exist. Doctors of my generation are, in my experience, extraordinarily resistant to this apparently self-evident advice. Rather than admit that they feel uncomfortable when warning of side effects in general, and sexual side effects in particular, they suggest that this information may itself precipitate impotence, and should therefore be evaded. The same rule should apply to all information of this kind; if we were patients ourselves, what would we expect to be told? Secrecy is always suspect, and rarely useful.

It is not possible or desirable to make patients responsible for decisions which they rightly consider to be our responsibility, but a start should be made in involving patients in more of these decisions if we want them to accept more active responsibility for their own treatment. This should begin with the simplest decisions of all: whether or not to continue follow-up and observation, and whether or not to initiate treatment with antihypertensive drugs.

An agreed informal contract is particularly important for the minority of patients who reject treatment, either from the start, or by systematic non-compliance. It should be made clear to them that a decision not to accept treatment need not be a decision to reject all supervision. Most will accept at least an annual check, with renewed negotiation if pressure rises substantially.

Economy

Simplicity of drugs and dosage is essential for high compliance. There are no major groups of antihypertensive drugs that require more than twice-daily dosage, and most people can now be controlled with once-daily dosage, often with two drugs in fixed combination. It should be remembered that the Veterans'

Administration trials, which obtained roughly 80% control and large reductions in cardiovascular morbidity and mortality, relied on only one pill a day of combined thiazide and reserpine. Family doctors are more aware than specialist doctors of the problems arising when patients on treble antihypertensive medication also have to take two, three, or even more other drugs concurrently to control other problems, such as diabetes or airways obstruction.

Three Stages of Follow-up

High blood presure and its management last for the rest of the patient's life. From the time that a single high pressure reading is obtained, to the time when organ failure or death make further control impossible or irrelevant, follow-up has three stages:

- a complex induction stage of baseline investigation, patient education, and initial trial of treatment
- a simple continuing stage of monitoring on a 3-monthly or other regular cycle, usually with healthy patients.
- an organ damaged stage in which treatment becomes complex again, new variables must be monitored, and patients begin to be ill.

The Induction Stage

There is so much to do in the induction stage that separation from long term follow-up is essential. If your appointment system is run fairly tightly, you are not likely to have more than 10 minutes even for induction consultations, so these meetings must be spread out over at least three visits, often five or six, ending at the point where a treatment plan has been formulated and begun, and thereafter need only be modified to achieve targets for pressure and other risk factors.

The main tasks of the induction stage are discussed in Chapter 12.

The Continuing Stage

Once a management plan has been agreed, follow-up visits have a smaller and more predictable content, usually possible within a 5-minute appointment time for the nurse, plus another 5–10 minutes with the doctor if targets are not reached or the patient wants to discuss any problems. In our experience, about one-third of patients attending need to see a doctor. We aimed at an eventual 3-month cycle, but patients were seen weekly for dosage changes until target pressures were attained, and monthly if, having achieved target control, this was subsequently lost.

Our default target pressure was 160/90 mmHg. In a few patients this cannot be attained without intolerable side effects, and you may have to settle for something higher, and try again later. Patients need to know what the target is, and should always be told their blood pressure values as they are measured.

All our patients saw a nurse for measurement of blood presure, weight, a check on smoking, and active questioning about possible medication side effects. Checklists for this were less useful than open ended questions. These interviews must be sufficiently private and personal to ensure that common problems of depression, sexual failure, and difficulties at work or at home can be elicited freely.

Control of smoking, unless it is attained quickly during the induction phase, fits awkwardly into schematic management. Although stopping smoking is in fact more important for most patients than controlling blood pressure, this may not be how they see it, and you may have to accept (for the time being) a contract for control of blood pressure without control of smoking. Similar ambiguities surround control of weight, blood cholesterol, and alcohol. Techniques for control of smoking are discussed in Chapter 7, and of alcohol, weight and blood cholesterol in Chapter 15. Other variables, for example gamma GT, MCV or peak expiratory flow rate may be added to the standard follow-up package for individual patients for whom there are special indications.

Patients should always be asked to bring all their current medication with them to every follow-up clinic. We found that few patients learned the names of their drugs despite encouragement to do so, and the most effective way to discuss individual drugs was to have them there on the table. Possible interaction of medication is easily forgotten unless this is done, and a computer list is more fallible than live patients with the tablets they are actually taking.

Formal tablet counts are not an effective way of monitoring compliance because patients who are systematically non-compliant soon get wise to them and others may be offended. If quantities prescribed are geared to consulting intervals, no formal count should be needed. The NHS rule that only 1 month's medication may be prescribed has not, in my experience, been enforced, and I always prescribed a 3-months' supply.

Five-Yearly Periodic Review

Several variables need monitoring occasionally, but less often than every 3 months. If patients were well controlled and felt well, we aimed to check urine for glucose and protein, and blood urea, creatinine, urate and posassium, once ever 5 years. We only did follow-up ECGs if patients had chest pain or 'indigestion'.

Drop-out Review

At the end of each follow-up clinic session, doctor and nurse spent 5 minutes going through the non-attenders, discussing reasons for default and what should be done about it. This was the main opportunity for continuing staff development and modification of the control programme in the light of experience. Once every 3 months, our nurse went through the whole card index of hypertensive patients, whether treated or observed, together with their GP records. Now, of course, she goes through a computer list, but the principle is the same. Errors were always found, and needed chasing up before rot set in.

We found it important to emphasize to all nurses new to this work that errors were expected events, not failures. Real failure, and the only cause for criticism, was denial or concealment of errors or failure to search for them.

The Organ-Damaged Stage

Sooner or later most treated hypertensives will develop evidence of organ damage, most commonly angina and claudication, often arrhythmias, sometimes heart failure presenting first with fatigue and then breathlessness, and occasionally early renal failure which will initially be asymptomatic. Many patients are likely to develop glucose intolerance or frank diabetes, which always implies progressive renal damage and accelerated atheroma. Management of these conditions is discussed in Chapter 18.

Monitoring of these complications can either be added to the standard tasks of the clinic, or dealt with separately at ordinary office sessions while continuing to monitor blood pressure at the clinic.

It is usually a mistake to remove anyone from the clinic completely, because some kind of follow-up is always needed, and general office sessions are rarely organized to recognize and discuss default.

Entries, Exits and Interruptions

Once a system is running, it must include provision for treated patients moving in from other practices, moving out, or being temporarily removed, for example by admission to hospital or travel abroad. In each case it is important that management be maintained.

Once high blood pressure is well controlled, there is usually no clinical evidence that it ever existed. Antihypertensive treatment started on inadequate criteria is so common that treatment may easily be lapsed by a critical family doctor seeing patients before their old GP records catch up with them. A dangerous rise in pressure may take as long as 6 months to reappear after treatment has lapsed, and the average delay in receiving a patient's previous medical record, containing the original evidence for treatment, is generally about 3 months. Patients transferring in should therefore continue in your own clinic on their old medication for about 6 months before even considering stopping medication. If medication is then stopped, continued 3-monthly monitoring remains essential for the first year, with annual checks thereafter. We continued treatment with placebo (ascorbic acid 250 mg twice daily) for at least some of this observation period, because the habit of regular pill taking is difficult to acquire and easy to lose.

Patients leaving the practice permanently or temporarily should be given a letter for any doctor who may see them, including the original criteria for treatment as well as details of current medication. Patients travelling abroad need to be reminded that you are as readily available for advice through an international telephone call as you are locally, and they may be wise to seek familiar advice before rushing into an unknown local facility.

Admission to hospital all too frequently leads to interrupted, revised, complicated or permanently lapsed treatment, often for no better reason than different prescribing habits, often without any written explanation or, occasionally, information of any kind. Most anaesthetists now aim to continue blood pressure control during the operative period; to withdraw antihypertensive drugs preoperatively from a moderate or severe hypertensive is as irrational as withdrawal of insulin from a diabetic[20], but it still happens.

Where medication is stopped, it may not be resumed before leaving hospital, and patients may not understand that a surgical house officer usually knows less about management of high blood pressure than their own family doctor. Difficulties also arise with medical departments, which may switch medication to whatever drugs their unit favours, without regard to your own practice policy, thus thoroughly confusing the patient.

It is particularly important to make sure that previous evidence of airways obstruction is made known to hospital staff, so that beta-blockers will not be used if they are contraindicated. Patients should take only one or two days' medication with them to hospital when they are admitted. If they go in with full containers these will only be thrown away and wasted; despite the poverty of the National Health Service, medication removed on admission is never (in my experience) returned to patients when they leave.

Annual Audit

We aimed to review progress of our clinic once a year, analysing men and women separately, on the following variables:

- What proportion of clinic patients is at or below target pressure (160/90mmHg)?
- How does the group mean pre-medication pressure (mean of the last three readings before medication began) compare with the current group mean pressure (mean of the last three available readings)?
- What proportion of clinic patients had a BMI of 30+ when medication began, and what proportion has it now?
- What proportion of clinic patients smoked when medication began, and what proportion smokes now?
- What proportion of medicated cases has been seen and reviewed within the last 4 months?
- What proportion of observed cases has been seen and reviewed within the past year?

I have called this an 'annual' review, but in fact we did it erratically, about once every 3 years, because without computerization the procedure was so laborious. Once data are computerized this should be easy, and should be a useful tracker for quality of care for annual reports.

The Clinic as a Social Group

One of the most precious advantages of concentrating cases in a clinic is that patients get to know one another as people with a shared problem. They then begin to educate each other, as already happens with diabetics; studies a generation ago showed clearly that diabetics got most of their knowledge (good or bad) from other diabetics, not doctors or nurses. It also means that patients can occasionally be invited as a group, to discuss organization of care or new developments in management of high blood pressure or associated risk factors.

To maximize compliance and minimize drop-out, most of the work involved in follow-up must be essentially educational: professionals educating patients through data about their bodies, patients educating professionals through data about their lives. The traffic should run both ways. When the news about erectile failure in men treated with thiazides first appeared in the medical press in 1981, I decided to explain this to all my treated patients, in case some were suffering unnecessarily and in silence, as in fact one was. More interesting, however, was the man who told me that, although he personally was unaffected, several other men in my clinic had had problems, but were now well aware of this complication, and had cured themselves by getting off the 'water tablets' which evidently caused this trouble, using other less embarrassing complaints to obtain the medical decisions they wanted. Patients think, talk, and, given the opportunity, share their experiences with each other, with more frankness than many doctors find possible.

Before the disintegration of Yugoslavia, hypertensive patients, and more recently patients with other chronic conditions, were encouraged to form and maintain their own clubs for mutual support and education[21] I know of no formal assessments of the effects of these on control and drop-out, but the idea was good, and its application appeared to be widespread and sustained.

Constraints on Innovation

It is important to understand the context within which work of this kind has had to evolve in most underfunded and understaffed public care systems, which are still the only means we have of reaching whole populations in most need of care.

A detailed study of 53 doctor-patient encounters at two Spanish social security clinics[22] showed an overall mean consultation time of 5.2 minutes. This was almost identical with findings in Aberdeen in 1976[23], which was probably representative of conditions throughout the UK at that time.

We have a little more time now, probably an average 7–8 minutes in most practices, but the pace remains hectic, particularly in poorer communities in greatest need. Few GPs working in these circumstances think full ascertainment and control of high blood pressure is possible on a population scale.

The 5.2 minutes in the Spanish study were divided (%) as follows:

health problems	17
diagnosis	14
psychological problems	13
administrative/bureaucratic tasks	13
health education	10
general chat	10
treatment	9
silence	6
social problems	4
greetings, courtesies etc.	4
total	100

How can organized proactive anticipatory care get off the ground in such conditions? The answer is to increase the time available for ordinary reactive consultations in general surgery sessions, by withdrawing follow-up cases from them and re-siting these in special clinics. Additional staff time must then be found for the clinics, but because diagnostic criteria and management protocols are reasonably well defined and easily quantified, every practice with a registered population can prepare its own body of evidence to support rational demands for new resources, which can then be put to responsible authorities. Because high blood pressure is such a common condition, local populations can be readily mobilized to support such demands.

Some kind of start, and some sort of progress on these lines is possible everywhere.

References

1. Mant D, McKinlay C, Fuller A *et al.* (1989) Three-year follow-up of patients with raised blood pressure identified at health checks in general practice. *Br Med J* **298**: 1360–2.

2. Kurji KH and Haines AP (1984) Detection and management of hypertension in general practices in north west London. *BR Med J* **288**: 903–6.

3. Sackett DL and Snow JS (1979) The magnitude of compliance and non-compliance. In: Haynes RB, Taylor DW, Sackett DL (eds) *Compliance in health care*, pp 11–25. Johns Hopkins University Press, Baltimore.

4. Ballard DJ, Strogatz DS, Wagner EH *et al.* (1988) Hypertension control in a rural southern community: Medical process and dropping out. *Am J Prev Med* **4**: 133–9.

5. Weingarten MA and Canon BS (1988) Age as a major factor affecting adherence to medication for hypertension in a general practice population. *Fam Pract* **5**: 294–6.

6. Degoulet P, Menard J, Vu H-A *et al.* (1983) Factors predictive of attendance at clinic and blood pressure control in hypertensive patients. *Br Med J* **287**: 88–93.

7. Haynes RB, Sackett DL, Taylor DW *et al.* (1977) Manipulation of the therapeutic regimen to improve compliance: Conceptions and misconceptions. *Clin Pharmacol Ther* **22**: 125–30.

8. Mushlin AI and Appel FA (1977) Diagnosing patient non-compliance. *Arch Intern Med* **137**: 318–21.

9. Finnerty FA and Mattie EC (1973) Hypertension in the inner city. I: Analysis of dropouts. *Circulation* **47**: 73–4.

10. Ettlinger PRA and Freeman GK (1981) General practice compliance study: Is it worth being a personal doctor? *Br Med J* **282**: 1192–4.

11. Horder JP and Moore G (1990) The consultation and health outcomes. *Br J Gen Pract* **40**: 442–3.

12. Ferran MM, Casabella AB, Parcet SJ *et al.* (1990) Educacion sanitaria en hipertension arterial: Evaluacion de un curso dirigido a hipertensos mal controlados. *Atencion Primaria* **7**: 40–4.

13. Inui TS, Yourtree EL and Williamson JW (1976) Improved outcomes in hypertension after physician tutorials: A controlled trial. *Ann Intern Med* **84**: 646–51.

14. Bass MJ, Buck C, Turner L *et al.* (1986) The physician's actions and the outcome of illness in family practice. *J Fam Pract* **23**: 43–7.

15. Kaplan SH, Greenfield S and Ware JE (1989) Assessing the effects of patient-physician interactions on the outcomes of chronic disease. *Med Care* **27**: S110.

16. Lassen LC (1991) Connection between the quality of consultations and patient compliance in general practice. *Fam Pract* **8**: 154–60.

17. Williamson JW, Aaronovitch S, Simonson L *et al.* (1975) Health accounting: An outcome-based system of quality assurance: Illustrative application to hypertension. *Bull N Y Acad Med* **51**: 727–38.

18. Green LW, Levine DM and Deeds S (1975) Clinical trials of health education for hypertensive outpatients: Design and baseline data. *Prev Med* **4**: 417–25.

19. Caldwell JR, Cobb S, Dowling MD *et al.* (1970) The dropout problem in antihypertensive treatment: A pilot study of social and emotional factors influencing a patient's ability to follow antihypertensive treatment. *J Chron Dis* **22**: 579–92.

20. Edwards WT (1979) Preanesthetic management of the hypertensive patient. *N Engl J Med* **301**: 158–9.

21. Kulcar Z (1991) Self-help, mutual aid and chronic patients' clubs in Croatia, Yugoslavia: Discussion paper. *J R Soc Med* **84**: 288–92.

22. Gervas JJ, Hernandez LM, Marti A *et al.* (1991) La comunicacion medico-paciente y la educacion para la salud. *Atencion Primaria* **8**: 202–5.

23. Buchan IC and Richardson IM (1973) *Time study of consultations in general*

practice. Scottish Health Studies No. 27. Scottish Home and Health Department, Edinburgh.

14

Referral and the Interface Between Primary and Secondary Care

In the UK, all specialists in public service practice only from hospitals, see only referred patients, are salaried rather than fee paid, and have had prolonged practical experience in specialized hospital departments. Elsewhere in Europe the picture is much more confused[1]; patients are still able to refer themselves to specialists, either directly to hospital departments, or indirectly by first seeking a private consultation outside hospital, and then being followed up by the same specialist in a hospital clinic. Specialists are generally paid by fees for each consultation, encouraging referral and retention of patients in hospital clinics for follow-up. The UK is almost alone in having virtually all specialist care filtered initially by GPs, although The Netherlands and Scandinavia are now moving rapidly towards this model. Direct access to specialists remains in Belgium, France, Germany, and throughout southern Europe. Referral correspondence in both directions, from GPs to specialists and from specialists to GPs, is still rudimentary in Spain, and in Italy seems non-existent.

A large majority of UK hospital based cardiologists and most GPs probably agree that specialist advice should not be needed for management of uncomplicated high blood pressure in middle or old age. Criteria for referral suggested by specialists at the large out-patient hypertension clinic at the Glasgow Western Infirmary[2] were as follows:

■ age < 40, diastolic pressure > 104 mmHg, or
■ age > 40, diastolic pressure > 114 mmHg, or
■ any abnormality relating to a cause or complication of high blood pressure, or
■ poor control or unacceptable side effects after 3 months with three or more antihypertensive drugs.

Audit of 298 consecutive patients referred to this Glasgow clinic from 1986 to 1988 showed that 69% were referred by family doctors, 23% were cross-referred from other hospital specialists, and 8% were referred from various other sources such as family planning clinics. Less than half (40%) of GP-referred patients met one or more of these criteria, so evidently fairly large numbers of GPs still pass responsbility to specialists even for routine care of uncomplicated high blood pressure in middle age.

Studies based, not on what GPs do, but on what they say are more optimistic. Whitfield, Grol and Mokkink[3] found that over 90% of samples of 371 English and 141 Dutch GPs said they would usually accept responsibility for management of moderately high blood pressure in the diastolic range 110–120 mmHg.

Appropriate Referral

Despite large differences between referral rates of individual GPs in the UK, virtually all of them lie within the range of 2–10% of all GP consultations. Because referrals have large cost implications, government tends easily to equate better practice with lower referral, but as Wilkin[4] has argued repeatedly, the real problem is to increase appropriate and reduce inappropriate referral, always allowing for necessary limits of competence and experience. There are three sets of problems: patients referred to specialists wastefully, patients retained in primary care dangerously, and patients unrecognized and neglected who have no care at all until they already have irreversible organ damage.

Sins of Poverty and Humility

Specialists generally assume that excessive referral for simple problems is simply an irresponsible shift of work-load. In general, the lazy GP is a myth, if that term implies a life of ease; although doubtless they exist, I have never actually met a GP who spent time on a golf course when he should have been seeing patients. On the other hand, GPs working at a rate that precludes a thoughtful approach to all but the most acute clinical problems remain common, particularly in areas of high morbidity and work-load. Having no idea how to change this situation, they make time by offloading what they can to other parts of the service. This is a problem of poverty of time and social imagination, not laziness.

Poverty begets humility; clinicians without time for clinical medicine soon lose whatever competence they once had. High referral rates thus become rational. Primary generalists should, as a general rule, be better placed than specialists, and more appropriately trained, to manage uncomplicated high blood pressure in middle and old age. A hospital out-patient clinic is the wrong place to be for any common condition whose care must be continued for a lifetime, and integrated with the management of all the many other problems that will occur in it.

Inappropriate referral wastes the creative resources of both specialists and patients. If specialists accept responsbility for management of uncomplicated high blood pressure in middle age, affecting 10–30% of the population depending on definition, they cannot specialize. They must either be pseudospecialists, with theoretical training but insufficient continuing experience of exceptional problems (what John Fry aptly called 'specialoids'), or delegate most of this work to inexperienced junior hospital staff in training, whose rapid turnover maximizes discontinuity and drop-out, and minimizes compliance.

Efficient management of high blood pressure depends on transformation of patients from their traditional role as passive consumers, to a new role as active and intelligent producers. Care sited in hospital out-patient departments rather than in primary care units where patients live makes this learning process more difficult. Patients are bigger and doctors are smaller in primary care than in hospitals, and that situation should create a better learning environment.

Having more complex puzzles to solve, few hospital specialists are really interested in high blood pressure. Except in a few innovative centres, district hospital cardiologists rarely have much more to offer than GPs, apart from more time, a bigger team, and easier access to laboratories and imaging departments, which are often over-used. The commonest problem in diagnosis is an insufficient number of readings, and the commonest problems in treatment are poor compliance and/or alcohol. Such difficulties should be more easily detected and overcome in primary than in secondary care.

Sins of Pride

A continuing deficiency in medical and nursing education is that we are seldom rewarded for honest confessions of ignorance, or for recognizing the limits of our competence and experience. Good clinicians at any level should take pride in their atuonomous creative work, but familiarity can lead to dangerous contempt.

As a rule of thumb, systolic or diastolic pressures at or over 200/120 mmHg must either be controlled quickly, with verification in days rather than weeks, or, if this is not possible, responsibility should be shared. This sharing need not always be with specialists; GPs in group practice tend, in my experience at least, grossly to under-use each other for consultation. The quickest and easiest remedy for the vanity that occasionally impairs the judgement of all clinicians with pride in their work is simply to discuss the case with a colleague after lateral referral.

Many GPs remain unaware of the rapid advances made in management of heart failure and arrhythmias during the past few years, and lack sufficient continuing experience to manage these conditions accurately with the new drugs available.

Very high pressures which cannot be controlled, even with triple therapy, are still common, and may not be solved even after referral to a district hospital specialist. In some of these cases tertiary referral to a regional centre may be necessary for ambulatory blood pressure monitoring.

Sins of Neglect

Patients with papilloedema and/or retinal haemorrhages and oedema represent an acute emergency requiring urgent referral to hospital, within hours not days, and virtually always need admission. Patients with headache, particularly children, must have their fundi examined. Not to do this, or to do this in adults without dilating pupils with a mydriatic (not usually necessary in children) is dangerously irresponsible. A medical centre without a dark place where fundi can be examined is equipped for malpractice.

More commonly, patients with high systolic pressures are still left untreated with antihypertensive drugs despite warning episodes of transient stroke or transient ischaemic attacks. They now usually get aspirin, but if diastolic pressures are low, systolic hypertension is still often ignored.

A study of medical deaths under age 50 in UK hospitals 10 years ago[5] showed that, of 105 who died from complications of high blood pressure, in about a quarter it had never been recognized, and in another quarter it had never been treated. This situation is probably improved today, but is certainly not abolished.

The Referral Process

In writing referral letters for these patients, five important points should never be omitted: specific reasons for referral, blood pressure measurements already recorded, investigations already performed, past antihypertensive medication and all current medication of whatever kind, and your plans for continuing responsbility.

You are unlikely to get a relevant answer if you do not pose a specific question. Even if you do, it may not be answered, but at least you have tried. All my referral letters were dictated in front of patients, so that they knew what I asked, and also what I had or had not said about them. This may help the consultation with the specialist to relate to the specific problems of your patient, and get more than a standardized response.

Inclusion of several past measurements will help a thoughtful specialist to assess whether pressure has risen rapidly and recently, or slowly over many years. This aspect, which must be important, is in my experience usually ignored, simply because no information is available.

Listing the results of investigations you have already done may hopefully avoid further waste of skilled time by repeating them. It should also help the specialist to sort out a diagnosis more fully during a first encounter, without having to recall the patient when results are available.

If you have already tried some types of antihypertensive medication and these have either not worked, or not been tolerated, say so; otherwise they are likely to be repeated. Review of other concurrent medication may reveal that referral is not necessary. Perhaps all you need to do is to stop concurrent non-steroidal anti-inflammatory drugs.

Finally, make clear your own plans for follow-up. If you simply want advice to help you to continue managing your patient, say so clearly. If your letter is dictated in front of the patient, this may help. If you want to share care, say so and suggest how responsibility might be divided.

References

1. Brearley S (1992) Medicine in Europe: Medical education. *Br Med J* **304**: 41–4.

2. Juncocsa S, Jones RB and McGhee SM (1990) Appropriateness of hospital referral for hypertension. *Br Med J* **300**: 646–8.

3. Whitfield MJ, Grol R and Mokkink H (1989) General practitioners' opinions about their responsibility for medical tasks: Comparison between England and The Netherlands. *Fam Pract* **6**: 274–8.

4. Wilkin D, Metcalfe DH and Marinker M (1989) The meaning of information on GP referral rates to hospitals. *Community Med* **11**: 65–70.

5. Whitfield AGW (1981) Young medical deaths: their cause and prevention. *Update* **22**: 1249–59.

15

Management Without Medication

Alcohol ■ Environmental stress ■ Relaxation training ■ Obesity ■
Does weight reduction work? ■ Is weight reduction feasible? ■ Can
weight control be harmful? ■ Insulin resistance and glucose intolerance
■ Vegetarian diet, dietary potassium and dietary fat ■ Dietary sodium
■ The history of low sodium diets ■ Is personal sodium restriction
feasible? ■ Can sodium restriction be harmful? ■ Conclusion on
sodium restriction ■ References

Traditionally, management by behavioural change has been seen as alternative or
adjunct to antihypertensive medication for controlling blood pressure alone, and
efficacy has been judged only in terms of pressure reduction. There is a case for
dietary change and relaxation techniques in controlling mild or moderate high
blood pressure as a single risk,[1] but the argument is much stronger and more
interesting if we consider control of all major risk factors for coronary heart
disease and stroke. Although some kinds of behavioural change, for example
stopping smoking, may be an added burden making other tasks of risk reduction
more difficult to bear, others, for example regular exercise, may make them
easier.

Despite rhetoric to the contrary, management of high blood pressure is all too
often equated in practice with prescription of antihypertensive drugs. Pressure
in this direction is inevitable because millions of pounds are used to promote
prescription, but nobody makes any profit from patient education[2]. Papers in the
Drug and Therapeutics Bulletin have done what they can to correct this.

In this chapter we will consider individually each of the main non-pharmacological measures that have been used to lower blood pressure in context with
other risk factors.

Alcohol

Alcohol is an important cause of high blood pressure, is probably a precipitating
factor for stroke, and is often linked with cigarette smoking. It is a major problem

in its own right, causing measurable liver damage, changes in red cells, or serious problems at work or in the home in at least 12% of most adult male populations which have been thoroughly studied in Britain, and less than half as much in women[3]. Alcohol consumption has predictably risen as its real price has, through government policy, been allowed to fall[4]. Official conscience has been eased by setting targets for the public to attain: the 25% of men now drinking to 'more than sensible limits' are to fall below 16% by the year 2005, and the similar 12% of women to fall below 8%.

Routine search for alcohol problems in all patients, by taking a concise but specific alcohol history ('How many drinks do you usually have on Mondays, Tuesdays?' etc.), and by checking with the spouse and entering the result in an accessible part of a structured record, will greatly improve the quality and accuracy of care, not only of high blood pressure, but all clinical problems.

Although the relationship of alcohol to high blood pressure, coronary disease and stroke is certainly important, it is not yet sufficiently precise to be entered into a risk equation. Where history or circumstantial evidence points to an alcohol problem, MCV and Gamma GT may give useful supporting evidence, but neither is by itself either specific or always sensitive, and most information comes (as usual) from the history[6,7]. MCV > 95 fl is suspicious and 100+ (with normal B_{12} values) almost certain. Alcohol is a much commoner cause of macrocytosis than B_{12} deficiency. MCV seems to be most useful with long standing alcohol problems, and returns to normal after about 3 months when drinking is controlled.

Gamma GT tends to be more sensitive in younger patients, but is often normal in severe, advanced, and very obvious alcoholics with a reduced functioning liver mass. Do not forget that it will be raised substantially by barbiturates and several other anticonvulsant drugs. With early alcohol problems gamma GT responds quickly to control.

In patients in whom either of these indicators are raised, they are very useful in informing and motivating the patient and providing feedback on achievement.

An occasionally useful alternative is measurement of blood alcohol (in a fluoride container), but the results are not easy to use without provoking confrontation. For the same reason I have never used a breathalyser; it has punitive and judgemental associations. However, other GPs have used them, apparently effectively.

Wallace and his colleagues[8] have shown convincingly that simple advice from GPs to people drinking too much alcohol is effective. Attitudes of despair, derived from experience of end-stage alcoholism, are unjustified. Our experience is that younger patients, or those with only the beginnings of a serious problem, respond well to advice and discussion, particularly if this is backed up by objective evidence of damage to health, or if blood pressure falls after a change in drinking patterns.

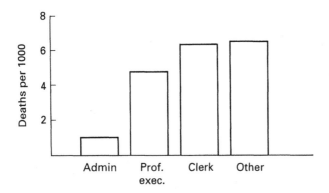

Figure 15.1: Percentage of men in Whitehall study dying from stroke in 10 years (age-adjusted) according to grade of employment[12]. (Reproduced with permission.)

Environmental Stress

Knowledge of stresses at work (or from unemployment) and in the family is essential to good management, and may sometimes suggest specific causes, either of high blood pressure itself, or more commonly, of poor compliance with treatment.

As most patients assume that stress is the cause of high blood pressure, previously undisclosed worries may be found easily simply by asking them if they can think of any possible causes in their lives. Such stresses are not usefully classifiable or measureable, because their effects depend above all on their meaning for patients, which in turn depend on their ideas about the world and how they fit into it[9]. Stress will therefore never be quantifiable for inclusion in a risk equation, for research or any other purpose.

There is now a large body of evidence suggesting that high coronary risk is related less to stress itself than to the socially determined combination of high stress with powerlessness to do anything about it. Displacement by either promotion or demotion in the social pile, or by migration from a familiar culture to a new one, consistently raises coronary mortality rates in many studies[10,11]. Stroke rates show an even closer association with social class (Figure 15.1)[12]. Some, but certainly not most, of this increased risk may be mediated through raised blood pressure.

Relaxation Training

At an individual level, stress can be tackled either by helping patients to understand the determinants of their powerlessness and thus in part to reduce it, or by helping them to adapt to it by learning a new set of physical responses. I know of no formal studies of the first technique, although it has been the main line I have tried to follow in my own practice, and I think it is likely to be most effective.

Individual teaching in relaxation techniques has been developed and evaluated by controlled trial in several centres, notably by Chandra Patel. In a randomized controlled trial she was able to show significant reductions in blood pressure persisting for 4 years after an initial training period[13], as well as a significant reduction in ischaemic events. Her technique depends on a combination of teaching, practice and feedback, given at eight weekly one-hour sessions, run jointly by a nurse and a doctor, to patients in groups of ten. Her treatment plan is given in Appendix 10. Similar techniques in another randomized trial failed to confirm her results for sustained reduction of blood pressure[14], but an independent beneficial effect on coronary risk remains an attractive possibility.

Obesity

Optimal body weight lies in the range of BMI 20–25. To use BMI, height needs to be recorded routinely at least once at age 20 or over, at a point in the record where it can be found easily.

Plotting mortality against BMI, there is a U-curve, with excess mortality for both very fat and very thin people. The upswing of the U-curve on the fat side becomes steep around BMI 30. BMI 26–29 can be regarded as cosmetic, 30+ as medical. Using that definition, which coincides with Garrow's[15] definition of clinical obesity, 17% of the Glyncorrwg population aged 20–70 was, or had at some time been, medically obese, at our last audit in 1989; the incidence is consistently higher in women than men. Like most industrial working class populations, we had more than average obesity. The national average for a BMI of 30+ is 8% for men and 12% for women. Again, the Secretary of State[5] has set a joint target for both men and women, to below 7% by the year 2005.

Blood pressure is positively associated with weight for height at all ages[16], and change in weight is more closely associated with change in blood pressure at younger ages[17]. Death rates from all causes are higher for fat people, and risks are less in those who can control their weight. Obesity has a much bigger effect on death rates in the young than in the old[18]. For people 10 kg (about 23 lb) or more overweight, death rates are 46% higher than average at ages 15–34, 30% at 35–49, and 18% at 50–65. Very fat people who survive over the age of 65 have an almost average life expectancy, although they may be very disabled. Their obesity is particulary resistant to treatment, and so, as with other risk factors, it is sensible to concentrate effort on the young and middle aged.

Does Weight Reduction Work?

Review of six intervention studies in 1980 suggested that weight reduction in obese hypertensive patients by energy intake restriction lowered blood pressure, at a rate of 3 mmHg systolic and 2 mmHg diastolic per 1 kg lost, up to 10 kg[19]. None of these studies used randomized controls. Surprisingly and disappointingly, a larger and much more powerful study than any of these, with a 4 kg loss in treated mild hypertensives and a loss of only 0.8 kg in untreated controls, showed no difference in either systolic or diastolic pressure[20]. Entry diastolic pressures were in the range 90–104 mmHg, and mean age was 47. This was confirmed by a further large study in Sweden in 1989[21].

The most likely explanations for these unexpected results are first, that patients over 40 may be already too old for high blood pressure to be reversible by weight control, and, secondly, that, as in sodium restriction, effects of weight reduction may be greater in more severe hypertension, with a threshold around 170/100 mmHg.

The first of these explanations is supported by a large Swedish study of military recruits with a BMI 30 at entry, compared with random controls. This showed strong correlation between weight changes and blood pressure (up as well as down), which was strongest of all in those with a history of obesity in childhood[22].

Anecdotally, some obese patients do attain blood pressure control for the first time when they lose weight substantially. This may be because they have an idiosyncratic response, not apparent in grouped trials, or it may be because the raised morale associated with successful weight loss leads to improved medication compliance. Either way, it is worth pursuing obesity aggressively in middle aged patients who respond badly to medication, but otherwise benefit is probably confined to patients under 40 years.

Is Weight Reduction Feasible?

Doctors tend to be nihilists about treating obesity. Most GPs accept that help with weight control is a part of their responsbility, but few believe that they can do this effectively[23]. Anorectic drugs are best avoided, so doctors trained to equate treatment with medication quickly lose confidence. Opinion is often based on experience of giant obesity (BMI 40+), which is extremely difficult to treat even by specialists with full teaching hospital facilities. Such experience is irrelevant to control of obesity around a BMI of 30, but it must be admitted that weight control is always difficult.

Experience is Glyncorrwg was that when, for about a year, we had a dietitian available in the practice, substantial and sustained weight loss was readily achieved, mainly through group work. The most effective method of weight reduction seemed to be a combination of diet and exercise, backed up by a specialized health worker (usually, but not necessarily, a dietitian), with initial personalized advice quickly moving to group work. Involvement of whoever did the cooking and shopping was essential.

Exercise not only improves virtually all risk factors for cardiovascular disease (discussed in Chapter 2), but probably improves compliance with advice on smoking. Advice from GPs appears to be effective, at least if it is linked with a community campaign[24].

When we reviewed all our treated hypertensive patients aged 40–64 in 1983, we found that 80% were above ideal weight, and one-third were medically obese (BMI 30). We also compared the BMI available for 72 of the original 98 patients identified by screening our whole community in 1968 with their BMI in 1981 or at exit by death or moving away. Results are shown in Table 15.1.

Table 15.1: Group mean body mass index in 98 screened hypertensive patients.

	Mean group BMI 1968–69	1981 or exit
Men	29.7	27.6
Women	33.0	30.2
Both	31.0	28.6

These reductions were obtained in different ways for men and for women. The women from time to time ran weight losing groups on a volunteer basis at our health centre, with good results, but always eventually expiring from cumulative problems of leadership and organization. We learned from experience that all self help groups must be expected to have a beginning, a middle and an end, that finding responsible volunteer group leaders within a community is an extremely delicate matter, and that getting rid of bad leaders is virtually impossible (because of their volunteer status).

We had a male group going for about a year, led by an experienced dietitian. Long term results were good, and many of these men have maintained good weight control ever since. The common assumption that only women are interested in, or successful at, weight control is wrong, but it is true that special effort is needed to set up and maintain male groups.

However, summarizing 25 years of effort by comparing group mean pre-treatment BMI with BMI at audit in 1989 in our 116 screened hypertensive cohort, there was little change; group mean BMI fell from 28.5 to 28.0. It is true that, without any attempt to control obesity, group mean BMI would have risen with age, so this effort was not entirely wasted.

Can Weight Control be Harmful?

Like sodium restriction, control of obesity is yet another burden for patients. Unless there is a past or family history of medical obesity or maturity onset diabetes, control of cosmetic obesity should be tackled only in patients under 40, or at the patient's request. Anorectic drugs have little to commend them for anyone, and are contraindicated in hypertension because all those currently available are likely to raise pressure.

Insulin Resistance and Glucose Intolerance

Figure 15.2 from the Framingham study[20], shows how the risks of cardiovascular disease increase by 60–80% with addition of glucose intolerance (not just frank diabetes) as a risk factor. Glucose intolerance is positively associated with high blood pressure and total blood cholesterol, as well as obesity and hyperinsulinaemia. Most cases are reversible by control of obesity, and onset of frank diabetes can, in many cases, be prevented by weight control in first degree relatives of diabetics[25]. Two-thirds of maturity onset diabetics can regain normal glucose tolerance after 6 months of dietary treatment alone[26].

As already discussed in Chapter 2, obesity and associated insulin resistance are probable causes of much, if not most, so-called primary hypertension, and clinically there is a large and obvious overlap between hypertensives and diabetics. In Glyncorrwg, about half our diabetics are hypertensives requiring treatment, and diabetes is a common complication of hypertension for which we should be permanently alert. The practical conclusion from this should be that, whether or not control of obesity (particularly central obesity) reduces blood pressure, it is likely to prevent diabetes and coronary heart disease, and is therefore worthwhile.

Vegetarian Diet, Dietary Potassium and Dietary Fat

A vegetarian diet reduces blood pressure substantially in normotensives[27,28] and greatly improves control of diabetes[29]. Some of this hypotensive effect probably arises from raised dietary potassium. Controlled trials of about 60 mmol added potassium daily have shown significant falls in blood pressure in 4 weeks in both normotensives[30] and moderate hypertensives[31].

Hunter-gatherer hypertension-free societies which consume ten times less salt than industrialized societies also consume much more potassium, both in fruit

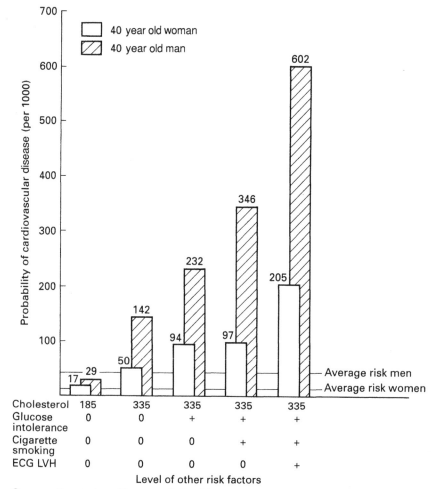

Cholesterol	185	335	335	335	335
Glucose intolerance	0	0	+	+	+
Cigarette smoking	0	0	0	+	+
ECG LVH	0	0	0	0	+

Level of other risk factors

Source: Framingham Monograph No. 28

Figure 15.2: Risk of cardiovascular disease in 8 years of systolic blood pressure of 165 mmHG according to level of other risk factors. Framingham study: 18 year follow-up.

and vegetables, and as a condiment prepared from wood ash. Our main normal dietary sources of potassium are fruit and vegetables, either raw, or cooked by some method other than boiling, which leaches out the potassium. Steaming, pressure cooking, or microwaving all conserve potassium without adding fat[32].

Another possible source is potassium chloride salt. This tastes very different from sodium chloride, but in Finland a mixed sodium-potassium salt has been developed which is more readily acceptable, and helps to raise the K : Na ratio, which may be how this hypotensive effect operates. This KCl/NaCl salt should be available through chemists or 'health food' shops, but may have to be specially ordered.

For prevention and treatment of high blood pressure, diabetes, and all their cardiovascular and cerebrovascular complications, a fully vegetarian diet has everything to commend it. It not only raises potassium, but also reduces intake of saturated fat (which raises both blood cholestrol and blood pressure), quickly and substantially[33], by mechanisms still poorly understood. On the other hand, polyunsaturated fats, including fish oils, seem to reduce blood pressue[34,35].

The now substantial cohort of young people in all social groups who have adopted vegetarianism should reap considerable health benefits when they reach middle age, and all research continues to reinforce the wisdom of their decision, except for convincing evidence of benefit from fish. For those like myself who intend to remain at least partial carnivores, an important, but so far untested, question is whether merely reducing meat and increasing vegetables and cereals may attract almost equal blessings. Until we have better evidence, it seems reasonable that quasivegetarianism may be a worthwhile and, for many people, a more feasible objective.

Dietary Sodium

Evidence in favour of sodium overload as a cause of high blood pressure has been discussed in Chapter 2. Here we are concerned with a different question: does reduction of dietary sodium cause a clinically useful fall in blood pressure, and if so, is it feasible as an adjunct to conventional therapy?

Sodium and potassium are discussed in this book in terms of SI units (millimoles). Conversion from grammes is as follows:

- 1 g NaCl = 17.1 mmol Na
- 1 g Na = 43.5 mmol Na
- 1 g KCl = 13.4 mmol K
- 1 g K = 25.6 mmol K

Surveys of British food habits have estimated average adult sodium intake at about 200 mmol/day[36]. Research studies on small populations have mostly shown lower intakes of around 150 mmol/day for men and 130 mmol/day for women. It is worth bearing in mind that big people eat more of everything than little people, and therefore eat more sodium; the average man is bigger than the average woman.

Even this lower estimate of 150 mmol is about 15 times the minimum physiological requirement, and three to six times the average for groups in Polynesia and parts of rural Africa and South America, which have no high blood pressure and no rise with age. However, this is about 50% less than the sodium load in northern Japan, 40% less than in Portugal, and 25% less than in Belgium, Australia and the USA.

Because monosodium glutamate is added to many processed foods to improve flavour (bringing Chinese take-away meals to monstrous sodium loads of 200 mmol or more per portion), because sodium nitrite is still used as a preservative, and because the entire food industry competes for instant flavour appeal, processed foods are now the main (and not always obvious) source of dietary sodium. One average sized potato contains 0.2 mmol sodium compared with 21 mmol in one cupful of instant mashed potato; one portion of branded fried chicken contains 75 mmol, and one portion of branded hamburger and chips contains 97 mmol[37].

The History of Low Sodium Diets

Before the advent of effective antihypertensive drugs in the 1950s, the only successful treatment for malignant hypertension was Kempner's rice and fruit diet. It worked, although most patients found it almost intolerable, and a few preferred to die, which without this treatment nearly all of them did within 2 years. Above a threshold of 10 mmol daily it was ineffective[38].

Severe sodium restriction has always been difficult, and with the advent of thiazide diuretics, which seemed to reduce sodium load by promoting excretion, English-speaking doctors quickly lost interest in dietary sodium restriction. The idea persisted in continental Europe.

Although the ground was prepared by Dahl's[39] persuasive arguments on causation based on his rats and crude between-society comparisons, the paper which first revived interest in sodium restriction as a treatment in Britain came from Australia[40]. Hypertensive hospital out-patients were studied, with a before-trial mean daily intake of 195 mmol sodium. Experimental subjects were given a target of 100 mmol/day, controls were given no dietary advice. Two years later the experimental subjects had a group mean diastolic pressure 7 mmHg less than the controls, and this was generally accepted as evidence that moderate sodium restriction was effective.

In fact, the experimental subjects only achieved a group mean daily sodium intake of 157 mmol, the design was not blind, and controls had their blood pressures measured less often than the experimental subjects, an obvious potential source of difference in pressure. The news of this treatment, so powerful that it worked even if it was less than half done, made rapid headway through international medical opinion. Advice on sodium restriction became essential to approved practice.

Since then there have been many trials of varying quality. Many of these, including two rigorous studies of genetically contrasted groups in the Glyncorrwg population[41,42], had completely negative results, despite truly heroic efforts by participating patients. However, meta-analysis of 68 crossover trials and 10 randomized controlled trials of salt reduction appear to vindicate sodium restriction[43], in line with meta-analysis of observation studies on populations by the same authors, discussed in Chapter 2. The conclusion of this meta-analysis is worth quoting:

'In people aged 50–59 years a reduction in daily sodium intake of 50 mmol (about 3 g of salt), attainable by moderate dietary salt reduction would, after a few weeks, lower systolic pressure by an average of 5 mmHg, and by 7 mmHg in those with high blood pressure (170 mmHg); diastolic pressure would be lowered by about half as much.'

Sodium reductions lasting 4 weeks or less (which included the Glyncorrwg trials) were generally not successful. The 33 trials lasting 5 weeks or more showed significant reductions, greater in older people and those with higher initial pressures. A continuing worry is that, in general, the most rigorous studies have shown the smallest effects.

Is Personal Sodium Restriction Feasible?

I know of no studies expressly designed to answer this question, but many who have conducted sodium restriction studies have expressed opinions on how easy or difficult it was for their experimental subjects. At one extreme Beard[44] reported little difficulty in getting patients to reduce sodium intake from 150 to 37 mmol/day for 12 weeks. He had no more drop-outs in his sodium restricted experimental subjects than in his unrestricted controls. His paper even refers to an 'elevation of mood' in his salt restricted subjects, who achieved sodium intakes within the range of hunter-gatherer populations among whom hypertension is unknown; 67% of them said they intended to carry on with the diet indefinitely.

Less remarkably, MacGregor[45], who ran several rigorous studies of sodium restriction on hospital referred hypertensive patients, found that 'moderate sodium restriction (reducing sodium intake to 70 mmol a day) can be quite easily achieved'.

Less fortunate researchers had serious difficulty in maintaining compliance even with 'moderate' sodium restrction. In the North Karelia coronary heart disease prevention project[32] normotensive and hypertensive random samples from the general population were studied intensively during a big whole-population campaign to reduce sodium load from an initial mean daily intake of 215 mmol for men and 171 mmol for women. Advice to reduce dietary sodium without specific advice on how to implement this resulted in no change at all after 1 year. After specific advice on methods was given, a 20% reduction was achieved. Hypertensives were given a 1-month trial of complete exclusion of salt from their food, and they achieved a 30–50% reduction in sodium load, but after the trial month original sodium loads were quickly regained. After 3 years of mass education, more intensive and on a bigger scale than anywhere else in the world, a general reduction of 20–50% was achieved, but this still left mean intakes higher than the average level in Britain, and more than twice the target levels of 'moderate restriction' studies.

Our experience of three sodium restriction studies in Glyncorrwg, involving middle aged hypertensives and relatively young people (minimum age 12) including my own family, was that compliance with our target (60 mmol/day) was very difficult for virtually all of us, although we achieved a group mean reduction to 50 mmol/day. Participants received sustained, simple and specific dietary advice from a dietitian, backed by specially written material and free specially prepared low sodium foods. Most of this would be impossible in ordinary practice. Asked what they thought about their 8-week experience of sodium restriction (four with added slow sodium tablets and four with placebo), all but one family said they found it difficult and unpleasant, were glad to return to normal eating, and that if they were hypertensive they would prefer lifelong medication, with any consequent risks, to such a diet. Only one couple said restriction was easy; but we knew (from one measurement of urinary sodium) that they had wholly failed to comply with the protocol.

It is difficult to reconcile these two views of how easy or difficult it is for people to reduce dietary sodium to 'more natural' levels of 30–80 mmol/day. Social selection is certainly important, and I find the negative studies of screened populations more convincing than positive studies of referred or volunteer patients, unless volunteers include a majority of the population (as in the Glyncorrwg studies). All our research team restricted their own sodium intake for a week before starting the trials, and all found it very difficult.

All the researchers I know of who have reported negative results have done so reluctantly. When they began their studies, they hoped and believed that sodium restriction would be effective for primary prevention; so I do not believe they are biased in their conclusion that sodium restriction below 80 mmol/day presents real difficulties to most patients. If it is so easy to restrict dietary sodium, why are there still so few published trials of high quality?

Can Sodium Restriction be Harmful?

Once we have overcome the problems of mass screening and ascertainment, the main obstacles to effective control of high blood pressure in populations is low compliance and high drop-out. Compliance falls and drop-out increases as we make greater and more complex demands on patients to make radical changes in their lives. Some of these, such as stopping smoking and reducing dietary fat, are necessary, effective, and backed by consistent evidence, although insistence on them may impair compliance with the easy, pill-taking part of the package.

Perfunctory advice to reduce salt, without verification or follow-up, is both harmless and ineffective. Serious advice, with specific recommendations, written back-up, follow-up and verification by measurements of 24-hour urine sodium, could be harmful if this competes with other more important personal tasks.

Salt restriction is likely to make other changes in diet more difficult. We found that, in their search for tasty food, salt-restricted patients increased their intake of fatty and fried foods.

Conclusion on Sodium Restriction

Accepting the conclusions of Law, Frost and Wald's meta-analyses, but taking into account considerable personal experience of the work entailed in both maintaining and verifying sodium restriction, three practical conclusions seem reasonable.

The first is that patients should be recommended to reduce, and eventually to eliminate, added salt from their diet, and advised of the high sodium content of some foods which few people consider in this regard, noteably cheese, milk, bread and virtually all other cereals, monosodium glutamate in take-away food, and sodium bicarbonate used in cooking. There is no hurry about this. The effect is gradual, and targets are much more easily achieved if a slow, decremental approach is adopted, aiming to reduce original intake by about 100 mmol day after the first year. By then most patients are likely to find they have become salt intolerant, compared with other people, and most find it easier to make the change as a whole family. Eating out becomes generally unpleasant. No rigorous study of adequate size has yet shown that such a decrementnal policy is in fact a more effective alternative to medication for control of mild hypertension in the diastolic range 90–104 mmHg, but if Wald's meta-analysis is correct, it should be. I see no justification on present evidence for medication in this range in people without either diabetes or organ damage, and no evidence that moderate, decremental sodium restriction would do anything but good.

Secondly, decremental sodium restriction by 100 mmol/day is probably an effective adjunct to medication, particularly with ACE inhibitors.

Finally, national food policies need to be adopted which apply this decremental approach to whole populations. The question may be tackled sooner in countries like Japan, China and Portugal where there are very high sodium intakes, than in the UK where the problem appears less urgent. Their very high sodium loads arise mainly from traditional methods of food preservation, many of which present other health hazards (notably for cancers of the oesophagus and stomach), and may therefore be more easily discarded.

In the UK, decremental reduction by 100 mmol/day is probably feasible within present food culture, providing this is done sufficiently slowly. The Health Education Council's[46] agreement with bakers reduced the salt content of bread by 12.5% and, as bread accounted for about one third of sodium load in the average UK diet, this was important. Collective action is therefore possible. Prepared foods account for most of the rest of dietary intake, if salt is not added in cooking or at the table, but decremental approaches here would probably be much more difficult. Salted and smoked fish, tinned foods, fast foods, and prepared foods generally need to be discouraged as part of a national food policy, which should defend the lower sodium intake we already have against further incursion by the American fast food industry and its imitators. Feasibility of such policies rests on how quickly taste adapts to lower sodium intakes within a wide range of ages and ethnic groups, and further evidence on this is urgently needed.

Wald's group estimate was that if population sodium intake were reduced by a mean 100 mmol/person/day, the incidence of coronary heart disease could be reduced by 30%, and of stroke by 39%, preventing 11 000 deaths a year under 65 years of age.

References

1. Andrews G, McMahon SW, Austin A *et al.* (1982) Hypertension: Comparison of drug and non-drug treatments. *Br Med J* **284**: 1523–6. See also correspondence from Johnston D and Steptoe A (1982) *Br Med J* **285**: 1046.

2. Andrews G (1984) On the promotion of non-drug treatments. *Br Med J* **289**: 994–5.

3. Wallace PG, Brennan PJ and Haines AP (1987) Drinking patterns in general practice patients. *J R Coll Gen Pract* **37**: 354–7.

4. Dunbar GC and Morgan DDV (1987) The changing pattern of alcohol consumption in England and Wales 1978–85. *Br Med J* **295**: 807–9.

5. Secretary of State for Health (1991) *The health of the nation: A consultative document for health in England.* HMSO, London Cm1523.

6. Beresford TP, Blow FC, Hill E *et al.* (1990) Comparison of CAGE questionnaire and computer-assisted laboratory profiles in screening for covert alcoholism. *Lancet* **336**: 482–5.

7. Skinner HA, Holt S, Sheu WJ *et al.* (1986) Clinical versus laboratory detection of alcohol abuse: The alcohol clinical index. *Br Med J* **292**: 1703–7.

8. Wallace P. Cutler S and Haines A (1988) Randomised controlled trial of general practitioner intervention in patients with excessive alcohol consumption. *Br Med J* **297**: 663–8.

9. Antonovsky A (1985) The life cycle, mental health and sense of coherence. *Isr J Psychiatry Relat Sci* **22**: 273–80.

10. Marmot MG and Syme SL (1976) Acculturation and coronary heart disease. *Am J Epidemiol* **104**: 225–47.

11. Marmot MG, Smith GD, Stansfield S *et al.* (1991) Health inequalities among British civil servants: The Whitehall II study. *Lancet* **337**: 1387–93.

12. Marmot MG, Rose G, Shipley M *et al.* (1978) Employment grade and coronary heart disease in British civil servants. *J Epidemiol Commun Health* **32**: 244–9.

13. Patel C, Marmot MG, Terry DJ *et al.* (1985) Trial of relaxation in reducing coronary risk: Four-year follow up. *Br Med J* **290**: 1103–6.

14. Montfrans GAV, Karemaker JM, Wieling W *et al.* (1990) Relaxation therapy and continuous ambulatory blood pressure in mild hypertension: A controlled study. *Br Med J* **300**: 1368–72.

15. Garrow J (1992) Treatment of obesity. *Lancet* **340**: 409–13.

16. Kannel WB (1980) Host and environmental determinants of hypertension: Perspectives from the Framingham study. In: Kesteloot H and Joossens J (eds) *Epidemiology of arterial blood pressure*. Martinus Nijhoff, The Hague, 265–77.

17. Miall WE, Bell RA and Lovell HG (1968) Relation between change in blood pressure and weight. *Br J Prev Soc Med* **22**: 73–80.

18. Seltzer CC (1966) Some re-evaluations of the build and blood pressure study 1959 as related to ponderal index, somatotype and mortality. *N Engl J Med* **274**: 254–9.

19. Amery A, Bulpitt C, Fagard R *et al.* (1980) Does diet matter in hypertension? *Eur Heart J* **1**: 299–308.

20. Kannel WB and Sorlie P (1975) Hypertension in Framingham. In: Paul O (ed) *Epidemiology and control of hypertension*, pp 553–92. Stratton Intercontinental Medical Books, New York.

21. Berglund A, Anderssen OK, Berglund G *et al.* (1989) Antihypertensive effect of diet compared with drug treatment in obese men with mild hypertension. *Br Med J* **299**: 480–5.

22. Sonne-Holm S, Sorensen TIA, Jensen G *et al.* (1989) Independent effects of weight change and attained body weight on prevalence of arterial hypertension in obese and non-obese men. *Br Med J* **299**: 767–70.

23. Cade J and O'Connell S (1991) Management of weight problems and obesity: Knowledge, attitudes and current practice of general practitioners. *Br J Gen Pract* **41**: 147–50.

24. Campbell MJ, Browne D and Waters WE (1985) Can general practitioners influence exercise habits? *Br Med J* **290**: 1044–6.

25. West KM (1978) *Epidemiology of diabetes.* Elsevier, New York.

26. Doar JWH, Wilde CE, Thompson ME *et al.* (1975) Influence of treatment with diet alone on oral glucose tolerance test and plasma sugar and insulin levels in patients with maturity-onset diabetes mellitus. *Lancet* i: 1263–6.

27. Rouse JL, Beilin LJ, Armstrong BK *et al.* (1983) Blood pressure-lowering effect of a vegetarian diet: Controlled trial in normotensive subjects. *Lancet* i: 5–9.

28. Rouse IL and Beilin LJ (1984) Vegetarian diet and blood pressure. *J Hypertens* **2**: 231–40.

29. Mann JI (1981) A high carbohydrate leguminous fibre diet improves all aspects of diabetic control. *Lancet* i: 1–5.

30. Khaw K-T and Thom S (1982) Randomised double-blind crossover trial of potassium on blood pressure in normal subjects. *Lancet* ii: 1127–9.

31. MacGregor GA, Smith SJ, Markandu ND *et al.* (1982) Moderate potassium supplementation in essential hypertension. *Lancet* ii: 567–70.

32. Henningsen N, Larsson L and Nelson D (1983) Hypertension, potassium, and the kitchen. *Lancet* i: 133.

33. Puska P, Iacono JM, Nissinen A *et al* (1983) Controlled, randomised trial of the effect of dietary fat on blood pressure. *Lancet* i: 1–5.

34. Iacono JM, Marshal MW, Dougherty RM *et al.* (1975) Reduction in blood pressure associated with high polyunsaturated fat diets that reduce blood cholesterol in man. *Prev Med* **4**: 426–43.

35. Norris PG, Jones CJH and Weston MJ (1986) Effect of dietary supplement-

ation with fish oil on systolic blood pressure in mild essential hypertension. *Br Med J* **293**: 104–5.

36. Bull NL and Buss DH (1980) Contribution of foods to sodium intake. *Proc Nutr Soc* **39**: 30A.

37. de Swiet M (1982) Blood pressure, sodium, and take-away food. *Arch Dis Child* **57**: 645–6.

38. Medical Research Council (1950) The rice diet in the treatment of hypertension. *Lancet* ii: 509–13.

39. Dahl LK (1972) Salt and hypertension. *Am J Clin Nutr* **25**: 231–44.

40. Morgan T, Adam W, Gillies A *et al.* (1978) Hypertension treated by salt restriction. *Lancet* i: 227.

41. Watt GCM, Hart JT and Foy CJ (1983) Effect of moderate dietary sodium restriction on patients with mild hypertension in general practice. *J Hypertens* **1**: 18–20.

42. Watt GCM, Edwards C. Hart JT *et al.* (1983) Dietary sodium restriction for mild hypertension in general practice. *Br Med J* **286**: 432–6.

43. Law MR, Frost CD and Wald NJ (1991) By how much does dietary salt reduction lower blood pressure? III: Analysis of data from trials of salt reduction. *Br Med J* **302**: 819–24.

44. Beard TC, Cooke HM, Gray WR *et al.* (1982) Randomised controlled trial of a no-added sodium diet for mild hypertension. *Lancet* ii: 455–8.

45. MacGregor GA, Markandu ND, Best FE *et al.* (1982) Double blind randomized crossover trial of moderate sodium restriction in essential hypertension. *Lancet* ii: 567–70.

46. Health Education Council (1986) Annual report 1985–6. HEA, London.

16

Antihypertensive Medication in General

The historical sequence ■ Effects on other risk factors ■ Evidence on iatrogenic impairment ■ Drug and disease interactions ■ Choosing and naming antihypertensive drugs ■ Five rules for starting, stopping and changing antihypertensive drugs ■ Economical prescribing

As a rule, systolic pressures sustained at or over 170 mmHg or diastolic pressures sustained at or over 110 mmHg over periods of days, or 100 mmHg over months, require control by medication. All effective drugs must have potential for harm as well as good, and although the possibility of harmful effects can be minimized by cautious and accurate prescribing, it cannot be eliminated. Our first task, therefore, is to ensure the probability of net benefit from medication by avoiding both benign neglect where there is controlled evidence to support medication, and hasty intervention where there is no such evidence.

Since thalidomide, patients have become more aware of risks of medication. In the UK at least, there is little evidence of pressure from patients for over-medication. Cardiovascular drugs account for about 17% of all prescriptions in the UK, but only 6% of prescriptions about which prescribers feel insecure or uncomfortable. This can be compared with antibiotics (12% of all prescriptions, 23% of uncomfortable prescriptions), and tranquilizers and hypnotics (8% of all prescriptions, 18% of uncomfortable prescriptions).[1]

The Historical Sequence

From time to time suggestions are made for a standard sequence of drugs, an optimal protocol that can be applied to all cases (stepped care). Such suggestions may be practical in a hospital out-patient setting or in other hitherto untreated populations, where there is a steady inflow of new cases, but they are not helpful to teams responsible for communities with established traditions of primary care. Every team inherits a population already including many people on a variety of antihypertensive drugs, reflecting whatever was in vogue when they started, as well as the prescribing habits of their various doctors. Even among contemporaries, it is usually difficult to get medical agreement even on a standard sequence of drug groups, let alone individual drugs.

One of the most difficult, but also most necessary, steps in management is to get patients to take medication regularly. Anything likely to disturb an established pattern is rightly viewed with suspicion, so otherwise obsolete drugs that are well tolerated and give good control can and should continue in use for 20 or 30 years, completely disregarding any standardized protocol.

Some older drugs have been prematurely discarded. Many of them were originally used in excessive dosage, in mistaken efforts to control blood pressure with a single agent, thus exaggerating their side effects and toxicity. This applies particularly to reserpine, which has almost disappeared from use, although in low dosage it remains a usually well tolerated, effective, and extremely cheap drug. There is little profit for pharmaceutical companies from sales of these unbranded older drugs, so they are no longer promoted, and may even be actively discredited by salesmen. Their long history, however, does at least ensure that we already have most of the bad news about them, in contrast to their more actively promoted successors.

Effects on Other Risk Factors

Because all hypertensive patients are at greatly increased risk for coronary heart disease, and because control of high blood pressure has had rather disappointing results in reducing this risk, the effects of antihypertensive drugs on other major coronary risk factors should be an important consideration in choice of medication. Thiazide diuretics have been particularly suspect in this respect, having small but significant adverse effects on glucose tolerance and total blood cholesterol, which increase with age and duration of treatment. Beta-blockers also mostly have small adverse effects on total blood cholesterol. Prazosin, on the other hand, seems to have quite a large favourable effect on blood total cholesterol.

Evidence on Iatrogenic Impairment

Impairments and risks associated with individual antihypertensive drugs are discussed in Chapter 17. A study in general practice by Jachuck[2] showed that, in 75 controlled hypertensives, none of their GPs was aware of any impairments associated with treatment, but 10% of patients admitted to adverse effects on direct questioning. When the same question was asked of close relatives and companions, perceived adverse effects rose to 75% of patients; 25% of these effects were described as mild, 45% as moderate, and 30% as severe. In their overall assessment of each patient's conditoon, 100% of GPs and 48% of patients thought this was improved, but 98% of relatives and companions thought it was worse since treatment. It is difficult to draw definite conclusions from this in the absence of a control group, but Jachuck's finding that relatives may be more ready to report apparent side effects than patients themselves, showed that trials could become more sensitive to these impairments if family opinions were included.

Several subsequent studies have sought to quantify iatrogenic impairment by antihypertensive drugs, usually in comparisons favouring newer against older drugs[3,4] but none have addressed their questions to families and friends, although these may be the best observers. In my experience, once patients are convinced that they need treatment, many, if not most, are reluctant to complain of side effects.

Doctors tend to be relatively insensitive to impairments caused by drugs they have prescribed, particularly if these are non-specific symptoms of tiredness, diminished libido, or just 'not feeling right'. This can be said with confidence because although doctors all over the world were prescribing thiazide diuretics on a colossal scale ever since these useful drugs came on the market in the late 1950s, the first report of a single case of impotence was not reported until 1977, and it was not until 1981 that the MRC controlled trial of treatment for mild hypertension showed impotence in 23% of men on thiazides, 13% of men on propranolol, and 10% on placebo after 1 year[5]. Evidently, we just did not want to know.

Drug and Disease Interactions

Antihypertensive treatment on a mass scale is directed mainly at people in middle and old age, liable to a host of other ailments also needing treatment. Patients are generally aware of the possibility of drug interactions, and, unless these are discussed with them specifically, may either choose their own uninformed priorities between medications for fear of precipitating chemical wars in their insides, or devise impossibly complex tablet timetables to avoid contact between potential adversaries.

The most important and frequently overlooked interaction with all antihypertensive drugs is with non-steroidal anti-inflammatory drugs (NSAIDs) operating through prostaglandin synthetase inhibition. Indomethacin raises blood pressure by a mean 19 mmHg systolic and 9 mmHg diastolic pressure in patients on diuretics or beta-blockers[6], almost eliminating their hypotensive effect. Remarkably little seems to have been written on this interaction in relation to the numerous alternative drugs in this group, and it is not clear from the more accessible literature whether this is mainly a true drug interaction, or an independent hypertensive effect. Most rheumatologists seem to think it is explained simply by sodium and water retention. Flurbiprofen has been proposed as a treatment for symptomatic hypotension, because of evidence that it raised blood pressure. The fact that indomethacin promotes closure of the ductus arteriosus, and is an effective medical treatment for patent ductus, is an indication of potent vascular effects usually forgotten in practice. Now that many NSAIDs are available without prescription, it is important to ask about them.

No antihypertensive drugs have any specific incompatibility with alcohol, although its periperhal vasodilator effect presumably augments the effect of other vasodilators. It is important to reassure patients that their medication is compatible with reasonable social drinking, otherwise they are likely to stop medication at weekends.

There are no important interactions between any commonly used antihypertensive and anticonvulsant or bronchodilator drugs, but of course beta-blockers should naver be prescribed without prior assessment of airways obstruction. Tricyclic, and probably all other effective antidepressent drugs, all tend to antagonize antihypertensive drugs, but otherwise there are no specific interactions I know of. Tricyclic antidepressants may promote cardiac arrhythmias, and should not be used in patients who already have these. The new and very expensive selective serotonin uptake inhibitors are an alternative for these patients; otherwise they seem to offer little proven advantage[7].

Choosing and Naming Antihypertensive Drugs

Within the main groups of antihypertensive drugs, it is important to agree within your team on one, or at most two, individual drugs and stick to them, so that what must at best be a confused situation does not become wholly incomprehensible.

Try also to agree on generic prescribing, generic recording, and generic discussion of drugs, so that the whole team begins to think pharmacologically rather than in terms of brand names and free lunches. There are already 52 different antihypertensive drugs listed in the current *British National Formulary* under their generic names. Is it really possible to think clearly about what you are doing, if you add another 96 brand aliases to these?

Five Rules for Starting, Stopping and Changing Antihypertensive Drugs

In the Glyncorrwg clinic, we found the following five rules useful.

■ Start and stop slowly.

Rapid reduction of pressure in even the most severe symptomless hypertension is a dangerous practice, even using drugs orally[8].

Nearly all side effects depend on dosage. Unless you start with the smallest possible dose, you will not find the fortunate minority of patients who respond well and may saddle them with a lifetime of marginal but unnecessary added risk. Start slowly, and add increments at weekly or monthly intervals until you either have control, or have to consider adding another drug.

Beta-blockers, methyldopa and clonidine can all cause severe rebound high blood pressure if they are stopped abruptly. Unless they are causing harm, all should be stopped decrementally over 2 or 3 days. Except for diuretics (which need only be given in low dose anyway) it seems wise to apply this rule to all antihypertensive drugs[9,10].

■ Always prescribe once- or twice-daily dosage.

The habit of regular medication is difficult for patients to acquire, and poor compliance is the commonest cause of poor control. All antihypertensive drugs mentioned in this book can be taken twice a day, and many once a day, without diminished control.

■ Make decisions on more than one reading.

If you get one unexpectedly high reading, do not immediately raise the dose or add another drug. Think and ask about possible causes (new anxieties, missed tablets, rushing to the appointment, a full bladder, a cold day) and get one or two more readings over the next day or two, before changing treatment.

■ Do not add new drugs unless you have to.

Few patients really need more than two antihypertensive drugs.

When you find yourself thinking about a third antihypertensive drug (which may be the fifth, sixth or seventh drug in a patient with other chronic problems such as airways obstruction, arthritis, peptic ulcer, diabetes or Parkinson's disease) check through other possible causes of failure: uncontrolled obesity, high alcohol intake, NSAIDs, or systematic failure to take drugs already prescribed.

■ Change one drug at a time.

If you change more than one drug at a time, there will be no way of identifying the real source of any change, good or bad. This means that fixed dose combinations, which may be very useful once blood pressure is under stable control, should not be used at the start. High prescription charges make this policy difficult to implement.

Economical Prescribing

All money represents somebody's labour, and should therefore never be wasted.

234

A patient taking bendrofluazide 2.5 mg twice a day costs the nation £5.11 a year ignoring prescription charges. If a second drug is required, you might add atenolol 100 mg a day, adding £8.79 to the annual cost, now totalling £13.90. The price of all four available proprietary brands of bendrofluazide has now fallen to generic cost, but the most expensive thiazide diuretic, indapamide (Natrilix) costs more than 28 times as much per tablet as bendrofluazide. If you believe that uncomplicated high blood pressure is best managed with ACE inhibitors, annuals costs at average dosage range from £156.82 for captopril (Capoten) to £273.75 for fosinopril (Staril).

Cautious prescribing tends also to be more economical. Although it might seem reasonable to assume that an energetic and comprehensive case finding programme for high blood pressure would increase prescribing costs for a population, in Glyncorrwg we found just the opposite. Based on data for the month of October in 1983 and again in 1985, Table 16.1 compares annual prescribing costs per 1000 population for drugs acting on the heart, diuretics and antihypertensives, between Glyncorrwg, a neighbouring village of similar social composition, and West Glamorgan as a whole. This was 15–17 years after we began screening and systematic case finding in Glyncorrwg, but before significant screening programmes had begun elsewhere.

Table 16.1: Annual prescribing costs per 1000 population for drugs acting on the heart, diuretics and antihypertensives: Glyncorrwg, a neighbouring village, and West Glamorgan, 1983 and 1985 (ratio to Glyncorrwg costs)

Year	Glyncorrwg		Neighbouring village		West Glamorgan	
1983	£4790	(1.00)	£6948	(1.45)	£6420	(1.34)
1985	£7495	(1.00)	£9750	(1.30)	£8628	(1.15)

Swales[11] pointed out that the cost of treating high blood pressure by the latest means available multiplies costs by more than 50 times, compared with the drugs on which the original Veterans' Administration and other classic trials were based. Therapeutic advances have been real, but few will believe that they match this price rise.

In the industrializing Third World, these differences are matters of life and death. In practice, continuing treatment for hypertension throughout South and Central America, with the singular exception of Cuba, is almost entirely restricted to a small minority of patients, who are all too often treated with whatever is the latest, most heavily promoted, and most expensive drug available. We are still discovering important new facts, not only about thiazides, but even aspirin. It takes at least 10 years to establish the main effects of new drugs.[12] It is therefore by no means certain that even this wealthy minority benefits as it thinks it does from early exposure to new remedies. Attending a conference on community control of hypertension in Bogota in 1984, I found neither generic thiazides nor reserpine of any kind available anywhere in Colombia. The conference was paid for by a company promoting ACE inhibitors, and I was told that suitably heavy prescribers for some companies had found themselves rewarded with free Volkswagens.

References

1. Bradley CP (1992) Uncomfortable prescribing decisions: A critical incident study. *Br Med J* **304**: 294–6.

2. Jachuck SJ, Brierley H, Jachuch S *et al.* (1982) The effect of hypotensive drugs on the quality of life. *J R Coll Gen Pract* **32**: 103–5.

3. Croog SH, Levine, S, Testa MA *et al.* (1986) The effects of antihypertensive therapy on the quality of life. *N Engl J Med* **314**: 1657–64.

4. Bulpitt CJ and Fletcher AE (1990) The measurement of quality of life in hypertensive patients: A practical approach. *Br J Clin Pharmacol* **30**: 353–64.

5. Medical Research Council Working Party on Mild to Moderate Hypertension (1981) Adverse reactions to bendrofluazide and propranolol for the treatment of mild hypertension. *Lancet* **ii**: 539–43.

6. Watkins J, Abbot EC, Hensby CN *et al.* (1980) Attenuation of hypotensive effect of propranolol and thiazide diuretics by indomethacin. *Br Med J* **281**: 702–5.

7. Edwards JG (1992) Selective serotonin uptake inhibitors. *Br Med J* **304**: 1644–6.

8. (1989) Severe symptomless hypertension [editorial]. *Lancet* **ii**: 1369–70.

9. Aylett M and Ketchin S (1991) Stopping treatment in patients with hypertension. *Br Med J* **303**: 345.

10. Burton R (1991) Withdrawing antihypertensive treatment. *Br Med J* **303**: 324–5.

11. Swales JD (1990) First line treatment in hypertension. *Br Med J* **301**: 1172–3.

12. Poulter N, Sever PS and Thom S (1990) Antihypertensive and adverse biochemical effects of bendrofluazide. *Br Med J* **300**: 1465.

Specific Antihypertensive Drugs

17

First line drugs: thiazide diuretics ■ Second line drugs: beta-adrenoreceptor blockers ■ Third line drugs: calcium-channel blockers ■ Third line drugs: angiotensin converting enzyme inhibitors ■ Last resorts

The historical order in which the main groups of antihypertensive drugs still in use first appeared is as follows.

■ Centrally acting (reserpine)	1949
■ Vasodilators (hydralazine)	1951
■ Thiazide diuretics	1957
■ Centrally acting (methyldopa)	1963
■ Centrally acting (clonidine)	1966
■ Beta-blockers (propranolol)	1966
■ Alpha-blockers (prazosin)	1976
■ Calcium channel blockers (nifedipine)	1979
■ ACE inhibitors (captopril)	1981

Rather than take them in this order, as in previous editions, it seems more practical to discuss them in terms of first, second and third line choices and last resorts, according to current consensus for management of moderate to severe hypertension, as set out in the current *British National Formulary*[1]:

- ■ first line: thiazide diuretics
- ■ second line: + beta-adrenoreceptor blockers
- ■ third line: + calcium–channel blockers or ACE inhibitors
- ■ last resorts: Vasodilators (hydralazine, minoxidil), alpha-adrenoreceptor blockers (prazosin), and centrally acting drugs (reserpine, methyldopa).

This consensus rests on the fact that all the more recent (second generation) major trials used thiazides and beta-blockers. Although ACE inhibitors and alpha-blockers have many theoretical advantages,[2,3] these are as yet unproved by large randomized controlled trials.[4] Recent evidence that beta-blockers add little if anything to the protective effect of diuretics, at least in the elderly, and may even reduce it, will increase pressure for a new consensus, which on currernt form seems likely to promote ACE inhibitors in their place.

First Line Drugs: Thiazide Diuretics

Thiazide diuretics inhibit reabsorption of sodium in the proximal segment of the distal tubules of the kidney. They have more antihypertensive effect than loop diuretics such as frusemide, which should not be used as antihypertensive agents.

Thiazides were the first easily used, well tolerated, and effective antihypertensive drugs available, coming into general use in the 1950s. Compared with potent but disabling ganglion-blocking drugs, and less powerful although more tolerable drugs like reserpine and hydralazine which preceded them, they seemed almost free from side effects. This reputation stuck, so the decision to use them is often made casually. About a quarter of the elderly population in the UK is now on continuous diuretic treatment, and even when iatrogenic symptoms are suspected, other less familiar drugs may be more likely to attract blame.

Generally, thiazides are at least as effective in lowering blood pressure as any more modern alternatives, lowering diastolic pressure by a mean 10–11 mmHg from a pretreatment mean of 100–120 mmHg.[5] They have four great advantages: they are well tolerated in the elderly; they have a long track record, so that we already have most of the bad news about them; they combine well with almost all other antihypertensive drugs, augmenting their action and often reducing their side effects; and they are cheap. Like many other antihypertensive drugs, we are still unsure exactly how they reduce blood pressure; some of their effect probably depends on sodium depletion, but they also have a vasodilator effect.

It is has long been known that they exert their full antihypertensive effect at lower dosage than that usually required for perceptible diuresis, greatly reducing potential side effects. It is pointless to give more than 2.5 mg twice a day of bendrofluazide, 25 mg once a day of chlorthalidone or hydrochlorothiazide, or 125 μg once a day of cyclopenthiazide. For bendrofluazide, the antihypertensive effect is identical 3 months after starting treatment at all doses from 1.25 to 2.5, 5, and 10 mg daily,[5] and the same was shown for cyclopenthiazide from 125 to 500 μg.[6] At low dosage, in both cases, biochemical side effects did not differ from placebo, despite a 10 mmHg fall in diastolic pressure. At a daily dose of 25 mg hydrochlorothiazide, drop-out of elderly patients from the recent MRC trial[7] was less than with placebo.

Patients are often told diuretics are 'water tablets', which may be helpful in sorting out the typical jumble of white tablets in unlabelled bottles. However, it is important to explain that although they do indeed promote water output, they have been prescribed for their direct effect on blood pressure, not to increase urine flow. If patients do not understand this, they may easily decide that since urine flow is all too free (particularly at night), they need not continue the tablets. Nocturnal frequency is not always caused by diuretics; nifedipine is a common culprit.

Use in Pregnancy and Lactation

Diuretics are contraindicated in pregnancy because they reduce placental blood flow, and may therefore provoke or exacerbate pre-eclampsia. They cross the placental barrier and appear in breast milk.

Contraindications

Thiazides are ineffective in patients with less than 20% renal function,[8] and may then precipitate renal failure. Frusemide is then a safer although less effective alternative.

Interactions with Other Drugs

Initiation of treatment with ACE inhibitors together with diuretics of any kind, can easily result in rapid and extreme hypotension and renal failure. For patients already on thiazides in whom ACE inhibitors are to be used, diuretic treatment should be stopped for a week before starting ACE inhibitors. Patients with heart failure, in whom diuretics must be maintained, should be admitted to hospital for cautious initiation of ACE inhibitors, under close supervision.

Thiazides reduce lithium clearance by 24%,[9] so they should not be used by patients prescribed this treatment for bipolar depression, or who are likely to be in the future. Thiazides also impair response to anticoagulants, and can precipitate bleeding when withdrawn.[10]

Side Effects

Diuretics have six important side effects: tiredness and depression, erectile failure, gout, glucose intolerance, reduction of blood potassium concentration, and raised blood total cholesterol.

Tiredness and depression, although rarely severe, are common side effects of diuretics, as well as all other antihypertensive drugs, with the possible exception of ACE inhibitors. Always ask about fatigue and depression at the first follow-up visit after starting any antihypertensive drug. Thiazides in fixed combination with other antihypertensive drugs, which simplify dosage and therefore improve compliance with established medication, should not be started in this way, because it is then impossible to sort out the source of early side effects.

Erectile failure is common, affecting 16% of men after 12 weeks of treatment in the MRC trial at high dosage (10 mg bendrofluazide).[11] Before starting this or any other antihypertensive drug, ask whether this is already a problem. Frequent or permanent erectile failure affects 5–10% of middle aged men in all placebo treated control groups so far studied. Only a minority are likely to have presented this already as a problem. Having thus established your point of departure, you should point out that this is a possibility with all antihypertensive drugs, and that if it occurs, you want to know so that alternative medication can be used. Loss of libido and erectile failure have also been reported with lipid lowering agents.[12]

The effect is quickly reversible when thiazides are stopped, and is probably much less common at the lower doses (which should always be used). No research studies seem to have been done on the effect of thiazides on sexual function in women. Other antihypertensive drugs also cause impotence occasionally, generally at a much lower rate.

Erectile failure is associated with raised blood pressure because of ischaemic nerve damage or peripheral atheroma, and is extremely common in longstanding diabetes. Failure from this cause is unlikely to improve without implant surgery or subcutaneous papaverine. Where permanent impotence occurs in patients on thiazides, ischaemia or diabetes are probable causes.

Gout is a common outcome of sustained thiazide treatment even at low dose, which almost always raise levels of blood urate, even if there is no symptomatic gout. Again, the effect is reversible. Alcohol overload may be an adjuvant cause, and reducing beer intake may be more effective as well as more rational than prescribing probenecid or allopurinol.

Glucose intolerance is a much more important side effect, as it is an independent risk factor for both coronary heart disease and stroke. Mean blood glucose levels generally begin to rise after 2 or 3 years of treatment, are more likely in the elderly[13] and impaired glucose tolerance in the elderly is roughly doubled even at low doses.[7] At higher doses, the attack rate for frank diabetes was about 9 per 1000 patient years of treatment in the MRC mild hypertension trial,[14] and in 40% of these glucose tolerance was still impaired after withdrawal of treatment. It seems unwise to start treatment with diuretics if they can be avoided in patients who are seriously overweight (BMI 30+), have a history of diabetes in first degree relatives, or already have diabetes, but there is often no reasonable alternative. As assiduous control of blood pressure is mandatory in diabetics to preserve kidney function, this often has to take precedence.

Although experts originally thought thiazide induced glucose intolerance was unlikely to carry the same risk as naturally occurring diabetes, failure of numerous trials to reduce coronary events despite good control of high blood pressure has led to growing suspicion that this may arise from promotion of insulin resistance. These fears have been confirmed by long term follow-up trials in Sweden, showing a sixfold prospective increase in non–insulin dependent diabetes over 10 years in thiazide + beta-blocker treated hypertensive patients compared with untreated controls.[15,16]

Both thiazides and beta-blockers consistently raise blood LDL cholesterol and triglyceride,[17] although not by large amounts. In the MRC mild hypertension trial,[14] mean blood total cholesterol in patients on thiazides rose by less than 1% after 3 years, but as those on placebo had a 2% fall, there could have been a true rise of almost 3%, which on a mass scale will have mass effects. In the MRC trial in the elderly,[9] low dosage thiazides produced no significant change in cholesterol levels.

Mean blood potassium levels fell from an initial 4.1 mmol/l to 3.6 mmol/l after 3 years in the MRC trial,[14] compared with a rise to 4.2 mmol/l for placebo treated controls. However, although mild hypokalaemia is a common consequence of diuretic treatment, no association was found between age-adjusted mortality and serum potassium levels in 3783 patients attending the hypertension clinic at Glasgow Western Infirmary,[18] and this risk seems to have been exaggerated in the past. Again, low dosage thiazides used in the MRC trial of treatment in the elderly[7] showed no change in potassium levels. Even the most carefully formulated slow release forms of potassium supplement, whether given alone or in fixed combination with diuretics, produce some mucosal gut damage in most young and healthy volunteers,[19] so they probably do more harm than good in most patients, particularly in the elderly.

Baseline electrolytes should be measured before starting antihypertensive treatment of any kind, but serious hypokalaemia is extremely unlikely in patients with uncomplicated hypertension who feel well. Routine potassium measurements during follow-up are probably not useful, certainly less so than continued clinical alertness to the possibility that fatigue in any patient may reflect hypokalaemia. Significant hypokalaemia is unusual even in the presence of heart failure.[20] Risks are greatly increased in patients also receiving digoxin.

Potassium-sparing diuretics (amiloride, triamterene, and spironolactone) were at one time often used, usually combined with thiazides, for hypertensive patients thought to be a high risk. In fact, even for these patients, the risks of potassium overload are probably much greater than any risks of hypokalaemia,[21] and I doubt if these drugs should ever be used for hypertension except in hospital.

Carlsen[5] found a significant rise in mean urate compared with placebo treated controls after 10 weeks on bendrofluazide 1.25 mg daily, but no significant change in any biochemical marker (potassium, creatinine, glucose, fructosamine, total cholesterol, apolipoprotein A and B, and triglyceride). McVeigh[6] found no change in any biochemical marker for cyclopenthiazide at a dose of 1.25 mg. All side effects occur more commonly and are more severe at the unnecessarily high doses used in all but the most recent trials of antihypertensive drugs, as well as in most current practice. Risks would be much less if thiazides were consistently prescribed at optimal levels, equivalent to doses of bendrofluazide 1.25 mg daily.

Despite academic consensus on low dosage, review of the formulations actually available, generic or branded, shows that obsolete production, marketing, and practice continue almost unchanged. The smallest available tablets are 2.5 mg for bendrofluazide and 50 mg for chlorthalidone, twice the fully effective dosage for blood pressure control. Cyclopenthiazide (Navidrex) is still available only as 500 μg, 3 years after published research showed that this was four times the optimal dose.

The doses of thiazides used in fixed dose combination with almost all other antihypertensive agents widely marketed and prescribed, must be used carefully to avoid unnecessarily high dosage. In general, manufacturers have included suitably small doses in their formulations, and made several dosage forms available to allow increases in other antihypertensive drugs without thiazide overload, but prescribers need to pick their way carefully through the bewildering variety of these options, and remember that these are even more confusing for patients.

Beneficial Side Effects

Thiazides produce a striking long term reduction in urinary excretion of calcium and thus reduce the risk of recurrent ureteric stone, a common companion of high blood pressure. Probably for the same reason, long term thiazide takers have greater bone density and fewer hip fractures than comparable non-takers,[22] and these differences are independent of body weight, ability to walk, or dementia.[23] Relative risk of hip fracture is halved after treatment for 6 or more years. Loop diuretics have no such effect.

Second Line Drugs: Beta-Adrenoreceptor Blockers

Beta-blockers block beta-adrenoreceptors by competitive inhibition in the heart, peripheral vasculature, bronchi, pancreas and liver. They thus impede links between nervous inputs and vascular response, but their mode of action in reducing blood pressure is still not fully understood.

Used alone, they reduce pressure slightly less than thiazide diuretics, but, as with other antihypertensive drugs, there is wide variability in individual response. The dose required for beta-blockade, shown by a slow heart rate or calm in the face of examinations, is usually less than the dose required for maximal reduction in blood pressure, and the full antihypertensive effect of beta-blockers may take 3 or even 4 weeks to appear.

Beta-blockers are better tolerated than their predecessors other than thiazides. Like thiazides, however, they often cause minor weakness, lethargy and depression, and probably reduce capacity for exercise. They are subjectively well tolerated in old age.

When they were first introduced in the mid–1960s, there were high hopes that they might break the causal sequence then widely believed to be operating in essential hypertension, and were therefore attractive as drugs acting closer to causes. They rapidly displaced methyldopa, which was often prescribed in huge doses of 2 g/day or more (thereby causing intolerable drowsiness). Compared with methyldopa, propranolol (the first beta-blocker) was well tolerated. Life was transformed for many patients, just as it had been before, when methyldopa rescued them from life on ganglion-blockers. Despite relatively short half-lives, the degradation products of most beta-blockers were pharmacologically active, so they need to be given only once or twice a day.[24,25] The slow release versions marketed by most companies are expensive and unnecessary.

They are a very effective treatment for angina, which in many patients coexists with hypertension. There were also reasonable hopes that beta-blockers might have a specific preventive effect on arrhythmias, preventing many sudden deaths from ischaemic heart disease. Up to the late 1970s, there was mounting but always inconclusive evidence that this might be so. Hopes were reinforced by good evidence that for the first few years after myocardial infarction, symptom free survival increased with propranolol, timolol, and metoprolol.[26–28] This effect is unproven for other beta-blockers, and disproven for some of them. There is also some evidence that, just as we all hoped, patients already receiving beta-blockers are about half as likely to die within 1 month of suffering a myocardial infarct.[30]

Side Effects

Despite improved prognosis once myocardial infarction occurs, probably through reduction in infarct size and stabilized heart rhythm, all major randomly controlled trials using beta-blockers, with or without thiazides, have failed to show expected falls in either all-causes mortality or mortality from coronary thrombosis, at least in middle age,[30] and both the MRC trial of antihypertensive treatment in the elderly[7] and the Swedish HAPPHY trial[31] showed significant reductions in stroke and coronary thrombosis only with diuretics, not with beta-blockers alone. Significant results with beta-blockers were found only when combined with thiazide diuretics. Indeed, it can be argued, consistently with this and other evidence, that beta-blockers abolish the benefits of thiazide diuretics, at least in the elderly, probably because of their known effect in reducing cardiac output.[32] Although a cardioprotective effect for 2 years after infarction seems to be real, where no infarction has yet occurred this seems to be outweighed by other effects, either increasing the incidence of infarction or increasing deaths from other causes, known or unknown.

Mechanisms for all these potential harmful effects abound. LDL cholesterol and triglyceride concentrations are consistently raised in patients taking either beta-blockers or thiazides, and protective HDL cholesterol is reduced.[17] The changes are small, but applied to the very large populations receiving these drugs, should not be dismissed. Like high dose thiazides, although to a smaller extent, beta-blockers also impair glucose tolerance, raising fasting glucose, plasma insulin and glycated haemoglobin[33,34]. Combined with thiazides, the effect is additive. They also suppress the tachycardia, although not the sweating, which many insulin dependent diabetics rely on to warn them of hypoglycaemic attacks, so their use in these patients can be tricky.

All beta-blockers cause bronchoconstriction in patients with hyper-reactive airways (asthma). This may be severe and has caused death in asthmatics. Asthma is therefore a contraindication to their use. Unfortunately we cannot assume that all asthmatics are known; many people with hyper-reactive airways either have no symptoms, do not report symptoms, or report them but are not recognized as asthmatic. The number of people with reversible airways obstruction will not be known until all patients with respiratory impairment have their peak expiratory flow rates measured routinely before and after a test dose of inhaled salbutamol, still very much a minority activity in UK practice, and in my experience even rarer abroad. In Glyncorrwg, we found that about one-fifth of all adults aged 20–74 had peak expiratory flow rate either 50% or more below their expected value for age, sex, and height, or improved by 15% or more after inhaling salbutamol. The proportion would probably be lower in a non-industrial population, but even so it seems likely that there is a much larger hypertensive population at risk of chronic or acute iatrogenic respiratory impairment than has been generally thought. I see no reason why this should not have contributed to mortality.

Suspicions persist that beta-blockers might be carcinogenic. Pronethalol, the first beta-blocker ever used, was quickly discarded because it caused malignant tumours in mice within 90 days.[35] Two later beta-blockers were found to be carcinogenic in animals by the Food and Drug Administration. These initial fears may be revived by the results of the MRC trial of antihypertensive treatment in the elderly,[7] which showed a significant excess of deaths from cancer in men treated with beta-blockers, independent of smoking history, but no increase in women. No similar results have been found in any other trial, and the unexpectedly high mortality in the intervention group (treated with thiazides and/or propranolol) at the tenth year of the Finnish trial discussed in Chapter 7[36] seems to have been attributable entirely to increased deaths from cardiovascular disease, accidents and violence, not to cancers.

Another possible factor which could explain the results of the Finnish trial would be sustained rebound increase in blood pressure after withdrawal of beta-blockade, but I know of no published evidence on this. Sudden withdrawal of beta-blockers can precipitate angina, and may cause a rise in blood pressure.

Oculomucocutaneous Syndrome

This serious and wholly unexpected side effect fortunately proved to be confined to practolol, although not before it had been used for several years on a mass scale. It consisted of a psoriasis-like rash, sore dry eyes with corneal scarring, conjunctival fibrosis, secretory otitis, sclerosing peritonitis, pleural adhesions and pericarditis, all of them irreversible in the worst cases. The mechanisms of this side effect are still not understood, so the possibility of similar effects with new formulations cannot be dismissed. Despite this risk, new molecular variants continue to appear, meeting commercial rather than clinical needs.

Minor Side Effects

Peripheral vasoconstriction often leads to cold hands and feet, and all patients need to be warned to wear gloves and good foot protection in winter. Although beta-blockers might in theory be expected to precipitate or worsen claudication, there is no evidence that this actually happens.[37] Peripheral vasoconstriction is less with beta-blockers with high intrinsic sympathomimetic activity (oxprenolol, pindolol, acebutolol and celiprol).

Sleep disturbance and nightmares are common, mainly with lipid soluble beta-blockers. Minor fatigue, depression or weakness affect about one-third of patients,[38] particularly those patients who have to do heavy physical work.

Beneficial Side Effects

Generally, beta-blockers reduce symptoms in angina, making them a particularly useful antihypertensive drug in this condition. This is often a good reason for choosing them, particularly in patients who have stopped smoking.

Use in Pregnancy and Lactation

Beta-blockers cross the placental barrier. They enter breast milk, but are not concentrated there. Most obstetricians prefer methyldopa despite its relatively high hepatotoxicity, but this seems to depend more on custom than evidence.

Contraindications

Beta-blockers reduce cardiac output and are therefore contraindicated by overt heart failure. Despite widespread fears when they were first introduced, they rarely precipitate heart failure *de novo*, even in the elderly.

Beta-blockade slows the heart, and second or third degree heart block is an absolute contraindication.

Even the most cardioselective beta-blockers are dangerous to asthmatics, and should rarely, if ever, be used for patients with any kind of airways obstruction.

Interactions With Other Drugs

Beta-blockers should never be used with the calcium-channel blockers, verapamil and diltiazem. They can be used in combination with all other commonly used antihypertensive drugs. Combinations with thiazides or other calcium-channel blockers seem particularly effective, as these counteract the cold extremeties so often caused by peripheral vasoconstriction in beta-blockade. In the MRC mild hypertension trial,[14] there was no benefit from beta-blockade in those who continued to smoke, suggesting that there might be a specific interaction.

Cimetidine greatly increases bioavailability of propranolol and metoprolol, but atenolol seems unaffected.[39]

Racial Differences in Response to Beta-Blockers

There is some evidence that blood pressure in black people, in the USA at least, responds less to beta-blockers or ACE inhibitors than in white patients.[40] The US Joint National Committee on Development, Evaluation and Treatment of High Blood Pressure[41] states, on unconvincing evidence, that black people respond better to diuretics and calcium-channel blockers.

Specific Beta-Blocking Drugs

The current *British National Formulary* lists 15 molecular variants of beta-blocking drugs. In general, they are equally effective in reducing blood pressure. I find it difficult to believe that any clinician can in practice select between them to optimize personal care. Each has its own market, based largely on the year when patients began treatment, or the persuasiveness of whichever sales representative got in first.

Labetolol combines alpha- and beta-blockade, which, according to its manufacturers, has some theoretical advantages. In practice it seems to offer no advantage.

Other beta-blockers are divisible in two main ways, according to solubility (and therefore body distribution) and according to cardioselectivity.

Lipid soluble beta-blockers cross the blood-brain barrier more easily and are therefore more likely to cause sleep disturbance, nightmares, and depressive symptoms. They include propranolol, metoprolol, and timolol (the only beta-blockers shown to reduce mortality and morbidity after myocardial infarction). Oxprenolol is also in this group, but seems to offer no particular advantage.

The most water soluble beta-blockers, ie least likely to cross the blood-brain barrier, are atenolol, nadolol and sotalol. Water soluble beta-blockers are excreted through the kidney; they can be used in renal impairment, but dosage usually needs to be reduced. No post-infarction cardioprotective effect has been shown for this otherwise more attractive group.

The most cardioselective beta-blockers are atenolol, betaxol, bisoprolol, and metoprolol. They have less effect on bronchial beta-receptors and therefore have less effect on airways resistance. Even so, their use in anyone with reversible airways obstruction is dangerous, and is never a risk worth taking, now that there are so many safer alternatives. They are useful for patients with moderate fixed airways obstruction, proven by measurement of peak expiratory flow rate before and after inhaled salbutamol.

All beta-blockers slow the heart (a useful indicator of compliance). Sotalol prolongs the QT interval and may be more likely than others to cause ventricular arrhythmias.

Reviewing all these advantages and disadvantages, atenolol looks like the best routine choice; it is less likely to cross the blood-brain barrier or to cause bronchoconstriction, and has been used in several large controlled trials.

Third Line Drugs: Calcium-Channel Blockers

Calcium-channel blockers impede transfer of calcium ions through the slow channel of active cell membranes, in particular cells in the conducting system and muscular syncytium of the heart, and in vascular smooth muscle. They reduce blood pressure about as effectively as other groups of antihypertensive drugs, but also depress conduction in the bundle of His, reduce heart output, and dilate peripheral vasculature. Like beta-blockers, they are all effective for treatment of angina. Occasionally, they can cause a paradoxical increase in severity of angina after the first dose, and their sudden withdrawal can cause rebound angina.

There are large differences between specific drugs in this group, greater than the differences between beta-blockers.

Although verapamil was originally promoted for treatment of arryhythmias and was generally used only by hospital specialists, it was later marketed widely as an antihypertensive drug for use by family doctors. Diltiazem has followed a similar course, promoted originally only for treatment of angina, but now being put forward for blood pressure control. I have never felt competent to use either. Combined with beta-blockers, both may easily precipitate heart failure. As there are safer alternatives, the easiest way to avert this combination is not to use them in the first place.

Nifedipine, nicardipine and amlodipine all relax vascular smooth muscle in the coronary and peripheral arteries, and have little effect on heart muscle or the conducting system. Nifedipine and nicardipine have short half-lives, and tend to cause flushing and headache unless prescribed in slow release form, which should be used routinely. Amlodipine has a longer half-life and can be given once a day in standard form.

All members of this group tend to cause symptoms from vasodilatation: flushing, headache, and often diuretic resistant ankle oedema. Although diuretics will not control this oedema, they may of course augment the antiphypertensive effect of calcium-channel blockadge. They may also cause menorrhagia[42].

Use in Pregnancy

All drugs in this group can inhibit contractions in labour, and nifedipine was toxic in pregnancy in animal studies.

Harmful Effects and Contraindications

Calcium-channel blockers should never be used in frank heart failure or when left ventricular function is known to be poor.[43]

Third Line Drugs: Angiotensin Converting Enzyme (ACE) Inhibitors[44]

ACE inhibitors inhibit conversion of angiotensin I to angiotensin II. They are effective, but with bigger differences between patients than for other agents; fall in pressure may be very rapid in some patients. ACE inhibitors should never be started in patients already on diuretics, because pressure may drop so quickly and so low that renal function is compromised; a 7-day wash-out period is wise.

Although experience of long term use is still limited, they may be marginally better tolerated than their predecessors. In a large trial comparing methyldopa, propranolol, and captropril (all with thiazides if necessary), drop-out from side efects was 8% for captopril, 13% for propranolol, and 20% for methyldopa.[45] Propranolol is probably less well tolerated than most later beta–blockers, and a smaller study comparing propranolol with atenolol, captopril and enalapril showed that all three were better tolerated, with no significant difference between them.[46] There was no significant difference in blood pressure control after 3 months' treatment in the 1986 trial. The proportions requiring added thiazides were 36% for captopril, 31% for methyldopa and 22% for propranolol.

The main known risk associated with ACE inhibitors is impairment of renal function. Renal fuction should always be checked before starting treatment, with measurements of blood creatinine and urea annually thereafter. A theoretical risk could be that, because regulation of blood flow through small brain arteries depends on angiotensin II, ACE inhibitors could increase the risk of intracerebral haemorrhage, despite good control of systemic pressure.[47] As far as I know, there is as yet no evidence of this possibility.

Their commonest unpleasant side effect is chronic and intractable dry cough, now said to occur in up to a quarter of all patients[48], more in women than men. There is no associated airways obstruction. It is usually worse on lying down, and onset is often delayed for weeks or months after starting treatment with any of the ACE inhibitors.[49] It seems to be caused by increased sensitivity in the cough reflex, which may depend in some way on prostaglandin metabolism.[50] It stops about a week after withdrawal and is dose dependent.[51]

Abdominal pain, angineurotic oedema, dizziness, headache, nausea and fatigue all occur occasionally in about 2–3% of patients, and lacrimation and rhinorrhoea have been reported.[52]

Inhibition of normal renin-angiotensin metabolism implies a worrying possibility, particularly in hot countries, that what would normally be a minor and self limiting diarrhoea might precipitate collapse, with acute dehydration and sodium depletion.[53] Patients should be warned that ACE inhibitors impede the normal mechanisms for correction of water and sodium depletion, and that if they develop diarrhoea this must be taken seriously, with immediately increased water and salt intake (one level teaspoonful of salt to each litre of water).

All ACE-inhibitors are contraindicated in aortic stenosis or other outflow tract obstruction.

Like virtually all other antihypertensive drugs, ACE inhibitors were originally introduced at much higher dosage than we now know to be optimal. The large doses of captopril first used often induced proteinuria and nephrotic syndrome, leukopenia and taste disturbances. All these are now rare. Combination with allopurinol may increase risk of leukopenia and is probably contraindicated.

Use in Pregnancy and Lactation

ACE inhibitors cross the placenta, have been associated with increased stillbirth rates in sheep and rabbits, and are contraindicated after the first trimester of pregnancy. In the USA, the Food and Drugs Administration has insisted that all ACE inhibitors be marketed with a boxed warning that they are contraindicated absolutely in the second and third trimesters, because of evidence of fetal damage, mainly to kidneys and the facial skeleton. There is no evidence of harm in the first trimester, so they are not contraindicated in women trying to conceive.

ACE inhibitors also appear in breast milk, but in extremely small quantities which are probably not significant.

Specific Indications

A major advantage of ACE inhibitors is their dramatic effect in improving prognosis in heart failure, which has transformed its management.[54,55] For hypertensive patients with evidence of impaired ventricular function this makes them an obvious choice.

They are also probably the best choice for control of high blood pressure in diabetics, a large group because of the good evidence justifying intervention from a diastolic threshold of 90 mmHg to conserve renal function.[56] ACE inhibitors do not impair glycaemic control[34] or lipid profile, and seem to reduce proteinuria independently of their effect on blood pressure in diabetic nephropathy.[57,58] They are probably better than nifedipine, although comparative evidence is not yet conclusive.[59]

First or Third Line Drugs?

Apart from this effect in heart failure, the main potential advantage of ACE inhibitors is that they do not have the marginally harmful effects on blood cholesterol and glucose tolerance known to occur with thiazides and beta-blockers. In the one-third of people of ACE inhibitors who have to take thiazides to obtain good blood pressure control, this argument is obviously weakened. Against this we must weigh the lack of evidence about their long term effects, bearing in mind that, as each new group of antihypertensive drugs was introduced, there were similar high hopes that they would solve all our problems. Generally speaking, these hopes have not been realized; there is no substitute for large, independently conducted long term controlled trials, and no such trial results are yet available for ACE inhibitors.

Some marketing of these drugs has implied that ACE inhibitors are a logical choice for first line treatment because they come closer to causes rather than effects, but the same was said of beta-blockers.

The much higher cost of ACE inhibitors is obviously important, but, on clinical grounds alone, a conservative policy seems justified, keeping ACE inhibitors as third line drugs until we have better evidence.

Individual ACE Inhibitors

The *British National Formulary* includes seven ACE inhibitors: captopril, enalapril, fosinopril, lisinopril, perindopril, quinapril, and ramipril. They are likely to be joined by trandolapril in 1993, as the effect of the good evidence of benefit in heart failure gathers momentum. We shall need a firm grip on our critical faculties.

Captopril was the first to be introduced in 1981, soon followed by enalapril, and these are the only ones on which there is extensive published experience. Although more side effects were reported for captopril, this was mainly, perhaps entirely, because of the unnecessarily high doses first used. Captopril seems to need twice-daily dosage, whereas enalapril is effective in a single dose daily.

It is difficult to see any convincing advantage for any of the more recent introductions. All except ramipril (which at equivalent dosage costs a bit less than captopril or enalapril) cost at least twice as much at average dosage.

Interactions with Other Agents

Although ACE inhibitors should never be started with patients already on diuretics, later introduction of adjuvant thiazide diuretics is necessary in about one-third of cases to get good control. Loop diuretics and potassium conserving diuretics are dangerous in combination with ACE inhibitors and should never be used.

ACE inhibitors can be used in cautious combination with all other antihypertensive agents, bearing in mind that blood pressure may fall rapidly, precipitating symptomatic hypotension.

Last Resorts

Alpha-Adrenoreceptor Blockers

Post-synaptic alpha-receptor blockers reduce blood pressure mainly by vasodilatation of both arterioles and veins. They are effective hypotensive drugs, with a greater effect on diastolic than systolic pressure, and have two important practical advantages.

They cause no deterioration in lipid profile, and may actually reduce plasma total cholesterol by about 9% and triglyceride by 16%, without reducing protective HDL cholesterol.[60]

Secondly, they substantially reduce outflow obstruction in benign chronic prostatic hypertrophy severe enough to cause symptoms, but not enough to justify surgery. This is a common situation in the age group mainly affected by high blood pressure, and well worth bearing in mind; the relief for many patients is quickly obvious. Prazosin may, by the same mechanism, cause urinary incontinence in women.[61] It is not a substitute for surgery where there is severe outflow obstruction; comparison of alpha–1 blockade with surgical prostatectomy showed 28% improvement in flow rate for medical versus 96% for surgical treatment, and 6% versus 45% improvement in symptom scores[62].

The great disadvantage of these drugs is that the first dose often causes syncope. This problem can be avoided by initiating treatment with a very small dose (500 µg of prazosin) given at night, after going to bed, with a gradual increase to a final 2–4 mg twice daily thereafter. Prazosin is available in a starter pack to make this procedure simple to follow. Patients should be warned of the possibility of syncope, and reminded that if they stop the drug, this initial procedure will have to be followed again. Even so, about 14% of patients still complain of faintness.[63] It may also cause water retention and ankle oedema.

Three drugs in this group are listed in the *British National Formulary*, prazosin, doxazosin and terazosin, of which prazosin is much the best documented and most widely prescribed. It makes a particularly good combination with beta-blockers, compensating for their side effects of peripheral vasoconstriction and raised lipids.

Vasodilators

Unlike prazosin, older and less selective vasodilators are ineffective alone, causing intolerable tachycardia. Used together with thiazides and/or beta-blockers, they can be very effective. There are four drugs listed in the *Formulary* in this group, hydralazine, diazoxide, nitroprusside and minoxidil, of which only the first is suitable for use in primary care.

Hydralazine was once popular in the USA, being one of the standard drugs in the Veterans' Administration trials, but was never used much in the UK. Its main disadvantage was development of lupus erythematosus in 10–20% of patients at doses over 200 mg daily.[64] This usually presented with widespread joint pains clinically indistinguishable from rheumatoid arthritis, with an onset months or years after starting the drug, and therefore easily misinterpreted. It is fully, although slowly, reversible by stopping the drug. Even below a 200 mg threshold this complication may occur in 1–3% of patients. Risk is much higher in slow acetylators, and in women. The test for acetylator status is easily performed (*see* Appendix 9), and should be done before starting treatment. Impotence is another common side effect.

Centrally Acting Drugs

This group of drugs reduces blood pressure through effects on catecholamine metabolism in the brain stem, with consequent risks of sedation, depression, and dry mouth. Three of these are still used in the UK, although all are now essentially obsolete: reserpine, methyldopa, and clonidine.

Reserpine came into general use in the 1950s, simultaneously with thiazide diuretics, with which it is usually combined. This combination was the main treatment available for community care of high blood pressure for about 20 years, and was the first line treatment in the Veterans' Administration trials, on which all responsible treatment policies were based throughout the 1970s.

Reserpine depletes brain stem catecholamines, and in the high doses originally used was a common cause of severe depression, which was sometimes suicidal. As well as a dry mouth and sometimes minor sedation, it often causes a stuffy nose. In combination with thiazides, it reduces blood pressure more than beta-blockers in combination with thiazide.[65] Providing daily dosage starts at 0.05 mg, and that a dosage of 0.3 mg is not exceeded, depression is in fact no more common than with other antihypertensive drugs which were available in 1980.[66, 67] As with thiazides, suitable tablets are simply not available for this policy to be pursued; the smallest simple formulation listed in the *Formulary* is now a 0.25 mg tablet, although a combined preparation with diuretic contains only 0.15 mg. Having long lost patent protection, no pharmaceutical multinational has much financial incentive to make it available or promote its use, even in poorer countries where it could be very useful.

This is a pity, because reserpine remains a useful drug in two particular circumstances. First, it may cause a dramatic response to antihypertensive medication in patients for whom nothing else seems to work. For the sort of patient for whom minoxidil or diazoxide, for example, are considered, reserpine may be a more effective and more tolerable alternative. Secondly, it is very cheap as well as effective; at current UK prices, one year's treatment with reserpine and thiazide costs about £8.58. If any Third World country ever follows Sri Lanka and Cuba in developing their own generic drug formularies, giving priority to patients rather than multinational companies, they should remember reserpine; severe high blood pressure and consequent stroke are common problems wherever poorer countries begin to industrialize.

The effects of reserpine appear slowly, and disappear slowly on withdrawal. It causes bradycardia, which, as with beta-blockers, gives a useful indication of medication compliance. A stuffed-up nose is a common side effect. Risk of depression should be discussed before prescribing it, and depressive symptoms should be sought actively throughout follow-up. Neither reserpine, nor any other centrally acting antihypertensive drug (including lipid soluble beta-blockers) should ever be used in patients who are already depressed, or with evidence of Parkinson's disease.

Methyldopa was introduced in 1963, and rapidly became the market leader, dominating treatment until beta-blockers overtook it in the mid–1970s. Although it is an essentially obsolete drug because of drowsiness in nearly all patients, and its relatively high liver toxicity, many elderly patients remain well stabilized on it.

For obstetricians, it remains the preferred treatment for hypertension in pregnancy, although it crosses the placental barrier.[68] It is probably a bit more effective than beta-blockers in reducing pressure, and there is no difference in maternal or fetal outcome.[69] Any substantial impairment in later brain function in the child has been excluded.[70] Any possible smaller, and therefore undetected, effect must be balanced against the high risk of fetal death and prematurity, as well as risks to the mother, of untreated pre-eclampsia.

Like reserpine, methyldopa acts by depleting brainstem catecholamines. It is effective in once-daily dosage, which should be given in the evening to concentrate drowsiness where it will be least troublesome; this simple fact remains ignored by most clinicians who still use it. At doses over 500 mg daily drowsiness is in my experience invariable, and is a serious risk for drivers.

Methyldopa causes measurable liver damage in about 3% of patients[71, 72], and should therefore be avoided in known heavy drinkers, anyone with raised gamma GT or other impaired liver function tests, or with gallbladder disease. It is an occasional cause of cholestatic jaundice; as about 20% of middle aged adults have asymptomatic gallstones, interpretation of jaundice in these patients can be difficult. Although it was widely used for elderly patients, this effect, together with drowsiness and a high risk of depression, make it a particularly inappropriate drug for this age group. About a quarter of elderly patients started on methyldopa stop within 6 months because of adverse side effects, mainly drowsiness.[73]

It interferes with many laboratory tests, causing misleading results unless you remember to mention its use on the request form. It interacts with major phenothiazines to produce a paradoxical increase in blood pressure, increases toxicity of lithium, and disturbs treatment of Parkinson's disease with L-dopa. At doses under 1 g daily, about 10% of patients develop a positive direct Coombs' test[74, 75], evidence of the first stage in an auto-immune process.

About 2% of all treated patients go on to develop an auto-immune haemolytic anaemia, which is usually reversible if treatment is stopped promptly.

If you do use methyldopa, measure baseline liver function tests before starting, never prescribe more than 1g daily (doses of 2 and even 3 g were once commonly prescribed), and check liver function and Coombs' test annually thereafter.

Clonidine came into use in 1966. It was fortunately never popular in the UK, but remains widely used elsewhere in Europe, especially in Germany where it was originally developed. It blocks catecholamines both centrally and peripherally, causing depression and fatigue in about half of all patients, but a more serious disadvantage is that blocked catecholamines accumulate. If the drug is then stopped, severe rebound hypertension follows.[76,77] Severe rebound hypertension has been reported occasionally after abrupt withdrawal of all anti-hypertensive drugs other than thiazides, ACE inhibitors, and reserpine, but clonidine is in a class of its own in this respect. This risk can be reduced by using the slow release preparation of this drug, but at very high cost.

References

1. British Medical Association and the Royal Pharmaceutical Society of Great Britain (1991) *British National Formulary No. 22*, p 72 Pharmaceutical Press, London.

2. Feher MD and Lant A (1991) First line treatment in hypertension. *Br Med J* **302**: 116.

3. Poulter N, Thom S and Sever P (1991) First line treatment in hypertension. *Br Med J* **302**: 116.

4. Ramsay LE and Yeo WW (1991) First line treatment in hypertension. *Br Med J* **302**: 352–3.

5. Carlsen JE, Kober L, Torp-Pedersen C *et al.* (1990) Relation between dose of bendrofluazide, antihypertensive effect, and adverse biochemical effects. *Br Med J* **300**: 975–8.

6. McVeigh G, Galloway D and Johnston D (1988) The case for low dose diuretics in hypertension: Comparison of low and conventional doses of cyclopenthiazide. *Br Med J* **297**: 95–8.

7. Medical Research Council Working Party (1992) Medical Research Council trial of treatment of hypertension in older adults: Principal results. *Br Med J* **304**: 405–12.

8. Reubi FC and Cottier PT (1961) Effects of reduced glomerular filtration rate on responsiveness to chlorothiazide and mercurial diuretics. *Circulation* **23**: 200–10.

9. Petersen V, Hvidt S, Thomsen K *et al.* (1974) Effect of prolonged thiazide treatment on renal lithium clearance. *Br Med J* **iii**: 143–5.

10. O'Reilly RA and Aggeler PM (1971) Impact of aspirin and chlorthalidone on the pharmacodynamics of oral anticoagulant drugs in man. *Ann N Y Acad Sci* **179**: 173–86.

11. Medical Research Council Working Party on Mild to Moderate Hypertension (1981) Adverse reactions to bendrofluazide and propranolol for the treatment of mild hypertension. *Lancet* **ii**: 539–43.

12. Bharani A (1992) Sexual dysfunction after gemfibrozil. *Br Med J* **305**: 693.

13. Murphy MB, Lewis PJ, Kohner E *et al.* (1982) Glucose intolerance in hypertensive patients treated with diuretics: A fourteen-year follow-up. *Lancet* ii: 1293–5.

14. Medical Research Council Working Party (1985) MRC trial of treatment of mild hypertension: Principle results. *Br Med J* 291: 97–104.

15. Skarfors ET, Lithell HO, Selinus *et al.* (1989) Do antihypertensive drugs precipitate diabetes in predisposed men? *Br Med J* 298: 1147–51.

16. Skarfors ET, Selinus I and Lithell HO (1991) Risk factors for developing non-insulin dependent diabetes: A 10-year follow up of men in Uppsala. *Br Med J* 303: 755–60.

17. Krone W and Nagele H (1988) Effects of antihypertensives on plasma lipids and lipoprotein metabolism. *Am Heart J* 116: 1729–34.

18. Robertson JWK, Isles CG, Brown I *et al.* (1986) Mild hypokalaemia is not a risk factor in treated hypertensives. *J. Hypertens* 4: 603–8.

19. McMahon FG, Ryan JR, Akdamal K *et al.* (1982) Upper gastrointestinal lesions after potassium chloride supplements: A controlled clinical trial. *Lancet* ii: 1059–61.

20. Sandor FF, Pickens PT and Crallan J (1982) Variations of plasma potassium concentration during long-term treatment of hypertension with diuretics without potassium supplements. *Br Med J* 284: 711–15.

21. Swales JD (1991) Salt substitutes and potassium intake: Too much potassium may be disastrous for some. *Br Med J* 303: 1084–5.

22. Wasnich R, Davis J, Ross P *et al* (1990) Effect of thiazide on rates of bone mineral loss: A longitudinal study. *Br Med J* 301: 1303–4.

23. Ray WA, Griffin MR, Downie W *et al.* (1989) Long term use of thiazide diuretics and risk of hip fracture. *Lancet* i: 687–90.

24. Morgan T (1976) Once-daily treatment of hypertension. *Br Med J* iii: 235.

25. Woolfson AMJ and Knapp MS (1976) Once-daily treatment of hypertension. *Br Med J* iii: 235.

26. Opie LH (1984) Drugs and the heart four years on. *Lancet* i: 496–501.

27. Breckenridge A (1982) Should every survivor of a heart attack be given a beta-blocker? *Br Med J* **285**: 37–9.

28. Olsson G, Lubsen J, van Es G-A *et al.* (1986) Quality of life after myocardial infarction: Effect of long term metoprolol on mortality and morbidity. *Br Med J* **292**: 1491–3.

29. Nidorf SM, Parsons RW, Thompson PL *et al.* (1990) Reduced risk of death at 28 days in patients taking a beta-blocker before admission to hospital with myocardial infarction. *Br Med J* **300**: 71–3.

30. MacMahon SW, Cutler JA, Furberg CD *et al.* (1986) The effects of drug treatment for hypertension on morbidity and mortality from cardiovascular disease: A review of randomized controlled trials. *Prog Cardiovasc Dis* **24 (Suppl 1)**: 99–118.

31. Wilhelmsen L, Berglund G, Elmfeldt D *et al.* (1987) Beta-blockers versus diuretics in hypertensive men: Main results from the HAPPHY trial. *J. Hypertens* **5**: 561–72.

32. Aursnes I (1992) Elderly patients with sustained hypertension. *Br Med J* **304**: 1054.

33. Houston MC (1988) The effects of antihypertensive drugs on glucose intolerance in hypertensive non-diabetics and diabetics. *Am Heart J* **115**: 640–56.

34. Pollare T, Lithell H, Selinus I *et al.* (1989) Sensitivity to insulin during treatment with atenolol and metoprolol: A Randomized, double blind study of effects on carbohydrate and lipoprotein metabolism in hypertensive patients. *Br Med J* **298**: 1152–7.

35. Paget GE (1963) Carcinogenic action of pronethalol. *Br Med J* **ii**: 1266.

36. Strandberg TE, Salomaa VV, Naukkarinen VA *et al.* (1991) Long term mortality after 5 years multifactorial primary prevention of cardiovascular diseases in middle aged men. *JAMA* **226**: 1255–9.

37. Solomon SA, Ramsay LE, Yeo WW *et al.* (1991) Beta-blockade and intermittent claudication: Placebo controlled trial of atenolol and nifedipine and their combination. *Br Med J* **303**: 1100–4.

38. Bai TR, Webb D, Hamilton M *et al.* (1982) Treatment of hypertension with beta-adrenoreceptor blocking drugs. *J R Coll Physicians Lond* **16**: 239–41.

39. Kirch W, Kohler H, Spahn H *et al.* (1981) Interaction of cimetidine with metoprolol, propranolol, or atenolol. *Lancet* **ii**: 531–2.

40. Zing W, Ferguson RK and Vlasses P (1991) Calcium antagonists in elderly and black hypertensive patients: Therapeutic controversies. *Arch Intern Med* **151**: 2154–62.

41. Joint National Committee (1988) The 1988 report of the Joint National Committee on development, evaluation and treatment of high blood pressure. *Arch Intern Med* **14**: 1023–38.

42. Rodger JC and Torrance TC (1983) Can nifedipine provoke menorrhagia? *Lancet* **ii**: 460.

43. (1991) Calcium antagonist caution [editorial]. *Lancet* **337**: 885–6.

44. Opie LH (1992) *Angiotensin converting enzyme inhibitors.* Wiley, New York.

45. Croog SH, Levine S, Testa MA *et al.* (1986) The effects of antihypertensive therapy on the quality of life. *N Engl J Med* **314**: 1657–64.

46. Steiner S, Friedhoff AJ, Wilson B *et al.* (1987) Antihypertensive therapy and quality of life: A comparison of atenolol, captopril, enalapril and propranolol. *J Hum Hypertens* **1**: 217–26.

47. Brown MJ and Brown J (1986) Does angiotensin II protect against strokes? *Lancet* **ii**: 427–9.

48. Goldszer RC, Lilly LS and Solomon HS (1988) Prevalence of cough during angiotensin-converting enzyme inhibitor therapy. *Am J Med* **85**: 887.

49. Berkin KE and Ball SG (1988) Cough and angiotensin converting enzyme inhibition. *Br Med J* **296**: 1279.

50. Fuller RW and Choudry NB (1987) Increased cough reflex associated with angiotensin converting enzyme inhibitor cough. *Br Med J* **295**: 1025–6.

51. Webb D, Benjamin N, Collier J *et al.* (1986) Enalapril-induced cough. *Lancet* **ii**: 1094.

52. Balduf M and Steinkraus Ring J (1992) Captopril associated lacrimation and rhinorrhoea. *Br Med J* **305**: 693.

53. McMurray, J and Matthews D M (1985) Effect of diarrhoea on a patient taking captopril. *Lancet* **ii**: 581.

54. SOLVD Investigators (1991) Effect of enalapril on survival in patients with reduced left ventricular ejection fractions and conjestive heart failure. *N Engl J Med* **325**: 293–302.

55. CONSENSUS Trial Study Group (1991) Effects of enalapril on mortality in severe congestive heart failure: Results of the Co-operative North Scandinavian Enalapril Survival Study (CONSENSUS). *N Engl J Med* **316**: 1429–35.

56. Parving HH, Smidt U, Anderson AR *et al.* (1983) Early aggressive antihypertensive treatment reduces rate of decline in kidney function in diabetic nepropathy. *Lancet* i: 1175–8.

57. Parving HH, Hommel E, Nielsen MD *et al.* (1989) Effect of captopril on blood pressure and kidney function in normotensive insulin dependent diabetics with nephropathy. *Br Med J* **299**: 533–6.

58. Apperloo AJ, de Zeeuw D, Sluiker HE *et al.* (1991) Differential effects of enalapril and atenolol on proteinuria and renal haemodynamics in non-diabetic renal disease. *Br Med J* **303**: 821–4.

59. Chan JCN, Cockram CS, Nicholls MG *et al.* (1992) Comparison of enalapril and nifedipine in treating non-insulin dependant diabetes associated with hypertension: One year analysis. *Br Med J* **305**: 981–5.

60. Leren P, Foss PO, Helgeland A *et al.* (1980) Effect of propranolol and prazosin on blood lipids: The Oslo study. *Lancet* ii: 4–6.

61. Thien T, Delaere KP, Debruyne FMJ *et al.* (1978) Urinary incontinence caused by prazosin. *Br Med J* i: 622–3.

62. Noble JG, Chapple CR and Milroy EJG (1991) Long term selective alpha-I adrenoreceptor blockade versus surgery in the treatment of benign prostatic hyperplasia. *Neurourol Urodynam* **10**: 296–8.

63. Brogden RN, Heel RC, Speight TM *et al.* (1979) Prazosin: A review of its pharmacological properties and therapeutic efficacy. In: Brogden RN (ed) *Antihypertensive drugs today*, pp 125–69. MTP, Lancaster.

64. Bing RF, Russell GI, Thurston H *et al.* (1980) Hydralazine in hypertension: Is there a safe dose? *Br Med J* **280**: 353–4.

65. Veterans' Administration Co-operative Group on Antihypertensive Agents (1977) Propranolol in the treatment of essential hypertension. *JAMA* **237**: 2303–10.

66. McMahon FG (1978) *Management of essential hypertension*, p 344. Futura, New York.

67. Veterans' Administration Co-operative Group on Antihypertensive Agents, (1982) Low dose versus standard dose of reserpine: a randomized, double-blind, multiclinic trial in patients taking chlorthalidone. *JAMA* **248**: 2471–7.

68. de Swiet M (1985) Antihypertensive drugs in pregnancy. *Br Med J* **291**: 365–6.

69. Fidler J, Smith V, Fayers P *et al.* (1983) Randomised controlled comparative study of methyldopa and oxprenolol in treatment of hypertension in pregnancy. *Br Med J* **286**: 1927–30.

70. Ounsted M, Moar V, Redman CWG *et al.* (1980) Infant growth and development following treatment of maternal hypertension. *Lancet* i: 705.

71. Hoyumpa AM and Connell AM (1973) Methyldopa hepatitis. *Am J Dig Dis* **18**: 213–22.

72. Sataline L and Lowell D (1976) Methyldopa toxicity. *Gastroenterology* **70**: 148–9.

73. Ramsay LE (1981) The use of methyldopa in the elderly. *J R Coll Physicians Lond* **15**: 239–41.

74. Carstairs K, Worlledge S, Dollery C T *et al.* (1966) Methyldopa and haemolytic anaemia. *Lancet* ii: 201.

75. Harth M (1968) LE cells and positive direct Coombs' test induced by methyldopa. *Can Med Assoc J* **99**: 277–80.

76. Goldberg AD, Raftery EB and Wilkinson P (1977) Blood pressure and heart rate and withdrawal of antihypertensive drugs. *Br Med J* i: 1243–6.

77. Reid JL, Wing LMH and Dargie HJ (1977) Clonidine withdrawal in hypertension: Changes in blood pressure and plasma and urinary noradrenaline. *Lancet* ii: 1171–4.

18

Refractory and Complicated Cases, and Hypertensive Emergencies

Professional causes of treatment failure ■ Patient causes of treatment failure ■ Management of high blood pressure complicated by other problems ■ High blood pressure with hypercholesterolaemia and/or obesity ■ High blood pressure with vascular damage ■ High blood pressure with chronic musculoskeletal pain ■ High blood pressure with airways obstruction ■ High blood pressure with recurrent depression or psychosis ■ High blood pressure with alcohol problems ■ High blood pressure with impaired renal function ■ High blood pressure with peptic ulcer ■ High blood pressure with diabetes ■ High blood pressure with gout ■ High blood pressure with impotence ■ Hypertensive emergencies

Even in the best run hospital blood pressure clinics, audit generally shows about 20% above target pressure. If drop-outs are included, and assumed to be uncontrolled, this proportion will be much higher. Drop-outs include those who collect repeat prescriptions, and are presumably taking their medication, but attend follow-up rarely or not at all.

Three professional errors and seven groups of patients account for most of these cases.

Professional Causes of Treatment Failure

■ Assumption that because a drug appears ineffective on its own, it will also be ineffective in combination.

No drug should be discarded as ineffective, if it has not been combined at least with a diuretic.

■ Failure to titrate medication against response to a point where side effects, or the risk of side effects, preclude higher dosage.

It is futile to add another drug, when dosage of the first is inadequate.

■ Inadvertent prescription of other medication which opposes the action of antihypertensive drugs.

The commonest of these are NSAIDs such as indomethacin, ibuprofen, and the myriad brand names that compete for the inflated aches and pains market. All these cause sodium retention and reduced glomerular flow, and there is probably little difference between them in these respects. Their use in non-inflammatory joint disease is in any case questionable, as there is good evidence that they accelerate damage in weight bearing joints (whether pharmacologically or through increased use is not yet certain), without giving more pain relief than can be achieved with other analgesics. Now that many of these are available across the counter without prescription, it is important to enquire about them specifically.

Other medication which can raise blood pressure includes oral contraceptives, parasympathomimetic amines used as anorectics, nasal decongestants, recreational or occupational stimulants, and carbenoxalone. All antideprssant drugs other than lithium oppose the action of hypotensive drugs to some extent, but depressive illness itself can be a cause of raised pressure. Phenothiazine drugs used for psychotic illness can interact with methyldopa to raise blood pressure.[1]

Patient Causes of Treatment Failure

■ Patients who persistently fail to take their medication.

About half of all patients in most published series show serious non-compliance 3 months after starting treatment, suggesting that initial non-compliance should be accepted as normal. Anyone having to take regular medication for an asymptomatic condition has to learn to remember to take tablets. This learning process can be helped by keeping medication simple, with the least possible number of drugs (including those prescribed for other problems), never giving more than twice-daily dosage, encouraging a regular routine, and enlistment of help from the spouse. If you explain that you know this is difficult initially, patients will be more likely to admit the problem rather than conceal it.

Formal tablet counts may be counterproductive because they imply unsympathetic assessment and invite falsification, but if prescriptions normally cover the whole interval before the next follow-up visit, and patients are asked always to bring their medication with them, a glance at the bottle is enough to estimate levels of compliance. Absence of bradycardia in patients on beta-blockers or reserpine suggests non-compliance. If readings are above target pressure, always ask about medication that day; repeated admissions that tablets have been missed that day suggest a compliance problem which needs to be explored sympathetically.

■ Male patients drinking 56, and female patients drinking 28 or more units of alcohol weekly.

Fifty-six units a week is roughly equivalent to 80 g alcohol a day, contained in four pints of beer, eight glasses of wine, or four double measures of spirits, bearing in mind that wines, and especially beers, have a widely varying alcohol content. In my experience this is the commonest cause of refractory hypertension in patients who have got past the initial learning phase on medication. Useful clues are smell of alcohol on breath, flushed face and palms, morning nausea, vomiting or diarrhoea characteristically on Mondays, unexplained work absence, and unexplained faint spells or syncope. Raised gamma GT and/or raised mean corpuscular volume are often present, but normal values do not exclude serious alcoholism, particularly in patients who have reached middle age. Alcohol is a much commoner cause of macrocytosis than B_{12} deficiency. Estimation of morning blood alcohol, using a fluoride tube as for blood glucose, may provide incontrovertible proof in patients who stoutly deny heavy drinking, but the results need careful handling to avoid destructive confrontation.

■ Patients exposed to intractable stress at home or work.

This may have a direct effect on blood pressure, and/or an effect on compliance or consumption of alcohol.

■ Patients who seem unable to tolerate virtually all antihypertensive drugs.

Previous records may show longstanding intolerance of most medication. If this seems to be happening try using a placebo as a learning exercise, for both you and the patient. If (say) 50 mg of ascorbic acid twice a day causes symptoms, this finding, and the fears underlying it, need to be discussed frankly but sympathetically before going further.

■ Patients in whom antihypertensive drugs initially seem effective, but later become ineffective.

The classic cause for this is acquired atherothrombotic renal artery stenosis or occlusion, possibly signalled by a renal bruit not previously audible. More commonly, use of older antihypertensive drugs (except diuretics and beta-blockers) can cause sodium and water retention, with expanded blood volume and therefore raised pressure. Adding a diuretic, or switching to one of greater potency, may restore control.

■ Patients with unrecognized secondary high blood pressure.

Rare causes of secondary hypertension such as aldosterone-secreting tumours or phaeochromocytoma are more likely to be detected as a result of an anomalous response to treatment than by routine investigation before treatment begins.

■ Patients who seem truly resistant to all commonly used antihypertensive drugs.

Uncontrolled systolic pressures over 200 or diastolic pressures over 120 mmHg must be controlled. If you cannot achieve this within 3 months your patient needs referral to a specialist with enough interest in hypertension to do more than repeat the routine investigations you have already performed. Responsible consultants exist in most, but not all, areas and may need an active search.

Most of these refractory patients have other problems in their lives, often too large to be readily revealed, which are affecting compliance. You are better placed to detect these than most specialists, and even after referral you may need to keep looking; discussion with the patient's partner or family may be helpful.

Everyone experienced in long term management of high blood pressure knows that, however difficult it may be in the first 2 or 3 years, most hyptertensive patients who persist with treatment eventually achieve control. In many cases this will be because they become able, with support and assistance, to reorganize their personal lives to include medication compliance. In others, perhaps low blood pressure begets lower blood pressure, just as high blood pressure begets higher blood pressure. A patient with a pre-treatment blood pressure of 210/130 mmHg who can achieve only 180/120 mmHg with medication is already at much lower risk, and will probably achieve full control eventually if you persist.

Management of High Blood Pressure Complicated by Other Problems

In 1992 I reviewed summarized histories of 154 men and 190 women from the Glyncorrwg population, living and dead, who met the criteria for mandatory antihypertensive medication advocated in this book (mean pressures at or over 160/100 mmHg under age 40, 170/105 mmHg at or over age 40, based on at least three readings on separate days, and/or exceptional risks [diabetes, existing vascular damage, and so on]). All were included in an intention to treat analysis, whether or not medication was actually started or maintained.

Of course, uncomplicated high blood pressure cannot really exist, any more than an uncomplicated pregnancy or sore throat, since all these conditions require a human vehicle, and no real person is uncomplicated. However, high blood pressure may occasionally be the only apparent medical problem requiring long term supervision and control, and its management may, in this traditional sense, appear uncomplicated.

Tables 18.1 and 18.2, showing the results of this review, illustrate how unusual this is, even on so narrow a definition. I searched for 12 chronic or recurrent problems whose existence inevitably affects rational management of high blood pressure; I could find only four men and 14 women without any of them.

Clearly, uncomplicated high blood pressure is exceptional. These complicating problems introduce competing, and sometimes conflicting, priorities, often more apparent to generalists than to specialists. They are dealt with here in descending order of male prevalence.

Table 18.1: Twelve chronic problems complicating high blood pressure in 154 consecutive men, Glyncorrwg 1961–91 (including 84 deaths to July 1992); mean age at diagnosis is 53, mean BP 183/108 mmHg before treatment; problems are listed in descending order of prevalence.

Complicating problem	No.	%
Total cholesterol >6.6 mmol/l	84	65*
Ischaemic event in same year as treatment started	66	43
Chronic joint pain	66	43
Airways obstruction	53	34
Body Mass Index 30+	47	30
Recurrent depression or psychosis	46	30
Alcohol problem	35	23
Impaired renal function	31	20
Peptic ulcer	26	17
Diabetes	23	15
Gout	19	12
Impotence	20	13
None of these problems	4	3

* % of 130 in whom total blood cholesterol had been recorded.

Table 18.2: Eleven chronic problems complicating high blood pressure in 190 consecutive women, Glyncorrwg 1961–91 (including 113 deaths to July 1992); mean age at diagnosis is 60, mean BP 196/106 mmHg before treatment; problems are listed in descending order of prevalence.

Chronic problem	No.	%
Total cholesterol >6.6 mmol/l	51	50
Ischaemic event same year as treatment	84	44
Recurrent depression or psychosis	83	44
Body Mass Index 30+	81	43
Chronic joint pain	75	39
Airways obstruction	46	24
Diabetes	18	9
Impaired renal function	14	7
Alcohol problem	12	6
Gout	11	6
Peptic ulcer	10	5
None of these problems	14	7

* % of 102 in whom total blood cholesterol had been recorded.

High Blood Pressure with Hypercholesterolaemia and/or Obesity

Over half of all men and women in whom it was sought had blood total cholesterols at or over 6.6 mmol/l, the limit generally recommended for mandatory medical intervention. Thirty per cent of men and over 40% of women were seriously obese, with a BMI of 30 or more. There is a substantial overlap between these two groups.

Whether either or both of these problems coexist with high blood pressure, blood pressure should be tackled first because it is usually easier to treat. The patient needs to understand from the beginning that this is only part of the whole risk. Cholesterol control, and attainment of desirable body weight (BMI 25) which should be the first step in cholesterol control, are difficult for most people. If you are doing first what can usually be done most quickly and effectively then aim for blood pressure reduction using antihypertensive drugs. Full control is often not possible until weight has been substantially reduced, but partial control sufficient to promote motivation should not be difficult.

Antihypertensive drugs such as prazosin, which generally reduces total cholesterol, should be considered first in these patients. Anorectic drugs, which generally raise blood pressure, should never be used.

High Blood Pressure with Vascular Damage

Although these data came from a population repeatedly screened for high blood pressure for over 20 years, over 40% of hypertensive men and women had evidence of vascular damage by the time of detection or within the same year.

If blood pressure is still high after evident organ damage, treatment is obviously late, but rarely too late for it not to be worthwhile. The situation after a stroke may be bad, but will be worse still after another one. Tablet for tablet, antihypertensive drugs are more effective in those who already have vascular injuries than in those at high risk but without demonstrable organ damage. It is rarely justifiable to withold treatment because you think it is already too late.

It is particularly important in this group not to ignore high systolic pressures because of reassuring diastolic pressures. Those who have been taught that systolic hypertension is merely the result of arterial ageing need to consider whether there is anything 'mere' about prematurely old arteries. All the evidence is that control of isolated systolic hypertension is no less effective than when diastolic pressures are also raised.[2]

For patients with angina, beta-blocking and calcium–channel blocking drugs have independent effects, both on blood pressure and chest pain, and are obvious first choices. Angina generally improves when blood pressure is reduced, however this is achieved. Patients with peripheral arterial disease and claudication also usually have better perfusion, and therefore less leg pain, when blood pressure is reduced, despite theoretical predictions to the contrary. For patients with heart failure, diuretics and ACE inhibitors have independent effects, both on blood pressure and systemic perfusion, and are likewise obvious first choices.

High Blood Pressure with Chronic Musculoskeletal Pain

Around 40% of Glyncorrwg hypertensive patients had chronic back or joint pain requiring frequent analgesics. As all NSAIDs raise pressure by about 10 mmHg, probably because of sodium retention, they largely negate the effects of antihypertensive drugs. Their use for non-inflammatory joint pains and headache, although common, is not rational.

In 1991 I audited all 94 hypertensive patients in Glyncorrwg, for whom full prescribing histories were available for the previous 12 months; 23 (24%) had had NSAIDs from the practice during that year, plus an unknown number who may have bought them over the counter.

Clearly there is a problem of prescribing inertia on the part of doctors, demand inertia from patients, and, perhaps most importantly, system inertia from computers generating repeat prescriptions. Bad habits are now magnified and perpetuated by repeat prescribing systems, to which doctors' signatures become generally uncritical appendages, legally required but thoughtlessly applied.

The solution may be a much more aggressive educational approach to patients, spelling out the nonsense of taking one drug to put pressure down while continuing another which puts it up by an equal amount. Patients need to know that by far the best routine analgesic for most of them is paracetamol (US=acetominophen). This will not raise blood pressure, nor will it ever conflict with anticoagulant or thrombolytic therapy, both likely to be used in this risk group. For the small number of patients with rheumatoid or other truly inflammatory arthritis, the disadvantages but continued necessity of NSAIDs may have to be accepted.

High Blood Pressure with Airways Obstruction

One third of hypertensive men and a quarter of hypertensive women in Glyncorrwg had significant airways obstruction, with peak expiratory flow rates averaging 50% of the value predicted for age, sex, and height. We had measurements for all our patients since 1975 because recordings of peak expiratory flow rate before starting treatment with any antihypertensive drug had been practice policy since that time. Many latent asthmatics were detected in this way.

This complication is important for two reasons. First, these patients must never be prescribed beta-blocking drugs. Rapid, unexpected deaths occasionally occur in young asthmatics whose disease has never previously seemed severe or caused serious concern. A fall in peak expiratory flow rate after beta-blockade may be profound and lethal. Emergency treatment for airways obstruction consequent on beta-blockade is with intravenous salbutamol or isoprenaline plus intravenous glucagon.[3]

Secondly, airways obstruction, often compounded by obesity, is a much more important contributor to ill health than mortality rates for specific respiratory diseases suggest.[4] This is partly because chronic lung diseases of all kinds tend to cause long term gross impairment rather than early death, but also because they contribute to heart failure. Probably by the same route, impaired lung function is an important predictor for stroke.[5]

Obese patients with airways obstruction and high blood pressure have a package problem, of which blood pressure is only one component. By far the most important question is whether they still smoke, as about two-thirds of our hypertensive men still did at detection. If the answer is 'yes', and pre-treatment pressure is less than about 200/120 mmHg, stopping smoking is more necessary and urgent than blood pressure control, and should also have priority over weight loss, inevitably to some extent a conflicting objective. All this needs to be made clear to patients, who need to understand that the purpose of treatment is risk reduction, not treatment of disease. Unless they understand this, they are likely to accept antihypertensive drugs as apparently simpler alternatives to behavioural change, which is then indefinitely postponed.

High Blood Pressure with Recurrent Depression or Psychosis

In 30% of Glyncorrwg men and 44% of women management was complicated by major depression, psychosis, or serious behavioural disorder before their final illness.

As explained in Chapter 2, depression is probably one cause of hypertension, and blood pressure is likely to fall (although not necessarily to normal values) as depression lifts. As explained in Chapters 12, 16 and 17, virtually all antihypertensive drugs may exacerbate depression, and the diagnosis of hypertension must itself add to the problems weighing down on these patients. Unless blood pressure is very high, 200/120 mmHg or more, it is almost always best to get depression under control first, before starting any antihypertensive medication. When medication does start, it will probably have to be added to antidepressant drugs. An ACE inhibitor combined with a diuretic is probably least likely to precipitate another depressive episode.

Assumptions about who will cope with antihypertensive treatment are so often wrong that it seems unwise to make judgements of this kind in any but the most extreme cases. Given reasonable professional support, in my experience most schizophrenics become accustomed to disciplined self-medication, and other people with long standing brain dysfunction also lead orderly lives as a condition for their survival. Both may therefore be exceptionally compliant patients. Even patients with major behavioural disorders may be easier to handle sympathetically when they are receiving treatment for a recognized physical disorder.

High Blood Pressure with Alcohol Problems

Almost a quarter of our hypertensive men and 6% of the women had present or past major alcohol problems, defined as intakes entailing high risk of liver damage, major alcohol related problems at home or at work, or objective evidence such as raised gamma GT or mean corpuscular volume. Although these objective indicators can be very important, particularly by giving feedback on improved health when drinking is reduced, the main way to find alcohol problems is simply to ask all patients at their first diagnostic assessment how much they drink each typical week, taking one day at a time from Monday to Sunday.

The known link between blood pressure and high alcohol intake needs to be spelled out for these patients, and distinguished from the entirely different link between cigarettes and mortality risk. Drinking less will usually reduce blood pressure, often enough to avoid antihypertensive medication. This is not true of smoking.

Where such routine questioning has not been done from the beginning, alcohol problems are likely to present as refractory hypertension.

High Blood Pressure with Impaired Renal Function

In the Glyncorrwg series, 20% of the hypertensive men and 7% of the women had impaired renal function (blood urea and creatinine concentrations both raised) some time during their management, mostly during their last years.

Raised blood pressure alone is hardly ever the cause of renal failure, but whatever the cause, the most important step in conserving renal function is assiduous control of blood pressure, aiming for target pressures around 150/70 mmHg.

Choice of medication is obviously limited, depending on degree of renal impairment. Residual function can be measured easily in general practice by estimating creatinine clearance, the technique for which is given in Appendix 8. Thiazide diuretics are ineffective in patients with less than 20% renal function[6] and can precipitate total renal failure. Spironolactone and other potassium conserving diuretics cannot be used because of the risk of hyperkalaemia. Frusemide is a safe alternative.

Beta-blockers, alpha-blockers, and calcium-channel blockers can all be used safely despite impaired renal function. ACE inhibitors are cleared through the kidney, and are therefore cumulative in renal failure unless the dose is reduced. They may reduce renal perfusion and thus exacerbate renal failure. All patients with seriously impaired renal function should be referred to the regional dialysis unit long before any question of dialysis arises, for assessment, advice on management, patient education on low protein diet,[7] and for subsequent monitoring, usually on an annual basis. With painstaking management of blood pressure and low protein diet, few ultimately need dialysis.

Steps must be taken to protect these patients from other drugs that can precipite gross renal failure in patients with relatively minor renal impairment. Tetracycline antibiotics are common offenders.

High Blood Pressure with Peptic Ulcer

Peptic ulcers were found in 17% of Glyncorrwg hypertensive men and 5% of the women, either before or after detection of high blood pressure. They are important mainly because they are a relative contraindication to use of aspirin or anticoagulants, both of which are ultimately needed by many hypertensive patients. Where there is also a history of gastroduodenal bleeding the contraindication is absolute. Records need to be labelled and, more importantly, patients need to be educated in the nature of this risk.

Cimetidine, but not ranitidine, interacts with anticoagulants.

High Blood Pressure with Diabetes

Diabetes coexisted with high blood pressure in 15% of Glyncorrwg men with hypertension and 7% of the women, nearly all were diagnosed as non-insulin dependent. The prevalence of diabetes is rising: because it is detected sooner, because populations are ageing (a 40% increase in diabetes is predicted in The Netherlands between 1990 and 2005 for this reason alone[8]), and because Indian and other south Asian migrants are much more prone to diabetes than Europeans.[9, 10]

In the UK today, no diabetic should die either directly from diabetes (ketoacidotic coma) or from its treatment (hypoglycaemic coma). Very few should now lose legs or feet from gangrene or leg ulcers, both of which have become less common as diabetics become better educated as to the nature of their disorder, and accurately supported in its management. Instead, most will now die from the macrovascular complications of diabetes,[11] coronary disease, stroke, and aortic embolism, and from microvascular renal damage. Long before death, they are likely to be impaired by erectile failure and retinal damage.

Both microvascular and macrovascular consequences can either be prevented or delayed by assiduous control of blood glucose,[12–14] monitored by glycosylated haemoglobin (HbA_1c) or fructosamine, and by assiduous control of blood pressure from a diastolic threshold of 90 mmHg at most.

By the time microvascular renal damage is detectable as more than trace proteinuria, it is already relentlessly progressive.[15] However, the rate of decline is critically dependent on blood pressure, throughout its range.[16–18]

It is hard to overstress the importance of good blood pressure control in these patients, and both practice staff and patients need to be continually reminded that resolute control, however difficult, is easier than the ultimate alternative, dialysis or transplant. This message should be easier to transmit in community care than in hospital practice, because patients are known personally and motivation should therefore be easier. If routine general practitioner care of diabetics still compares badly with routine hospital care,[19] routines must be changed. Diabetics need to be recognized as the group at highest risk of coronary disease, stroke, and all the consequences of hypertension, who could benefit most from diligent care. One of the most important aspects of their management, a high carbohydrate, low fat, leguminous diet[20], is equally appropriate for all hypertensive patients; in fact so much of the continuing care of diabetics overlaps with care of hypertensives that in Glyncorrwg we merged the two clinics.

Used with care in the presence of even minimal renal failure, ACE inhibitors are of proven value in conserving diabetic renal function, even after proteinuria becomes measurable.[21] Beta-blockers may mask hypoglycaemic symptoms in diabetics, and are therefore best avoided. All diuretics tend to impair glucose tolerance after 2 or 3 years.[22] There is persuasive evidence that iatrogenic impairment from this cause is substantial, with a possible sixfold increase in the incidence of diabetes for hypertensives treated with thiazides compared with controls.[23] However, it is virtually impossible to avoid their use altogether. The most important practical step is to keep dosage to a minimum in all cases, not only in diabetics. Frusemide can precipitate ketoacidotic coma in insulin-dependent diabetics and should be used cautiously, if at all, outside hospital.

Microvascular retinal damage is associated with increased retinal vascular perfusion,[24] independently promoted both by raised blood glucose and by raised blood pressure.[25–27] Like diabetic nephropathy, prevention and control of diabetic retinopathy probably depend on careful control of blood pressure.

Autonomic neuropathy is common in diabetics, so it is worth measuring standing as well as seated blood pressure routinely. If standing pressure is substantially lower than seated pressure, it should be used for all monitoring thereafter.

High Blood Pressure with Gout

Gout complicated treatment in 12% of Glyncorrwg hyptertensive men and 6% of women. Much of this was caused by thiazide diuretics, often in excessive dosage. When episodes of gout continue with low doses of thiazides, allopurinol must be added to the medication list.

Others were caused by continued high alcohol intake; use of allopurinol for these patients should be avoided if possible, as an acutely painful toe is surely a useful message to the patient, which we should not interrupt.

High Blood Pressure with Impotence

Erectile failure was recognized in 13% of Glyncorrwg hypertensive men; the true prevalence was probably at least 50% more. Although many of these will be consequences of depression, marriage failure and/or alcohol, vascular causes are common, particularly in diabetics.

It is important to ask all male patients about this before starting antihypertensive drugs, so that a clear baseline is established, and the possibility of impotence caused by antihypertensive medication can be more easily recognized. Virtually all such drugs have been incriminated, although thiazide diuretics carry the highest risk. In all cases, the effect is reversible. The possibility and reversibility of this side effect should be mentioned before drugs are prescribed.

By middle age, many couples adjust surprisingly well to this situation, or claim to do so. Where morning erections still occur, skilled advice from an experienced marriage counsellor is likely to be helpful; addresses are available from the Family Planning Association. Where morning erections are absent, referral for an internal erectile prosthesis should be considered. For many diabetics these are very successful.

Hypertensive Emergencies

In the UK at least, virtually all hypertensive emergencies will be admitted to hospital, and transferred to the care of hospital physicians. Initial treatment decisions will usually be taken by junior staff. However, antihypertensive treatment should usually be initiated before admission, unless this is likely to cause further delay.

In the present understaffed and overworked state of most hospitals, safe transfer of responsibility depends more than ever on a well documented history, much easier if this is computer-held. This should include representative values for blood pressure and other baseline measurements over several years, a full account of recent medication and of whatever may have been tried and failed, a brief account of major complicating factors both clinical and social, and enough interest to telephone the next day to ensure that all these messages have been effectively received.

Evidence even of the most transient cerebrovascular damage makes blood pressure control extremely urgent, as such damage can never be assumed to be fully reversible. Distinction between hypertensive encephalopathy (reversible) and stroke (irreverisble) is difficult even with full hospital resources, and impossible outside hospital. There may be good arguments for keeping most non-hypertensive (or controlled hypertensive) stroke patients at home, at least for the first 24 hours. There is little evidence that any medical interventions, in hospital or out, are of value during this time; CT scans are unreliable in the first 2 or 3 days. Survival depends on good nursing (which should be available from the home nursing service), and the nature and extent of the brain lesion. Sensible decisions can be taken the following day, when it should be easier to see what is probable or possible.

This is not true of stroke with uncontrolled hypertension. Blood pressure must then be reduced urgently, with hourly charting and frequent control of medication which would be difficult or impossible at home. Uncontrolled hypertension with stroke in a conscious patient is an indication for immediate admission.

Similar arguments apply to left ventricular failure associated with high blood pressure, and to unstable angina. ECG evidence of infarction often lags behind pathology, about 20% of even major infarctions are painless, and dangerous arrhythmias are likely at any time within the first few days. Left ventricular failure associated with high blood pressure should be assumed to indicate present or impending myocardial infarction until proved otherwise. Such proof depends on evolving evidence from ECGs and enzymes, available only in hospital and therefore outside the scope of most UK family doctors. Except in elderly patients who specifically request home care, in full knowledge of consequent absence of good facilities for resuscitation, home care of these conditions is now obsolete.

This does not mean that initial domiciliary management of suspected coronary thrombosis is unimportant. Early and effective control of pain and anxiety are essential, and can greatly reduce the risk of subsequent complications, including arrhythmias. We now have good controlled evidence, not only that early thrombolytic treatment can almost halve the 3-month mortality of myocardial infarction, but that well organized family doctors can deliver this to 61% of patients within 2 hours of the onset of symptoms, compared with only 1% for specialists or their junior staff initiating thrombolysis after admission to hospital.[28]

In all hypertensive emergencies, diastolic pressure should be reduced to below 90 mmHg, if possible further, within 24 hours, but not within 24 minutes. Rapid but safe reduction of blood pressure depends on not exceeding the rate at which autoregulation of brain perfusion can adapt.[29, 30] This in turn depends on age, level of untreated pressure, and how long this has been sustained; older people, and those who have had very high pressures for years rather than months, are more vulnerable to rapid falls in pressure.

Low dose aspirin, 300 mg daily or thereabouts, will reduce platelet aggregation and reduce net mortality risk by at least 15% in all four groups: malignant hypertension, stroke,[31] myocardial infarction, and unstable angina,[32] and should be started in all patients with very high uncontrolled pressure, unstable or prolonged angina, or transient cerebral ischaemic attacks, unless potential benefits appear outweighed by a history of serious gastrointestinal bleeding, or suspected cerebral haemorrhage.

In myocardial infarction, the benefits of early aspirin and thrombolytic treatment with streptokinase are additive.[33] There is no evidence yet on whether this is true also for anistreplase, which, unlike streptokinase, can be given before hospital admission by slow intravenous injection over 5 minutes. In stroke, the small increase in mortality from haemorrhagic stroke is far outweighed by reduction in mortality from thrombotic stroke, which is much commoner. The two types of stroke cannot be reliably distinguished without a CT scan, and on present evidence net benefit from early aspirin treatment probably should not be delayed to make this distinction, at least while less than half of all health districts in England and Wales have scanning facilities available.[34]

These conclusions are based on studies which excluded people with a clear history of peptic ulcer, present in 17% of hypertensive men in Table 18.1. Even very low doses of aspirin promote both gastrointestinal ulceration and bleeding, an effect which seems not to be dose dependent. This injury seems to be prevented by enteric coating,[35] although this will delay effects on platelet aggregation, which are measurable within 5 minutes of an oral dose of uncoated aspirin.[36]

To initiate rapid but safe control of blood pressure in the presence of apparent cerebrovascular or retinal damage, GPs should use whatever antihypertensive medication they are most familiar with, other than ACE inhibitors. As hypertensive emergencies must by definition entail a possibility of new renal damage of unknown extent, ACE inhibitors should not be started for the first time in such circumstances.

All the commonly used antihypertensive drugs except ACE inhibitors have at one time or another been commonly used in hospitals for hypertensive emergencies, and none seem to have such outstanding advantages as to make any of them a best choice for anyone with little experience in their use.

For left ventricular failure, with or without chest pain or other evidence of infarction, intravenous morphine or diamorphine is still the most rapidly effective initial treatment, not only giving quick relief of dyspnoea, but also often reducing blood pressure substantially. Other antihypertensive medication can then be given after response to morphine has been assessed. Morphine is safe providing the injection is given slowly, and previous airways obstruction can be excluded. Such exclusion may be difficult or impossible in a patient seen for the first time, or in unfamiliar patients seen without their records, although the patient's partner or family will know if the patient has often suffered a bad chest. As Tables 18.1 and 18.2 show, serious airways obstruction is common. Even small doses of morphine may be fatal in asthmatics.

The next step in acute heart failure is normally injection of a loop diuretic such as frusemide. Although ACE inhibitors are very effective for heart failure itself, apart from their hypotensive effect, the temptation to use one before transfer to hospital should be resisted; combination of ACE inhibition with a loop diuretic may lead to a catastrophic fall in pressure, with collapse and/or renal failure.

References

1. Westervelt FB and Atuk NO (1974) Methyldopa-induced hypertension. *JAMA* **227**: 557.

2. SHEP Cooperative Research Group (1991) Prevention of stroke by antihypertensive drug treatment in older persons with isolated systolic hypertension. *JAMA* **265**: 3255–64.

3. Harries AD (1981) Beta-blockade in asthma. *Br Med J* **282**: 1321.

4. Carpenter, L, Beral V, Strachan D *et al.* (1989) Respiratory symptoms as predictors of 27-year mortality in a representative sample of British adults. *Br Med J* **299**: 357–61.

5. Strachan DP (1991) Ventilatory function as a predictor of fatal stroke. *Br Med J* **302**: 84–7.

6. Reubi FC and Cottier PT (1961) Effect of reduced glomerular filtration rate on responsiveness to chlorothiazide and mercurial diuretics. *Circulation* **23**: 200–10.

7. Locatelli F, Alberti D, Graziani G *et al.* (1991) Prospective, randomised, multicentre trial of effect of protein restriction on progression of chronic renal insufficiency. *Lancet* **337**: 1299–304.

8. (1992) Diabetes practice: The information gap [editorial]. *Lancet* **339**: 97–8.

9. Simmons S, Williams DRR and Powell MJ (1989) Prevalence of diabetes in a predominantly Asian community: Preliminary findings of the Coventry diabetes study. *Br Med J* **298**: 18–20.

10. McKeigue PM, Shah B and Marmot MG (1991) Relation of central obesity and insulin resistance with high diabetes prevalence and cardiovascular risk in south Asians. *Lancet* **337**: 382–6.

11. Rosengren A, Welin L, Tsipogianni A *et al.* (1989) Impact of cardiovascular risk factors on coronary heart disease and mortality among middle aged diabetic men: A general population study. *Br Med J* **299**: 1127–31.

12. Chazan BI, Balodimos MC, Ryan JR *et al.* (1970) Twenty-five to 45 years of diabetes with and without vascular complications. *Diabetologia* **6**: 565–9.

13. McCance DR, Hadden DR, Atkinson AB *et al.* (1989) Long-term glycaemic control and diabetic retinopathy. *Lancet* ii: 824–7.

14. Brinchmann-Hansen O, Dahl-Jorgensen K, Sandvik L *et al.* (1992) Blood glucose concentrations and progression of diabetic retinopathy: The seven year results of the Oslo study. *Br Med J* **304**: 19–22.

15. Viberti GC, Jarrett RJ, Keen H (1982) Microalbuminuria as a predictor of clinical nephropathy in insulin-dependent diabetes mellitus. *Lancet* i: 1430–2.

16. Parving HH, Smidt U, Anderson AR *et al.* (1983) Early aggressive antihypertensive treatment reduces rate of decline in kidney function in diabetic nephropathy. *Lancet* i: 1175–8.

17. Parving HH and Hommel E (1989) Prognosis in diabetic nephropathy. *Br Med J* **299**: 230–2.

18. Parving HH, Hommel E, Nielsen MD *et al.* (1989) Effect of captopril on blood pressure and kidney function in normotensive insulin dependent diabetics with nephropathy. *Br Med J* **299**: 533–6.

19. Hayes TM and Harries J (1984) Randomised controlled trial of routine hospital clinic care versus routine general practice care for type II diabetes. *Br Med J* **289**: 728–30.

20. Mann JI (1981) A high carbohydrate leguminous fibre diet improves all aspects of diabetic control. *Lancet* i: 1–5.

21. Bjorck S, Mulec H, Johnsen SA *et al.* (1992) Renal protective effect of enalapril in diabetic nephropathy. *Br Med J* **304**: 339–43.

22. Murphy MB, Lewis PJ, Kohner E *et al.* (1982) Glucose intolerance in hypertensive patients treated with diuretics: A 14-year follow up. *Lancet* ii: 1293–5.

23. Bruce R, Stevenson JC, Oliver MF *et al.* (1990) Thiazide diuretics, beta-blockers, and coronary heart disease. *Lancet* **335**: 1534–5.

24. Patel V, Rassam S, Newsom R *et al.* (1992) Retinal blood flow in diabetic retinopathy. *Br Med J* **305**: 678–83.

25. Knowler, WC, Bennett PH and Ballintine EJ (1980) Increased incidence of retinopathy in diabetics with elevated blood pressure. *N Engl J Med* **302**: 645–50.

26. Klein R, Klein BEK, Moss SE *et al.* (1984) The Wisconsin epidemiological study of diabetic retinopathy. II: Prevalence and risk of diabetic retinopathy when age at diagnosis is less than 30 years. *Arch Ophthalmol* **12**: 520–6.

27. Klein R, Klein BEK, Moss SE *et al.* (1984) The Wisconsin epidemiological study of diabetic retinopathy. III: Prevalence and risk of diabetic retinopathy when age at diagnosis is 30 or more years. *Arch Ophthalmol* **12**: 527–32.

28. GREAT group (1992) Feasibility, safety, and efficacy of domiciliary thrombolysis by general practitioners: Grampian region early anistreplase trial. *Br Med J* **305**: 548–53.

29. Wollner L, McCarthy ST, Soper NDW *et al.* (1979) Failure of cerebral autoregulation as a cause of brain dysfunction in the elderly. *Br Med J* **ii**: 1117–18.

30. Mitchinson MJ (1980) The hypotensive stroke. *Lancet* **i**: 244–6.

31. SALT Collaborative Group (1991) Swedish Aspirin Low-dose Trial (SALT) of 75 mg aspirin as secondary prophylaxis after cerebrovascular ischaemic events. *Lancet* **338**: 1345–9.

32. RISC Group (1990) Risk of myocardial infarction and death during treatment with low dose aspirin and intravenous heparin in men with unstable coronary artery disease. *Lancet* **336**: 827–30.

33. ISIS–2 (Second International Study of Infarct Survival) Collaborative Group (1988) Randomised trial of intravenous streptokinase, oral aspirin, both, or neither among 17187 cases of suspected acute myocardial infarction: ISIS–2. *Lancet* **ii**: 349–60.

34. Sandercock P (1988) Aspirin for strokes and transient ischaemic attacks: No panacea. *Br Med J* **297**: 995–6.

35. Murray FE, Cole AT, Hudson N *et al.* (1992) Possible low-dose-aspirin-induced gastropathy. *Lancet* **339**: 1058–9.

36. Carpenter AL and Carvalho J (1990) Early public use of aspirin in the face of probable ischaemic chest pain. *Lancet* **335**: 163.

19

High Blood Pressure in Childhood and Adolescence, and the Origins of Adult Disease in Childhood

Measurement of blood pressure in childhood ■ Immediately serious hypertension in childhood ■ Should primary high blood pressure in childhood be treated? ■ Possible childhood origins of adult high blood pressure ■ Can adult hypertension be prevented by control of obesity in childhood? ■ Can adult hypertension be prevented by control of dietary sodium in childhood?

This chapter deals with three important themes: how not to miss the once in a lifetime case of immediately serious, almost always secondary, hypertension in childhood; what to do about children with blood pressures relatively high for their age group, virtually all primary, without immediate risk; and what to do about possible origins of adult hypertension in childhood. As before, we are discussing detection and management in general practice. Availability of skilled back-up by hospital based specialists is assumed.

Measurement of Blood Pressure in Childhood

The considerable difficulties of guaranteeing accurate and representative measurement of arterial pressure in adults are much greater in childhood[1]. A full range of child-size cuffs is essential, which means at least three different sizes to cover the age range 5–15 years. Table 19.1 shows the cuff sizes proposed by a WHO expert committee[2].

Table 19.1: Appropriate cuff sizes for various applications proposed by a WHO expert committee.

Subject	Bladder width (cm)	Bladder length (cm)
Newborns	2.5–4.0	5.0–10.0
Infants	6.0–8.0	12.0–13.5
Children	9.0–10.0	17.0–22.5

Under 4 years of age a Doppler ultrasound recorder with earphones and an acoustic head are essential to pick up a systolic signal, and diastolic pressure cannot be reliably measured at all. Measurement of blood pressure under 5 years is a research exercise requiring special training and experience. Although there is every reason why GPs interested in longitudinal population studies should undertake this work, it has no meaningful connection with current clinical practice.

In Glyncorrwg our research team recorded systolic pressures monthly in a cohort of infants and followed them annually from 1977 for 10 years. We confirmed what everyone else working in this field already knew: blood pressure in infancy and childhood is far more variable than in adults, so that many more readings have to be taken to characterize an individual as ranking high or low in a population distribution. Artefacts related mainly to cuff size and method of picking up the systolic signal can introduce huge measurement errors, and children examined in schools are subject to very large effects from apprehension which may not be obvious. For example, I examined 15 11-year-old children in the last school clinic we held. None were in an obviously distressed state. Three had diastolic pressures over 90 mmHg confirmed by two replicate readings, using a random zero sphygmomanometer. We followed them up at the health centre a week later with the results given in Table 19.2.

Table 19.2: Means of two blood pressure recordings in three primary schoolchildren.

Mean school reading (mmHg)	Follow-up health centre reading (mmHg)
158/126	108/56
137/105	108/54
154/94	90/56

A further problem complicating clinical measurements of blood pressure in later childhood is that normal blood pressure relates to stature more than to age[3]. Children in any given age band show a wider dispersion of stature (weight for height; BMI is not an appropriate measure for children) than adults, because they vary so much in development. Around the time of the adolescent growth spurt, usually between the ages of 12 and 17, children change so dramatically that ranking for blood pressure is absurd unless development is taken into account as well as stature.

Immediately Serious Hypertension in Childhood

A sustained blood pressure of say 145/95 mmHg in a child of 12 is unusual enough to require careful follow-up and some elementary investigations, but is not a medical emergency. Unless it is found to rise higher over the next few days or weeks, it is not in the category considered here. Alarm bells should ring for children at roughly the same thresholds as for adults; systolic pressures over 200 mmHg and diastolic pressures over 120 mmHg require intensive follow-up and urgent control within days, not weeks.

Clinical hypertension in childhood is almost always secondary hypertension; primary ('essential') hypertension probably begins in childhood or adolescence, but is not then a clinical problem[4]. Of children with a sustained diastolic pressure >120 mmHg, 95% have an identifiable cause of secondary hypertension[5]. Secondary hypertension in childhood is overwhelmingly renal: acute glomerulonephritis, renin secreting tumours, renal malformations already approaching end-stage renal failure, occasionally nephroblastoma (Wilms' tumour), though this usually presents as a mass in the flank rather than as raised blood pressure alone.

Coarctation of the aorta usually presents during the first year of life, but children who survive to the second year without symptoms generally seem healthy, and tend to be picked up from investigation of a systolic murmur. Blood pressure is not necessarily very high; it is the difference between arm and leg pressures which is important.

Headache is a common symptom in childhood. It is usually migrainous, often accompanied, or for several years preceded by, spells of abdominal pain. Pallor during the attack is usual, and initial visual spectra are frequently present if asked for, although children hardly ever describe these on their own initiative. Even with a classic history of migraine (a symptom rather than a disease) all children complaining of headache should have a careful examination of both optic fundi (nearly always easy with large pupils of childhood), and all should have their blood pressure measured.

Unfortunately these elementary rules are often ignored in practice, sometimes because no dark area has been made available for fundoscopy, although all this usually needs is imagination and a tin of blackboard paint. Although dangerously high blood pressure in childhood is rare, when it does occur it seems usually to be overlooked until organ damage is already advanced, and often irreversible. Three children aged 11–12 admitted to the Hospital for Sick Children at Great Ormond Street with neurovascular damage were found to have previously unrecorded blood pressures of 270/180, 280/190 and 190/110 mmHg at 10 weeks, 9 months and 4 years respectively after their first presentation with morning headache[6]. Two became permanently blind, one was left with permanent gross visual field defects, and one became paraplegic. All had renal hypertension.

Should Primary High Blood Pressure in Childhood be Treated?

The report of the United States Task Force on childhood hypertension[7] suggested that infants and children with sustained blood pressures above the 95th centile for age required a complete medical history and examination to determine the cause and to develop an appropriate follow-up programme. As blood pressure in childhood is such an unstable measurement, huge populations are required to establish what these centile values are. Ironically, the figures were finally determined, not by studies in the USA, but by a multicentre study in Cuba, former East Germany, Hungary and the former USSR[3]. 95th centile thresholds are shown in Table 19.3.

Table 19.3: 95th centile values for raised blood pressure by age.

Age group	Threshold (mmHg)
Boys and girls 12–14	130/80
Boys 15–16	140/85
Girls 15–16	135/80
Values must be replicated on at least three occasions on separate days	

In American clinical practice, experts in this field suggested[8] that these children be considered:

'. . . legitimate candidates for sustained drug treatment. . . . There is some preliminary information from studies with certain pharmacologic agents over the course of 5–7 years that major adverse effects due to these drugs are generally uncommon. That is not to say that adverse reactions do not occur in this population, but to indicate that the incidence and effects noted do not differ significantly from those observed in adults.'

That such a suggestion could be put forward seriously in our present state of ignorance (little has changed since 1981) seems extraordinary. Nothing is more dangerous than aggressive, underemployed specialists with potent drugs, an available patient and a rational strategy, lacking only the empirical evidence of randomized trials which are the only conceivable justification for treatment. A 20-year follow-up of young Czechs, aged 14–26 with arterial pressures at or over 170/100 mmHg and not treated, showed that only 17% had progressed to higher pressures, none had retinopathy, and one-third had diastolic pressures <90 mmHg[9].

The USA Task Force report stimulated detection programmes of some kind in school medical services in many parts of Britain, presumably leading to referrals to district hospital paediatricians for investigation and assessment. Very few of these will have had clinically severe high blood pressure (nearly all secondary) which could be controlled by antihypertensive drugs with ultimate benefit to the

281

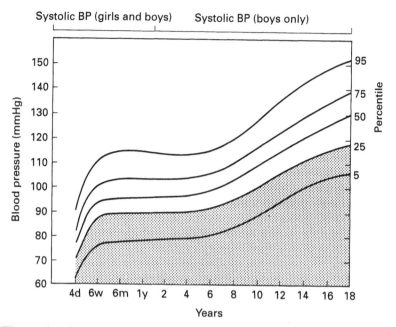

Figure 19.1: Centile distribution of blood pressure from birth to 18 years. Derived from measurements up to 12 months at the Brompton Hospital, London[10] and from 18 months onwards from centres in Miami, Muscatine and Rochester, USA[11].

patient. By 'severe', I mean severe in terms of adult ranges of pressure. Nearly all 'cases' found will have been children with more or less stable primary high blood pressure, but 'high' in the relative sense of centile deviance from their age group.

The truth is that we simply do not have the evidence to justify any programme of long term medication for any of these children. Weight reduction and perhaps reduction in dietary sodium are the only interventions likely to help them. These are probably best organized on a group rather than an individual basis, because children will only change their behaviour if they have group support. To tell these children and their parents that they are at high risk would, on present evidence, be untrue and irresponsible. There is in any case no need for this, since control of obesity and reduction of sodium load are justifiable targets in their own right.

Figure 19.1 shows a centile distribution for boys and girls from 4 days to 18 years old.

This chart is only a rough guide, because it does not allow for differences in stature and development, and because, even with the greatest care, different research programmes on similar populations show as much as 10 mmHg difference between the same centile lines for systolic and diastolic pressures[11].

Possible Childhood Origins of Adult High Blood Pressure

High ranking for blood pressure in infancy tends to be associated with high ranking for blood pressure years or decades later, the phenomenon known as 'tracking'. This is hardly surprising, because most other characteristics also show tracking: weight for height, skinfold thickness, airways reactivity, reading proficiency, or aggressive personality. Blood pressure increases with age throughout childhood, and is also closely associated with growth (represented by height), obesity (represented by weight for height and skinfold thickness), and development (represented by Tanner sexual development staging)[12]. Since rankings for height and obesity do not vary randomly between periodic measurements in a cohort (and we would be very surprised if they did), why should we not expect blood pressure to behave this way also?

Stability of ranking for blood pressure in a cohort could be represented in two ways; as an expected tendency for successive rankings to resemble one another, or as an unexpected tendency for successive rankings to differ. Both tendencies are important, and both are obscured by the true variability of blood pressure around its mean value, and by immense measurement difficulties, particularly in young children.

All this must be said because, although the idea that adult high blood pressure begins in childhood is strategically important and biologically plausible, it is not necessarily true. Even if it is true, origins in childhood do not exclude critical influences at later stages of growth and physiological adaptation. There are other nodal points in development, notably adolescence and the early reproductive years, which are no less likely as starting points for the development of high blood pressure. There is also the possibility of cumulative maladaption to sustained environmental pressures of many kinds. None of these possibilities exclude others. Almost the only thing we can be sure of is that high blood pressure rarely begins in the age group in which it is usually recognized, from 40–65, although even here there are surprises, with rapid individual rises in pressure over a few years for no obvious reason.

Longitudinal studies of blood pressure and other risk factors for coronary disease have been made in cohorts of children in Britain[10, 13], in The Netherlands following early initiatives by de Haas[14], and in the USA in Boston[15] and in the Bogalusa study in Louisiana[16], a sort of childhood Framingham. The USA and West European studies have been reviewed by Labarthe[17]. Another multicentre longitudinal study of 19 000 children born in 1964 began in Budapest, Moscow, Kaunas (Lithuania), East Berlin, Havana, and Ulan Bator (Mongolia) in 1975[18].

Studies in Dunedin, New Zealand[19] are of particular interest because they measured socioeconomic correlates of blood pressure in a cohort of more than 1000 children at birth, and at 3 and 7 years of age. Surprisingly, no associations were found with socioeconomic status, maternal intelligence, maternal or paternal education, breast feeding, or language development or observed behaviour in the child. Several USA studies have shown that the divergence between blacks and whites, which is a social as well as racial difference, develops only after 7 or 8 years of age, and really spreads out during and after adolescence.

All these studies show tracking of blood pressure, increasing from unimpressive correlation coefficients of 0.2–0.3 at 2 years to adult correlations by age 20. Zinner, for example, found that 65% of children with initial systolic pressures more than one standard deviation above the mean and 70% of children with initial systolic pressures more than one standard deviation below the mean remained in the same rank 4 years later[15].

Studies of blood pressure in over 4000 randomly sampled children aged 5–7 in the nine towns of the British Regional Heart Study showed that children share the same geographical (and essentially social) distribution of blood pressure as their parents, with higher mean population pressures and much higher adult cardiovascular mortality in industrial than affluent residential areas[20].

A succession of important papers from David Barker has explored connections between prenatal and infant growth and adult blood pressure, glucose tolerance, fibrinogen and Factor VII levels, coronary heart disease and airways obstruction[21–28]. These studies deploy impressive evidence that impaired growth during gestation and the first year of life is a critical determinant of all these variables in middle aged adults. Correlation of blood pressure with birth weight has been confirmed in 5–7 year-old children by other studies[29].

As impaired fetal and infant growth have always been associated with poverty, the next obvious step is to link this evidence with social class data. David Barker has done this, and claims that the effect he has found is independent of social class. This may well be true, if by social class we simply mean the rather clumsy categories used by the Registrar General for mortality analyses since before the First World War, but I find this unconvincing. Many other studies have confirmed that mortality from all causes, and from most specific causes, is more closely related to income than to social class; this does not mean that social class is unimportant, but that income is a better measure of it than the Registrar General's categories. Poverty, and the social dislocation and powerlessness it entails, seem to be bad for all human development[30], and are no doubt more damaging to growing children than to grown adults. The exact biological pathways through which they operate are of interest, but, like contaminated water supplies in the 19th century, we need not wait to understand all of them before taking action against some of them.

Can Adult Hypertension be Prevented by Control of Obesity in Childhood?

All cross-sectional studies show an association between obesity and blood pressure in childhood. The effect of weight is independent of age and height[31]. White

American children in the upper third of the distribution of blood pressure are about 15 kg heavier than those in the bottom third, and 1 hour after an oral glucose load their blood glucose is about 0.82 mmol/l (15 mg/dl) higher. After controlling for weight, there is still an independent association of blood pressure with blood glucose, particularly in children with evidence of peripheral insulin resistance. These associations may be smaller in black children.

Several controlled intervention studies are under way in different parts of the world to test the hypothesis that control of obesity in childhood may prevent later onset of hypertension. The short term results so far available suggest that both blood pressure and blood cholesterol fall in intervention groups, and it is reasonable to suppose that this could eventually lead to a substantial fall in coronary and stroke risk. As both high blood pressure and obesity are strongly inherited, we cannot assume that obesity control will necessarily have the full effect we hope for, but it is certainly reasonable to act now on the assumption that it will.

Can Adult Hypertension be Prevented by Control of Dietary Sodium in Childhood?

Although rigorously designed and carefully performed studies in young teenage children have failed to show any significant association between urinary sodium output (the only way to measure intake) and blood pressure[32], a small positive association has been shown in infants[33]. Average North American and West European diets contain far more sodium than is necessary, and big reductions are probably possible if undertaken slowly. It is still likely, despite the weakness of experimental evidence so far available, that excess dietary sodium sustained over years rather than weeks interacts with genetic factors as the principal cause of primary hypertension. If this is so, it is also likely that this effect occurs mainly in childhood, and may be more easily reversible at that time by reduction in sodium load.

Where such a reduction can be made easily, without obstructing other measures for which there is better experimental support (reduction in dietary fat, for example), it should certainly be done. Contrary to most of our assumptions, snack foods and added table salt have not accounted for most teenage sodium intake in studies so far available. Table 19.4 shows the percentage distribution of various sources of dietary sodium in the diet of 200 USA high school students aged 15–17, with an average daily sodium intake of 170 mmol for boys and 110 mmol for girls[34]. This reflects USA eating patterns, in which bottled sauces largely replace added table salt, but it emphasizes the large contribution from bread and other cereal products. As these form a large part of most fibre–rich diets, there is potential conflict between fibre promotion and sodium reduction.

The most important contribution to reduced sodium load in childhood would be a return to free school meals with planned menus aimed at a realistic compromise between teenage tastes (which may change) and health needs.

Table 19.4: Percentage distribution of various sources of sodium in adolescent diets in the USA

Food group	% of total sodium intake
Cereals	30
Meat, fish, eggs	21
Sauces, dressings, etc	19
Fruit and vegetables	16
Snack foods	6
Added table salt	<1
Other	7

References

1. de Swiet M, Dillon MJ, Littler W *et al.* (1989) Measurement of blood pressure in children. *Br Med J* **299**: 497.

2. World Health Organization (1978) *Arterial hypertension.* Technical Report series 628. WHO, Geneva.

3. International Collaborative Group (1987) *International collaborative study on juvenile hypertension.* Hungarian Institute of Cardiology, Budapest.

4. de Swiet M and Dillon MJ (1989) Hypertension in children. *Br Med J* **299**: 469–70.

5. Still L and Cottom D (1967) Severe hypertension in childhood. *Arch Dis Child* **43**: 34–9.

6. Hulse JA, Taylor DSI and Dillon MJ (1979) Blindness and paraplegia in severe childhood hypertension. *Lancet* **ii**: 553–6.

7. Blumenthal S, Epps RP, Heavenrich R *et al.* (1977) Report of the National Heart, Lung and Blood Institutes Task Force on blood pressure control in children. *Paediatrics* **59**: 797–820.

8. Kotchen JM and Kotchen TA (1981) Correlates of high blood pressure in adolescents. In: Onesti G and Kim KE (eds) *Hypertension in the young and the old.* Grune and Stratton, New York.

9. Widimsky J and Jandova R (1980) Long term prognosis in juvenile hypertension: Condition after 20 and 28 years. *Cas Lek Cesk* **119**: 1185.

10. de Swiet M, Fayers P and Shinebourne EA (1980) Value of repeated blood pressure measurements in children: The Brompton study. *Br Med J* i: 1567–9.

11. Berenson GS, Voors AV and Webber LS (1981) Hypertension in the young: Measurement and criteria. In: Onesti G and Kim KE (eds) *Hypertension in the young and the old*. Grune and Stratton, New York.

12. Tanner JM (1962) *Growth at adolescence*. Blackwell, London.

13. Darby SC and Fearn T (1979) The Chatham blood pressure study: An application of Bayesian growth curve models to a longitudinal study of blood pressure in children. *Int J Epidemiol* **8**: 15–21.

14. van der Haar F and Kromhout D (1978) *Food intake, nutritional anthropometry and blood chemical parameters in three selected Dutch schoolchildren populations*. Veenman and Zonen BV, Wageningen, The Netherlands.

15. Kass EH, Rosner B, Zinner SH *et al.* (1977) Studies on the origin of human hypertension. *Postgrad Med J* **53**: 145–52.

16. Berenson GS, McMahan CA, Voors AW *et al.* (1980) *Cardiovascular risk factors in children: The early natural history of atherosclerosis and essential hypertension*. Oxford University Press, Oxford.

17. Labarthe DL (1983) Blood pressure studies in children throughout the world. In: Gross F and Strasser T (eds) *Mild hypertension: Recent advances*, pp 85–96. Raven Press, New York.

18. Török E (1979) The beginnings of hypertension: Studies in childhood and adolescence. In: Gross F and Strasser T (eds) *Mild hypertension: natural history and management*. Pitman, London.

19. Simpson A, Mortimer JG, Silva PA *et al.* (1981) Correlates of blood pressure in a cohort of Dunedin seven-year-old children. In: Onesti G and Kim KE (eds) *Hypertension in the young and the old*. Grune and Stratton, New York.

20. Whincup PH, Cook DG, Shaper AG *et al.* (1988) Blood pressure in British children: Association with adult blood pressure and cardiovascular mortality. *Lancet* ii: 890–3.

21. Barker DJP, Osmond C, Golding J et al. (1989) Growth *in utero*, blood pressure in childhood and adult life, and mortality from cardiovascular disease. *Br Med J* **298**: 564–7.

22. Barker DJP, Winter PD, Osmond C et al. (1989) Weight in infancy and death from ischaemic heart disease. *Lancet* **ii**: 577–80.

23. Barker DJP (1990) The fetal and infant origins of adult disease. *Br Med J* **301**: 1111.

24. Barker DJP, Bull AR, Osmond C et al. (1990) Fetal and placental size and risk of hypertension in adult life. *Br Med J* **301**: 259–62.

25. Barker DJP (1991) The intrauterine origins of cardiovascular and obstructive lung disease in adult life. *J R Coll Physicians Lond* **25**: 129–33.

26. Barker DJP, Godfrey KM, Fall CHD et al. (1991) Relation of birth weight and childhood respiratory infection to adult lung function and death from chronic obstructive airways disease. *Br Med J* **303**: 671–5.

27. Barker DJP, Meade TW, Fall CHD et al. (1992) Relation of fetal and adult growth to plasma fibrinogen and Factor VII concentrations in adult life. *Br Med J* **304**: 148–52.

28. Hales CN, Barker DJP, Clark PMS et al. (1991) Fetal and infant growth and impaired glucose tolerance at age 64. *Br Med J* **303**: 1019–22.

29. Whincup PH, Cook DG and Shaper AG (1989) Early influences on blood pressure: A study of children aged 5–7 years. *Br Med J* **299**: 587–91.

30. Power C, Manor O and Fox J (1991) *Health and class: the early years*. Chapman and Hall, London.

31. Voors AW and Berenson GS (1981) Search for the determinants of the early onset of essential hypertension. In: Onesti G and Kim KE (eds) *Hypertension in the young and the old*, pp 43–56. Grune and Stratton, New York.

32. Cooper R, Liu K, Trevisan M et al. (1983) Urinary sodium excretion and blood pressure in children: Absence of a reproducible association. *Hypertension* **5**: 135–9.

33. Hofman A, Hazebroek A and Valkenburg HA (1983) A randomized trial of sodium intake and blood pressure in newborn infants. *JAMA* **250**: 370–3.

34. Ellison RC, Capper AF, Witschi JC *et al.* (1986) Sources of sodium intake in adolescents (abstract 174). *CVD Epidemiology Newsletter (American Heart Association) no. 39.*

20

High Blood Pressure in Young Adults

Experience in Glyncorrwg ■ Secondary hypertension ■ Comparison with normotensive controls ■ When, whether and how much to treat ■ Most causes of hypertension in youth are known ■ Inheritance ■ Obesity ■ Alcohol ■ Oral contraception ■ Associated cardiovascular risks ■ A policy for young adult hypertensives ■ Antihypertensive medication in youth

This is a far more serious and immediate clinical problem than childhood hypertension, because there is much more of it about, and just as little evidence on which to base a responsible policy. There is scarcely even a descriptive literature relating to whole unselected populations, let alone controlled trials.

We know that by age 20 most people who will later be recognized as hypertensive are already following a relatively stable track along the top centiles of distribution of blood pressure within their age group. Failure of antihypertensive treatment to reduce substantially the coronary risk may be partly attributable to late intervention, after vascular changes have become less reversible, so logically we should try to detect and treat such cases in their early 20s. Teenagers are probably not a suitable target group, partly because their pressures are less stable and readings are therefore poorly predictive[1,2], and partly because they have too many other things on their minds.

Measurement of blood pressure in young adults, although required by the 1990 Contract to be carried out every 3 years from April 1991, is still not established practice. As recently as 1991 at least one authority still denied the value of routine measurement of blood pressure under 35 years[3]. In 1974, in seven randomly sampled London practices, Heller and Rose[4] found blood pressure recorded in only 10% of men and 18% of women aged 20–39 years. In 1982, in 23 randomly sampled London general practices, Kurji and Haines[5] found blood pressure recorded in 28% of men and 61% of women aged 30–39. By 1986, in 5123 randomly sampled men in Scotland, Smith and Tunstall-Pedoe[6] found blood pressure recorded in 52% of GPs' records for males aged 40–44 years, rising to 74% of those aged 55–59 years. This study showed that even in the age group 40–44 years, young women were more than twice as likely to be detected as men.

Experience in Glyncorrwg

From the complete screen for high blood pressure begun in Glyncorrwg in 1968 and maintained for the following 18 years, in a total population around 2000 (at any one time) we found 25 men and 16 women with systolic pressures at or over 160 mmHg, or diastolic pressures at or over 100 mmHg, on the mean of three consecutive readings on separate days[7]. All readings were with a random zero sphygmomanometer and outsize cuffs where appropriate. Five-year detection rates estimated from our data were at least 26/1000 for men and 18/1000 for women in the age-group 20–39 years, so high arterial pressure in young adults is much commoner than has been generally supposed.

Practices with less stable populations would have to run a shorter cycle to achieve similar detection rates; some inner city practices have an over 30% annual turnover. In the absence of a screening or case finding programme with high response, most of these cases will not be detected until they are aged over 40.

Secondary Hypertension

Virtually the only thing we are taught about high blood pressure in young adults is that it usually has a secondary cause, meaning not one of the common known causes (obesity, alcohol, oral contraception or amphetamine abuse), but one of the rare classic causes. Causes of secondary hypertension were sought in all our cases in Glyncorrwg, including estimations of urine vanillylmandelic acid at periods of peak pressure or acute symptoms, plasma potassium, urea and creatinine, and searches for bacteriuria and signs of coarctation or renal artery stenosis. No such abnormalities were found except for one adolescent with end-stage renal failure from ureteric obstruction undetected in infancy, in whom the presenting sign was not hypertension but proteinuria.

Obviously classic causes of secondary hypertension do occur, but even in this age group they are rare.

Comparison with Normotensive Controls

We compared these young hypertensives with randomly sampled controls matched for age and sex from the same population, who had never had recorded blood pressures in this range; these were not strictly 'normotensive', as they included those with borderline high pressures. All survivors, including out-migrants, were followed up in 1989. Some characteristics of these 41 people are compared with controls in Table 20.1.

Table 20.1: Characteristics of 41 hypertensives aged under 40 in Glyncorrwg, 1969–1989, compared with matched controls

	Men		Women	
Group mean values	25 cases	25 controls	16 cases	16 controls
Age at diagnosis or match	31.6	31.9	33.3	33.4
Mean blood pressure at diagnosis (three readings)	165/110	128/79	172/107	124/78
Mean blood pressure at follow–up in 1989, or before death	148/89	134/79	145/86	131/78
Initial BMI	28.4	26.3	26.9	22.8
BMI 1989	29.4	27.4	27.6	23.5
Initial smokers	17	18	8	7
Smokers in 1989 or at death	8	10	6	7
Alcohol problem ever recorded	14	15	5	1
Non-fatal cardiovascular events	10	2	4	1
Deaths all causes	5	2	1	0

Our most dramatic findings were the immediately high risk for men, and the large excess of men over women. Ten of these 25 men suffered non-fatal first cardiovascular events at a mean age of 40.2 years, on average less than 9 years after diagnosis. The five male deaths in hypertensives occurred at a mean age of 47.8. Four were cardiovascular, and although the fifth died of perforated diverticulitis aged 40, he had already had one coronary thrombosis. One control died of alcohol poisoning and the other of motor neurone disease at a mean age of 49.5. The only woman who died was drowned while drunk, but she had had a large myocardial infarct one year earlier at age 49. The differences in mortality are statistically significant, and in morbidity highly significant.

Almost twice as many men as women were hypertensive. This confirms the findings of epidemiologists who have studied whole young populations[8], but conflicts with medical folklore, which still assumes a large female excess.

When, Whether and How Much to Treat

Group mean blood pressures at follow-up in 1989 (or calculated from the last three readings before death) are given in Table 20.1 on an intention to treat basis, including people who refused treatment or were relatively non-compliant. Although in isolation a group mean pressure of 148/89 mmHg may not look too bad, it is higher than the control by 14/10 mmHg. In this still very energetic age group, I found the allegedly minor side effects of most antihypertensive drugs poorly tolerated, and was reluctant to push them hard enough to cause symptoms. ACE inhibitor drugs only became available towards the end of this experience, but, although they certainly cause less and fewer side effects than beta-blockers or calcium–channel blockers, they are not always well tolerated in this age group, nor do they always give optimal control, even together with diuretics.

However, I push harder now than I did when we first detected these cases. Five male and six female hypertensives in this data set were never treated with antihypertensive drugs; four because pressure fell when a cause was removed (one had a renal transplant and three stopped oral contraception), four because patients refused, and three because no treatment programme was ever organized (one of these died of intercurrent disease soon after diagnosis, and the other two both had predominant alcohol problems). The other 20 men and 10 women started antihypertensive medication at mean ages 35.5 and 40.8 respectively.

Many patients were observed for long periods before starting medication, especially in the early 1970s. It is difficult to believe today that a consultant physician could advise against medication for a 38-year-old man with a blood pressure sustained at 194/126 mmHg in 1960. His treatment began 6 years later, when I found another consultant to approve it; in those days we still believed specialists must know best. Both morbidity and mortality were much higher in the first than the second half of my 21 years' experience from first complete screen in 1968 to follow-up in 1989. I have no doubt at all that this was because I was initially slow to intervene energetically in this age group, mainly because of a lack of appropriate evidence on which to base policy at that time.

Although failure to treat energetically is a burden on conscience, so is any decision to put a young man or woman on continuous medication for 50 years or more, without evidence of the full consequences of this assault on normal biochemistry. Worries about not treating seem to me to be about equal to worries about treating; whatever you do may have more serious consequences in young people, because long term risks are higher, both for intervention and non-intervention. Three of our young male hypertensive patients had treatment withdrawn on a trial basis. One attained normal pressures when his alcohol intake (average 10 pints of beer daily) was drastically reduced, and has never needed medication since. Another was able to stop medication after more than 10 years of good control, without any serious rise in pressure although his pressures are now again borderline and my guess is that he will eventually have to resume medication. Another is attempting, so far successfully, to control blood pressure through weight reduction alone.

Risks of non-intervention are less in women, although much of their advantage will disappear if young women continue to smoke even more than their male contemporaries.

Most Causes of Hypertension in Youth are Known

Although the numbers of patients studied in our Glyncorrwg study are small, they are complete, and drawn from a defined population, so it seems reasonable to draw three important conclusions.

First of all, once blood pressures in the adult population are fully known, as they will be by applying policies of screening or case finding over 5–10 years, accurate family data should be available for most patients. Nearly all young hypertensives seem to have a family history of high blood pressure in at least one first degree relative, so the vulnerable group can be defined.

Secondly, within that vulnerable group, alcohol and obesity stand out as powerful accelerating factors. Both are reversible, not easily, but with less difficulty and with greater chances of success in young adults than in the middle aged.

Finally, careful monitoring of oral contraception at 3-monthly intervals, as well as the choice of lowest dose combined preparations, should substantially reduce the incidence of hypertension in young women.

As yet we do not know all the causes of primary hypertension, but we already seem to know enough to make nonsense of the category. Not only is hypertension not essential, most of it is not even primary, but secondary to known and reversible causes acting against a fairly well defined (although certainly polygenic) genetic background.

Inheritance

Precise blood pressure measurements were available for parents and/or siblings for eight male and six female young hypertensive patients in Glyncorrwg. Seven of the eight men and five of the six women had one or both parents and/or a sibling with hypertension above our threshold for treatment.

Obesity

As expected[9,10], our young hypertensive patients were substantially more obese than controls. Mean BMI at ascertainment was 28.4 for males compared with 26.5 for controls, and 26.9 for females compared with 22.8 for controls; differences were highly significant for males $(0.01>P<0.001)$, and significant for females $(0.5>P<0.10)$.

Obesity increased equally in all groups over the 20 years or so of follow-up, despite sustained medical advice but without help from a dietitian. Group mean BMI in hypertensive men rose from 28.4 to 29.4, and in controls from 26.4 to 27.4. However, many of these men had family histories of both obesity and high blood pressure, and without some attempt at dieting their weight gains might have been much worse. Mean BMI in hypertensive women rose from 26.9 to 27.6, and in controls from 22.8 to 23.5. Two women but no men had extreme weight problems (BMI 39.1 and 42.0).

Alcohol

High alcohol intake, both acute[11] and chronic[12,13], is a known cause of high blood pressure. I know of no data on age differences in susceptibility, but it is reasonable to assume that this effect may be maximal in young men, who often drink very heavily especially before marriage, and that it may be more easily reversible then than later.

We found evidence of present or past excessive alcohol intake (stated intake >36 units a week, and/or raised MCV or gamma GT) in 14 of our 25 young male hypertensives, an impressive figure until we examined records for male controls; 15 of 25 had similar evidence. The extent of alcohol problems in this age group was surprising, but probably typical of other geographical areas of declining heavy industry. Mean stated intake was higher in the hypertensive group, but the difference was not impressive. However, the effect of reduced drinking in the hypertensives was obvious; perhaps genetic factors make some respond more than others. I have little doubt that alcohol is both a common and important cause of hypertension in young people, and its reduction is an equally important treatment, often obviating the need for antihypertensive medication.

Although five of our hypertensive women drank more than 36 units of alcohol a week, only two had serious alcohol problems, and in both cases blood pressure fell when drinking was reduced, although one still needed antihypertensive medication.

Oral Contraception

Oral contraceptives have long been recognized both as an occasional cause of severe hypertension, and as a common cause of a relatively small, but epidemiologically highly significant, rise in pressure[14], whose potential mass effects could be considerable. Occasionally oral contraceptive induced hypertension may become irreversible and even lethal[15].

From careful analysis of recorded associations between individual arterial pressures and oral contraception prescription and withdrawal, it appeared to be a probable sole cause in three patients studied in whom pressure fell permanently after stopping oral contraception, and a probable contributory cause for another three whose blood pressures fell on withdrawal, but subsequently showed a sustained rise.

Cases reported here were associated with 50 μg oestrogen combined pills, mostly before this risk was recognized; it remains to be seen whether 30 μg pills are safer, but as the progestogen component may carry a greater hypertensive risk than the oestrogen component[14], all cases still need careful follow-up at not less than monthly intervals. Even with structured A4 records, computerized recall and repeat prescribing, and a relatively vigilant team, we found it difficult to ensure that women who had stopped taking the Pill because of a rise in pressure did not resume it, even when they and practice staff were apparently aware of the risk.

Associated Cardiovascular Risks

We gave all our young hypertensive patients repeated advice and support on associated or causal risks for coronary disease, particularly smoking. Controls were given similar advice at routine consultations, but this was generally less systematic, sustained, reinforced, or motivated, unless they had respiratory symptoms. The proportion of stated smokers among the young male hypertensives fell from an initial 17/25 to 8/25, and in controls from 17/25 to 10/25. Smoking in women was virtually unchanged, starting at 8/16 in hypertensives and 7/16 in controls, and ending at 6/16 and 7/16 respectively.

For blood cholesterol, too few controls had contemporary measurements to allow valid comparisons, but attempts to reduce risk were generally not successful.

A Policy for Young Adult Hypertensives

An active search for young hypertensives, for men from age 20 when growth is complete, and for women from the beginning of sexual activity, seems just as important as an active search in middle age. An active call-up policy is justifiable for the offspring of hypertensive parents, or the younger siblings of known hypertensives.

Multiple readings and follow-up for at least 3 months before starting any medication are essential. People under 40 years with mean pressures at or over 160/95 mmHg should be asked for a detailed account of their normal drinking habits through the week, checked with any partner, who should be involved at some stage in the inception of treatment, whether or not this includes medication. MCV, gamma GT, and triglyceride may be raised, and, if so, will fall when intake is reduced, allowing good educational feedback. Height and weight should be measured, and plans agreed for change towards desirable body weight (BMI 25). Fasting lipids should be measured (to include tirglyceride), both to assess coronary risk and give feedback on results after reducing dietary fat, and to assess triglyceride as a fairly consistent indicator of high alcohol intake. Cigarette smoking should be assessed and, if the patient agrees, a plan made for giving up, with priority for stopping smoking if there seems to be conflict with weight targets.

Antihypertensive Medication in Youth

Although some harmful side effects develop quickly within a month or two of starting antihypertensive medication, in general risks are related to the number of years drugs are taken. A man of 30 years, starting on a thiazide diuretic and a beta-blocker, may receive them continuously for another 45 years or more, but the best evidence we have on long term side effects covers only 11 years for thiazides and 10 years for propranolol.

There are as yet no randomized controlled trials of the balance between risks and benefits for antihypertensive medication in this age group, sustained over decades. Even if trials were to start now, there would have to be a lapse of at least 20 years before sufficient end-points could accumulate to demonstrate any advantage for treatment. On the other hand, we have good reasons to believe that early control of blood pressure may be more effective than treatment in middle age, particularly in preventing atheroma and consequent coronary heart disease.

If we have to use drugs, which of them carry least risk and have fewest harmful side effects for such prolonged use? ACE inhibitors seem an obvious choice, but they usually require concomitant diuretics to obtain good control at low dosage, and the long term effects of diuretics are worrying. Prazosin is attractive because of its effect on blood cholesterol. The fatigue so often associated with beta-blockers, which is more frequent in younger and more physically active patients, and the cholesterol raising effect of at least some of them, make them a poor choice in this age group. Nifedipine seems to be well tolerated, but again it usually needs a thiazide.

Whatever drug you choose, complete absence of symptomatic side effects is essential if you are to expect long term compliance. My guess is that most of these patients will in future be treated with ACE inhibitors, combined with the smallest possible dose of diuretic if necessary. This can only be justified if the diagnosis is made carefully, after repeated measurements during at least 2 or 3 months' observation before medication, and after serious efforts have been made to control obesity and alcohol intake.

References

1. International Collaborative Group (1987) *International collaborative study on juvenile hypertension*. Hungarian Institute of Cardiology, Budapest.

2. Widimsky J and Jandova R (1980) Long term prognosis in juvenile hypertension: Condition after 20 and 28 years. *Cas Lek Cesk* **119**: 1185.

3. Morrell DC (1991) Role of research in development of organization and structure of general practice. *Br Med J* **302**: 1313–16.

4. Heller RF and Rose G (1977) Current management of hypertension in general practice. *Br Med J* i: 1442–4.

5. Kurji KH and Haines AP (1984) Detection and management of hypertension in general practices in north west London. *Br Med J* **288**: 903–6.

6. Smith WCS, Lee AJ and Crombie IK (1990) Control of blood pressure in Scotland: The rule of Halves. *Br Med J* **300**: 981–3.

7. Hart JT, Edwards C, Haines AP *et al.* (1993) Screen-detected high blood pressure under 40: A general practice population followed for 21 years. *Br Med J* **306**: 437–40.

8. Miall WE and Chinn S (1973) Blood pressure and aging: Results of a 15–17 year follow-up study in South Wales. *Clin Sci Molec Med* **45**: 23–33s.

9. Wadsworth MEJ, Cripps HA, Midwinter RE *et al.* (1985) Blood pressure in a national birth cohort at the age of 36, related to social and familial factors, smoking, and body mass. *Br Med J* **291**: 1534–8.

10. Bjorntorp P (1985) Obesity and the risk of cardiovascular disease. *Ann Clin Res* **17**: 3–9.

11. Beevers DG (1977) Alcohol and hypertension. *Lancet* ii: 111–14.

12. Arkwright PD, Beilin LJ, Rouse I *et al.* (1982) Effects of alcohol use and other aspects of lifestyle on blood pressure levels and prevalence of hypertension in a working population. *Circulation* **66**: 60–6.

13. Puddey IB, Beilin LJ and Vandongen R (1987) Regular alcohol use raises blood pressure in treated hypertension subjects. *Lancet* i: 647–51.

14. Weinberger MH and Weir RJ (1983) Oral contraceptives and hypertension. In: Robertson JIS (ed) *Handbook of hypertension. Vol 2: Clinical aspects of secondary hypertension*, pp 196–207. Elsevier, Oxford.

15. Zech P, Riffle G, Lindner A *et al.* (1975) Malignant hypertension with irreversible renal failure due to oral contraceptives. *Br Med J* iv: 326–7.

21 High Blood Pressure in the Elderly

Measurement of blood pressure in the elderly ■ Progression of blood pressure in the elderly ■ Risks of high blood pressure in the elderly, and risks of antihypertensive treatment ■ Initiating and continuing treatment in the elderly ■ Benefits of treatment initiated in the elderly ■ Antihypertensive medication in the elderly ■ Is reduction of pressure ever dangerous in the elderly? ■ When and how to continue treatment ■ When and how to stop ■ Control of other cardiovascular risk factors in the elderly

About half the people treated for high blood pressure in Britain are aged 65 or over. High pressures and their lethal or disabling outcomes are much commoner in this age group, but so are some of the risks of medication, and deaths from other more unpleasant causes.

In the past few years we have at last achieved good controlled trials of inception of antihypertensive medication in this age group on which to base policies. However, even more than in younger patients, it is difficult to apply evidence derived from these trial populations to decisions about individuals. Elderly people vary enormously in their biological rather than chronological ages, in their accumulated burdens of diverse organ damage, and their reasonable fears of other causes of death.

Measurement of Blood Pressure in the Elderly

Despite suggestions that measurement error is necessarily greater in the elderly[1], indirect measurements of arterial pressure approximate more closely to intra-arterial pressures in elderly than in younger subjects[2].

As with diabetics, it is worth measuring standing as well as seated blood pressure in elderly patients, in whom autonomic impairment is common. If standing pressure is substantially lower than seated pressure, it should be used for all monitoring thereafter.

Progression of Blood Pressure in the Elderly

In industrialized populations whose group mean pressures rise with age, group mean diastolic pressure begins to fall in the age range 60–80 years, in men more than in women. This tendency is seen in both cohort and cross-sectional studies, so it is not just an effect of early deaths in men with high diastolic pressures[1]. Group mean systolic pressure, however, continues to rise, flattening out in men from about 70 years onwards. From age 80, both systolic and diastolic pressures tend to fall in both sexes[2].

Risks of High Blood Pressure in the Elderly, and Risks of Antihypertensive Treatment

Up to about age 70, all prospective studies show a positive association between blood pressure and cardiovascular mortality, particularly from stroke. Contrary to traditional teaching, even in the elderly, this association is closer with systolic than with diastolic pressure[3]. The Framingham study showed continued associated mortality risk up to age 76, but in a British study of apparently healthy men aged 70–89, neither systolic nor diastolic pressure showed any association with survival[4]. Other evidence from several countries[5–9] confirms that, from a threshold somewhere around 70 years, obviously depending more on individual biological than chronological age, neither systolic nor diastolic pressure has much prognostic significance.

The explanation for this seems to be that in whole free living populations there is a J-curve for all-cause mortality in relation to both systolic and diastolic pressures, with raised mortality at very low as well as very high pressures[7,10]. Low pressures over the age of 70 are likely to be associated with previous myocardial infarction, atrial fibrillation, heart failure, cancer, and many other terminal illnesses with accompanying weight loss. Since none of these, with the occasional exception of coronary thrombosis, can actually be caused by low blood pressure, the J-curve is not a valid argument against controlling high blood pressure in old age.

Elderly patients already complaining of transient spells of vertigo and ataxia are particularly likely to be started on antihypertensive medication, although arrhythmias are in fact much more likely causes of these symptoms than high blood pressure. Such 'wee turns' should be investigated with a long lead II ECG, followed by referral for ambulatory ECG monitoring.

However, there is no doubt that reduction in arterial pressure can be harmful if it occurs too fast for autoregulation of brain perfusion to adapt[11]. Many strokes seem to be precipitated by hypotension caused by extracranial events such as heart failure and arrhythmias, gastrointestinal haemorrhage, or multiple pulmonary emboli[12], and there seems no reason to doubt that incautious prescription of antihypertensive drugs can act in the same way. The answer is always to start with the smallest possible dose of single drugs, with slow incremental titration against blood pressure response at intervals of at least 1 week. True hypertensive emergencies (in the sense that reduction of pressure is an over-riding priority) are rare at any age.

Initiating and Continuing Treatment in the Elderly

It is important to remember that the clinical problems associated with initiating antihypertensive treatment in the elderly differ from those of continuing treatment originally begun in middle age or youth. As whole populations become more completely screened, decisions to start or withhold treatment in the elderly should become less frequent. Few develop hypertension as a clinical problem for the first time in old age, and most of those who need treatment should already be having it.

Benefits of Treatment Initiated in the Elderly

There have now been five major randomized controlled trials of antihypertensive treatment initiated in the elderly: the European Working Party on High Blood Pressure in the Elderly (EWPHE) multicentre hospital trials[13], Coope's multicentre trial in UK general practice[14], the US Systolic Hypertension in the Elderly Program (SHEP)[15], the STOP-Hypertension trial in Sweden[16] and, most recently, the MRC trial of antihypertensive treatment in the elderly[17]. New multicentre trials of treatment for systolic high blood pressure are now starting in Europe and China, and a large age 80+ trial is now at the planning stage, but these five trials already give a wealth of evidence on which to base rational management policies.

Contrary to most expectations, certainly to my own, all this evidence vindicates aggressive treatment, even of moderately raised blood pressure, much more convincingly than trials in middle age.

The 43% reduction in all-causes mortality in patients aged 70–84 at entry in the Swedish STOP trial is particularly striking. The SHEP trial confirmed that isolated systolic hypertension carries a high risk, and that this risk is reduced by treatment. Together with the MRC trial, these justify routine consideration of antihypertensive medication from a threshold of 160/90 mmHg sustained through three readings on separate days, in people aged 65–84. However, 'consideration' means just what it says: consider it, and share these considerations with your patients to reach joint decisions.

Although a majority of all patients with severe dementia have degenerative disease of the Alzheimer type[18], most demented men under age 75 have multi-infarct dementia[19]. Antihypertensive medication has not been shown to improve cognitive performance over relatively short periods, but iatrogenic impairment is certainly unlikely[20]. Once common in my local population, multi-infarct dementia seems almost to have vanished since we achieved virtually full control of hypertension in the sixth and seventh decades. The numbers are small and the observation uncontrolled, but it is at least encouraging.

Antihypertensive Medication in the Elderly

Elderly people in general are much more likely than younger people to get serious unwanted side effects, even from correct medication[21], and are more likely to make mistakes and to be targets for thoughtless repeat prescribing, often by a variety of unco-ordinated agencies. Even more than in younger patients, the rule should be to keep medication simple, and prescribing under one roof.

Thiazide diuretics are almost always a best first choice for treatment of high blood pressure in the elderly. Although glucose tolerance is much more often impaired in old people, and diabetes should be actively sought in all patients considered for antihypertensive medication, the benefits of thiazides in low dosage probably outweigh their risks in this age group, even when glucose tolerance is already impaired. Low dose thiazides in the MRC trial were very well tolerated, as already discussed in Chapter 17, and unlike the MRC trial for the middle aged, thiazides used alone reduced coronary as well as stroke mortality.

If thiazides do not control pressure, beta-blockers are usually well tolerated if reversible airways obstruction has been excluded, and they have been widely accepted as the natural second line drug for this age group. However, evidence from the MRC trial suggests that they are almost completely ineffective in reducing net risk; all of the substantial reductions in stroke and coronary mortality in that trial seemed attributable to diuretics rather than beta-blockade, and it now seems likely that beta-blockers used in combination with thiazides actually abolish benefit from thiazides, perhaps because of reduced cardiac output[22]. Blood levels of beta-blockers are much more variable in the elderly, and many weeks of trial and error may be needed to find an optimum dose.

Methyldopa is effective in a single evening dose, when its hypnotic effect may be welcome. With a starting dose of 125 mg it is tolerated by about three-quarters of all elderly patients[23]. Postural hypotension is an increased risk in the elderly, particularly in diabetics, so it is probably best to avoid prazosin. Nifedipine is usually well tolerated, and like beta-blockers is useful for concomitant angina. Reserpine is very effective in combination with thiazides, but depression needs to be actively sought throughout follow-up. However, with all antihypertensive drugs of whatever group, it is prudent to look actively for depression in all elderly hypertensive patients at every follow-up visit.

ACE inhibitors have been introduced too recently to give any substantial trials experience in this age group. In view of their usefulness in heart failure, elderly patients presenting with hypertensive heart failure are likely to be treated with them, as well as with a diuretic. Elderly people are likely to have impaired renal function, so it is particularly important to assess this first by measuring blood urea and creatinine. If renal function is impaired, ACE inhibitors should not be used. If urea and creatinine levels are normal, start with a very low dose of ACE inhibitor, and stop diuretics for a wash-out period beforehand. Diuretics can be re-introduced later. All this will require either unusually close supervision at home, or admission to hospital.

Is Reduction of Pressure ever Dangerous in the Elderly?

Contrary to all expectation, John Coope's trial[14] showed no difference in additional symptoms between cases treated with beta-blockers (atenolol) and diuretics, and untreated controls. The authors, rightly sceptical of this result, wondered whether an administered questionnaire on side effects might be too coarse an instrument to perceive additional symptoms in an age group in which virtually everyone has aches, pains and weakness, even without medical intervention. However, this result did seem to exclude any very dramatic symptomatic impairments in elderly patients.

Despite its low dosage, the MRC trial showed more symptoms in those on thiazides than on placebo, particularly for impaired glucose tolerance (more than doubled), gout and skin disorders (each increased fourfold), muscle cramps (increased fivefold), and nausea and dizziness (each increased sevenfold). However, losses to follow-up (withdrawn because of side effects or dropped out) over 5.5 years were only 48% for the diuretic group, compared with about 53% for those on placebo, suggesting that few of these side effects were severe. Tables in the USA Systolic Hypertension in the Elderly Program[15] showed high rates for symptomatic side effects, but these were not commented on either in the text, or in editorial commentaries in the main journals.

When and How to Continue Treatment

Where control of hypertension has been achieved in middle age there is seldom any need for change in treatment through the seventh decade, unless angina requires treatment in its own right (usually with a beta-blocker or nifedipine), or blood pressure falls after myocardial infarction. Over the age of 70, however, long term medication begun in middle age should be systematically reviewed. Around this time there are important physiopathological changes, including a sharp fall in creatinine clearance and slowed hepatic metabolism which may cause higher plasma concentrations of many drugs despite unchanged dosage. Adverse drug reactions of all kinds have been shown to occur in about 4–10% of patients at age 25, rising to 7–12% at 60 and 21–24% at 80[24,25].

As the risks of overdosage and adverse side effects rise, doses required to achieve an antihypertensive effect seem usually to fall. Control of high blood pressure generally becomes easier over time, and excessive reduction occurs more often as patients grow older. Occasionally it may be possible to stop treatment in the seventh decade altogether, without return to pre-treatment pressures, but in my experience all of these have eventually returned to their original pressures within a year, unless the initial assessment of high blood pressure was suspect. Where a trial of no treatment is undertaken, it is prudent to substitute a placebo during 6 months of regular observation before finally discarding all medication. If treatment has to be resumed, the hard learned habits of regular medication will then be unimpaired. More often review leads to reduction in dosage, or a change to simpler medication. In the light of recent evidence, I can see little justification for continuing beta-blockers in old age, unless they are necessary to control angina.

A dangerous time for all hypertensives, but particularly for the elderly, is transfer to a new doctor. Confronted by an unknown patient, with a currently normal pressure, before the previous GP's record is available, or with a record suggesting previously casual supervision, it is easy to assume that treatment is no longer necessary now, and possibly never was. All too often this is true, but follow-up a week or two later is not enough to endorse this decision. Dangerous levels of pressure may take as long as 3 months to return, particularly after withdrawal of beta-blockers. It is prudent to maintain any treatment that is well established until the original criteria for diagnosis are available with the arrival of the previous medical record. *Per contra*, if your patient is leaving your practice, a letter giving the original diagnostic criteria and current medication should be given to the patient to hand to the next family doctor. Patients should be, and occasionally are, aware of the original mean pressure on which the decision to start treatment was based; make sure your patients have this information, in writing.

When and How to Stop

There are three situations in which treatment in the elderly should stop.

The first is when it should never have been started. Critical evaluation of the criteria on which the original decision appears to have been made often shows no valid indication for treatment, and this is particularly frequent in the elderly.

The second is when treatment is getting too easy. If smaller doses maintain pressure below target levels, they should be reduced further and eventually stopped. A common reason for this is onset of heart failure.

The third is when treatment is getting too difficult. All the achievements of geriatric medicine notwithstanding, people still die of old age, and we are no longer forbidden to record senility as a cause of death. There are few old people on antihypertensive drugs who would not feel a little better without them. Needless to say, this is a decision to be taken jointly with patients and sometimes their carers, but initiative in discussing it may need to come from the family doctor.

The most difficult dilemma is presented by brain failure. Where dementia is of gradual and relentless progression, without the relapses and remissions of multiple infarcts, antihypertensive drugs should be stopped. Prolonged survival with Alzheimer's disease is worse than death from stroke, and prolonged survival after stroke with dementia is unusual. Association of hypertension with multiple brain infarcts must be assumed to be causal and therefore worth treating to the bitter end.

Control of Other Cardiovascular Risk Factors in the Elderly

All the non-pharmacological interventions that reduce blood pressure, or reduce other causes of cardiovascular risk, apply also to elderly people. Although the case for mass screening of risk factors is even weaker in this than in younger age groups[26], if you cross these bridges as you come to them, most elderly people present useful opportunities for discussion of reversible risks within ordinary consultations, and respond at least as well as the middle aged to thoughtful advice.

Elderly people who have led active, healthy lives, need encouragement to maintain their activities, and occasionally protection from their anxious offspring, particularly if these live far away. For example, lifelong cyclists over 75 years have a ten times lower than average incidence of coronary heart disease[27], although they are probably at higher risk of road accidents. People who have smoked, eaten and drunk dangerously deserve encouragement to consider the benefits of changing their habits in later life, since all evidence refutes the view that it is then too late to make any difference. Although many elderly people will persist in that view, and should be left alone if that is their wish, most people over 70 years who survived a myocardial infarction at the John Radcliffe Hospital in Oxford appreciated, and largely followed, advice to stop smoking, reduce weight and dietary fat, and increase regular exercise[28]. Sodium restriction seems to be more effective in elderly people than in youth, and increases the effect of thiazide diuretics.

References

1. Spence JD, Sibbald WJ and Cape RD (1978) Pseudohypertension in the elderly. *Clin Sci Molec Med* **55**: 399s–402s.

2. Berliner K, Fujry H, Lee DH *et al.* Blood pressure measurement in obese persons: Comparison of intra-arterial and auscultatory measurement. *Am J. Cardiol* **8**: 10–17.

3. Kannel W and Gordon T (1978) Evaluation of cardiovascular risk in the elderly: The Framingham study. *Bull N Y Acad Med* **54**: 573–91.

4. Anderson F and Cowan NR (1976) Survival of healthy older people. *Br J Prev Soc Med* **30**: 231–2.

5. Hodkinson HM and Pomerance A (1979) The clinical pathology of heart failure and atrial fibrillation in old age. *Postgrad Med J* **55**: 251–4.

6. Evans JG, Prudham D and Wanless I (1980) Risk factors for stroke in the elderly. In Barbagallo-Sangiorgio G and Exton-Smith AN (eds) *The ageing brain*. Plenum, London, 113–26.

7. Miall WM and Brennan PJ (1981) Hypertension in the elderly: The South Wales study. In: Onesti G and Kim KE (eds) *Hypertension in the young and the old*. Grune and Stratton, New York, 277–84.

8. Haavisto H, Geiger V, Mattila K *et al.* (1980) A health survey of the very aged in Tampere, Finland. *Age and Ageing* **13**: 266–72.

9. Langer RD, Ganiats TG and Barret-Connor E (1989) Paradoxical survival of elderly men with high blood pressure. *Br Med J* **298**: 1356–7.

10. Coope J, Warrender TS and McPherson K (1988) The prognostic significance of blood pressure in the elderly. *J Hum Hypertens* **2**: 79–88.

11. Wollner L, McCarthy ST, Soper NDW *et al.* (1979) Failure of cerebral autoregulation as a cause of brain dysfunction in the elderly. *Br Med J* ii: 1117–18

12. Mitchinson MJ (1980) The hypotensive stroke. *Lancet* i: 244–6.

13. Amery A, Brixho P, Clement D *et al.* (1985) Mortality and morbidity results

from the European Working Party on High Blood Pressure in the Elderly. *Lancet* i: 1349–54.

14. Coope J and Warrender TS (1986) Randomized trial of treatment of hypertension in elderly patients in primary care. *Br Med J* **293**: 1145–51.

15. SHEP Cooperative Research Group (1991) Prevention of stroke by antihypertensive drug treatment in older persons with isolated systolic hypertension. *JAMA* **265**: 3255–64.

16. Dahlof B, Lindholm LH, Hansson L *et al.* (1991) Morbidity and mortality in the Swedish Trial in Old Patients with Hypertension (STOP-Hypertension). *Lancet* **338**: 1281–4.

17. MRC Working Party (1992) Medical Research Council trial of treatment of hypertension in older adults: Principal results. *Br Med J* **304**: 405–12.

18. Kay DWK, Bergman K, Foster EM *et al.* (1970) Mental illness and hospital usage in the elderly: A random sample followed up. *Comp Psychiatr* **2**: 26–35.

19. Bergman K (1980) Dementia: Epidemiological aspects. In: Barbagallo-Sangiorgio G and Exton-Smith AN (eds) *The ageing brain*, pp 59–69. Plenum, New York.

20. Bird AS, Blizard RA and Mann AH (1990) Treating hypertension in the older person: An evaluation of the association of blood pressure level and its reduction with cognitive performance. *J. Hypertens* **8**: 147–52.

21. Williamson J and Chopin JM (1980) Adverse reactions to prescribed drugs in the elderly: A multicentre investigation. *Age and Ageing* **9**: 73–80.

22. Aursnes I (1992) Elderly patients with sustained hypertension. *Br Med J* **304**: 1054.

23. Ramsay LE (1981) The use of methyldopa in the elderly. *J R Coll Physicians Lond* **15**: 239–41.

24. Seidl LG, Thornton GF, Smith JW *et al.* (1966) Studies on the epidemiology of adverse drug reactions. *Bull Johns Hopkins Hosp* **119**: 299–315.

25. Hurwitz N (1969) Predisposing factors in adverse reactions to drugs. *Br Med J* i: 536–9.

26. Beaglehole R (1991) Coronary disease and elderly people: No mass treatment of risk factors yet. *Br Med J* **303**: 69–70.

27. Robertson HK (1977) Heart disease in lifelong cyclists. *Br Med J* **ii**: 1635–6.

28. Cohen DL and Fowlie S (1992) Changing lifelong habits of elderly people. *Br Med J* **304**: 1055–6.

Appendix 1
Educational Leaflet for Patients

What you Need to Know about your High Blood Pressure

Your blood pressure has been found to be high enough to need further investigation and perhaps medication, probably for the rest of your life. That is a long time. Spend a few minutes reading this leaflet carefully, and then read it again to make sure you understand it. Then get your partner to read it and discuss it together. Next time you see the doctor or nurse, discuss any points which are not clear to you.

Everyone's blood is under pressure, otherwise it would not circulate. If the pressure is too high it damages the walls of your arteries, increasing the risk of coronary heart disease, heart failure, stroke, retinal bleeding or detachment, and kidney failure. High blood pressure itself is not a disease, but a treatable cause of these serious diseases. All these effects are very much increased if you also smoke or have diabetes.

Unless it has already caused damage, high blood pressure seldom makes you feel unwell. It can be very high without causing headaches, breathlessness, palpitations, faintness, giddiness, or any of the symptoms which were once thought to be caused by high blood pressure. You may have any or all of these symptoms without having high blood pressure, and you can have dangerously high blood pressure with none of them.

The only way to know what your blood pressure is, is to measure it with a manometer when you are sitting quietly. Because blood pressure varies so much from hour to hour and from day to day, this measurement must be done at least three times to work out a true average, before taking big decisions like starting or stopping treatment.

Mechanisms

The level of blood pressure depends on how hard your heart pumps blood into your arteries, on the volume of blood in your circulation, and on how tight your arteries are. The smaller arteries are sheathed by a spiral muscle, to make them wider or narrower according to varying needs in different activities. In people with high blood pressure something goes wrong with this mechanism, so that the arteries are too tight. The heart then has to beat harder to push blood through them. This tightening up may result from nervous or chemical signals, chiefly from the brain, the larger arteries, and the kidneys.

Causes

The causes of transient rises in blood pressure are well understood, but these are not what we mean by high blood pressure. High blood pressure is important only when it is maintained for months or years; it is a high average pressure which is important, not occasional peaks. The causes of such long term rises in pressure are not fully known, but we do know that it runs in families. This inherited tendency seems to account for about half the difference between people; the rest seems to depend on how people live and what they eat, in childhood as well as adult life. We do not know enough about this to be able to prevent most cases.

One cause we do know is being overweight, particularly in young people. Weight reduction is a sensible first step in treatment. Weight loss depends mainly on eating less fat and oil, meat, sugar and alcohol, and more fruit, vegetables, cereal foods and fish. Of all these, eating less fat and oil is by far the most important. Some dietary changes have other good effects as well as helping weight loss. There is good evidence that eating less fat reduces blood pressure, apart from any effect on weight. These changes in diet will also reduce the risk of coronary heart disease by lowering blood cholesterol.

Another known cause is excessive alcohol (more than 8 glasses of wine or 4 pints of beer a day). Again, the biggest effect is in young people. Limiting alcohol to not more than half this level often brings high blood pressure back to normal without any other treatment.

Stress

Blood pressure rises for a few minutes or hours if you are anxious, angry, have been hurrying, have a full bladder, or if you are cold, so blood pressure measured at such times is not reliable, but none of these things seem to be the cause of permanently raised blood pressure. High blood pressure seems to be just as common in peaceable, even tempered people without worries as it is in excitable people with a short fuse, but feeling pushed at work or home may be an important cause in some people, if not for everyone. The word 'hypertension' is used in medical jargon with exactly the same meaning as 'high blood pressure'. This does not mean that feeling tense necessarily raises blood pressure, nor does it mean that everyone with a high blood pressure feels tense. Training in relaxation certainly lowers blood pressure for a while (it falls profoundly during normal sleep), and may have a useful long term effect on high blood pressure in people who learn how to 'switch off' at times during the day, but there is no evidence that treatment by relaxation is an effective or safe alternative to drug treatment in people with severe high blood pressure.

Salt and Sodium

Table salt is sodium chloride; it is the sodium which is important in blood pressure. Among people who eat food with about 20 times less sodium than a typical Western diet, high blood pressure is unknown, and even very high blood pressure can be controlled by reducing sodium intake to this low level. The diet required for this consists of rice, fruit and vegetables and is difficult to maintain for most people.

The usual British diet contains more salt than needed, and it does no harm to reduce sodium intake by not adding salt to cooked meals, by reducing or avoiding high sodium processed foods (sausages, sauces, tinned meats and beans, and canned foods generally), Chinese take-aways (which contain huge quantities of sodium glutamate) and strong cheeses. Milk and bread also contain surprisingly large amounts of salt.

There is no convincing evidence that the roughly one-third reduction in sodium intake you can achieve by these changes is an effective alternative to drug treatment for severe high blood pressure. However, people with blood pressure high enough to need drugs may manage on a lower dose if they reduce sodium intake, and very heavy salt eaters should certainly try to cut down. There is much better evidence that reducing fat in your diet reduces blood pressure, as well as reducing blood cholesterol. You may find it difficult to reduce fat and salt at the same time.

Smoking

Smoking is not a cause of high blood pressure, but if you have high blood pressure already, your risk of a heart attack is increased threefold by smoking up to about 50 years of age, and doubled after that age. Heart attacks in people under 45 years occur almost entirely in smokers.

Smoking is a very powerful risk factor in its own right, not only for coronary heart disease and stroke, but also for cancer of the lung, bladder, and pancreas, and for chronic obstructive lung disease. Unlike all other risk factors, it also affects your family and friends, through passive smoking.

When should High Blood Pressure be Treated with Drugs?

High blood pressure should be treated with drugs if there is already evidence of damage to the arteries, brain, heart, eyes or kidneys, and in all diabetics. Otherwise it should be treated only if the average blood pressure (averaged from at least three readings on separate days) is at or over about 170/100 mmHg. You do not need to know what these figures mean, but you should know what, in your own case, they are, just as you should know your own height and weight. This threshold (plus or minus 5 either way) is based on evidence from large scientific trials in Britain, Australia, Scandinavia and the USA, which have shown worthwhile saving of life in many thousands of treated cases compared with untreated controls. Most of the benefit has been in reduced incidence of strokes, heart failure, and kidney damage; the effects on coronary (heart) attacks have been much smaller. Benefits are greatest in people with highest pressures. More important ways to prevent coronary attacks are to stop smoking, reduce blood cholesterol, and maintain regular exercise.

Drugs for High Blood Pressure

People with severe high blood pressure are likely to live longer if their blood pressure is reduced by drugs than if they are left untreated, but they seldom feel better and sometimes feel worse. Their tendency to high blood pressure is permanent and is not affected by any treatment now available, so treatment must nearly always continue for the rest of their lives. The aim of all present treatment of high blood pressure is not to cure this tendency, but to prevent its consequences by holding blood pressure down; if drugs are stopped, blood pressure nearly always rises again, although this may take several months.

People with blood pressure averaging 175/105 mmHg or more nearly always need medication to control it, which usually has to be continued for the rest of their lives. All drugs used for high blood pressure cause unpleasant side effects in some people, although the newer ones are generally easier to live with than the older ones. If you think your drugs are upsetting you, say so; there are many alternatives. Tiredness, depression, and failure of erection are common side effects of most drugs in common use, and if any of these happen, make sure you tell the doctor or nurse; they will clear up soon after your drugs are changed. If you have any wheezing or asthma, some blood pressure lowering drugs can be dangerous. Do not try to alter your medication yourself.

Remembering to take tablets is difficult for many people. Take them at set times, and ask your partner to help you learn the habit of regular medication. Do not stop them because you are going out for a drink; all drugs used to control high blood pressure can be taken with a reasonable amount of alcohol. Some drugs used for back and joint pains can interfere with the effect of drugs for blood pressure, and you should ask the doctor about these if you take them. The contraceptive pill can raise blood pressure very seriously, and women with high blood pressure should discuss other methods of birth control.

Follow-Up

Always bring all your tablets (not just those for high blood pressure) with you when you see the doctor or nurse for follow-up, so that both of you know exactly what you are taking. If your blood pressure does not fall despite apparently adequate medication, think about your weight or your alcohol intake. Follow-up visits will be frequent at first, perhaps once a week until your blood pressure is controlled to about 160/90 mmHg or less. After that most doctors like to check blood pressure every 3 months or so; never go longer than 6 months without a check.

Appendix 2
A Weight Reducing, Cholesterol Lowering Diet for High Blood Pressure and/or Non-Insulin Dependent Diabetes

This diet was designed for people with high blood pressure, diabetes, or high blood cholesterol, or who are simply overweight, but anyone following it will be healthier for it. Diets are easier to follow if the whole family joins in.

Six Golden Rules

- eat less fat
- eat less sugar and other high energy food
- stop nibbling between meals but do not miss meals
- eat more vegetables of all kinds, and bread and fruit
- take regular exercise
- measure your weight honestly and regularly on accurate scales.

Eat Less Fat

Fats (which include oils, cream, and the concentrated fat of cheeses, chocolate, and all fried foods) are not only the most concentrated form of energy, but also the main source of blood cholesterol (which narrows and hardens arteries) and your own excess body fat. The main way people become overweight in the first place, and therefore become more likely to have high blood pressure, diabetes, or high blood cholesterol, is because they are eating too much fat. There is also good evidence that a low fat diet can reduce blood pressure almost as much as medication.

Some kinds of fat raise cholesterol much more than others. In general, fat from farmed animals, both on meat and in it, and as milk, cream, butter, hard margarines and cheese, are saturated fats, which raise blood cholesterol. The biggest source of fat for most people is fried food in general, and chips in particular. Biscuits and cakes contain large amounts of fat as well as sugar, and should be reduced as far as possible. Processed and convenience foods often conceal large amounts of saturated fat which are not obvious; sausages may contain over 50% fat, and there are huge amounts in burgers. If you take off the skin, poultry contains much less fat than other meat. Most vegetable oils (including corn, olive, sesame and sunflower oil but not peanut or coconut oil) and fish oils are unsaturated fats, which help to reduce blood cholesterol. Fatty fish (mackerel, herring, trout and salmon), all seem to have a protective effect on the heart.

Your aim should be to reduce fat to about 25% of total energy intake. This is about one-third less than the average British intake now. An easy way to start is to use semi-skimmed instead of whole milk (it takes a few days to get used to the new taste), eat less and leaner meat and cut off the fat, cook by grilling, steaming or microwaving rather than frying, and do not automatically spread butter or margarine on all your bread.

Calories and Energy

Your body needs fuel to work, as well as other sorts of food for maintenance and repairs. This fuel part of food we call energy is measured in calories. Do not let the advertisers kid you that if you eat more energy-containing foods, you will feel less tired; you would probably feel a lot more energetic if you ate less energy! Reducing energy intake begins with eating less concentrated energy food (fats, sugars including sweet drinks, and alcohol). All these put in large amounts of energy, without making you feel full.

Nibbling between meals can add a lot more surplus energy to your diet, and one of the first things to do is to stop this. Do not be tempted to go over the top, and miss meals altogether. If you do, you will either eat even more at the next meal to make up for it, or you may even develop an obsessive hostility to all eating (anorexia nervosa). This happens mainly in young people and it can be very dangerous. In general, crash diets which aim at very rapid weight loss through some kind of starvation are ineffective in the long run, and despite the claims of advertisers, are often harmful to health.

Beneficial Foods (Fibre)

Reducing fats and sweet foods is easier if you replace these by foods which, weight for weight, contain less energy: all vegetables and fresh fruits, bread, rice and potatoes. These are generally more bulky and need more chewing, so that overeating is more difficult. Plant foods contain varying quantities of indigestible residues, usually called fibre, although they include liquid gums which are not fibrous at all, but equally valuable.

These residues slow down absorption of food from your gut, so your pancreas does not have to work so hard to produce insulin. This makes for better control of diabetes, and may actually prevent diabetes in people who are overweight and/or have a family history of diabetes. They also help to prevent constipation and piles, gall-stones and diverticulitis, and may help to prevent bowel cancer.

Huge amounts of added fibre, usually bran, can cause colic and even intestinal obstruction in obsessive weight losers who rush into crash diets. Plant foods in general, and pulses (beans, peas, and lentils) in particular, produce a lot of gas during digestion in the gut, and this has to go somewhere. This seems to be less of a problem when your gut gets used to its new diet, so start slowly and do not overdo it.

Exercise

Even if the balance between energy intake and energy output stays the same (because exercise increases appetite), increased energy throughout reduces blood pressure and blood cholesterol in everyone, improves control of blood glucose in diabetics, improves efficiency of the heart even in heart failure, and nearly always gives a greater general sense of optimisim and well-being which makes dieting much easier. Avoid static exercises like press-ups or weight lifting. Beyond middle age, avoid competitive sports or extreme trials of endurance. Do what you enjoy, and stop when you are tired.

Weight Monitoring

Weigh yourself once a week. Bathroom scales are accurate only to about the nearest 1 lb or 0.5 kg. As you should plan to lose weight at a steady rate of about half a pound a week, bathroom scales may easily either fail to register this loss, or may kid you that you have lost it when in fact you have gained weight. Accurate feedback on your progress is essential, so for this you need good balance arm scales, either at your doctor's surgery, at a chemist, or at a weight-loss group. Weigh at roughly the same time of day, and with more or less similar clothing.

Appendix 3
A Low Sodium, Low Fat Diet for Refractory High Blood Pressure, with Procedure for Measuring 7-Day Sodium Output

If your high blood pressure is poorly controlled, a big reduction in sodium intake may bring it down. This is especially true for people taking ACE inhibitor drugs, which may be ineffective unless sodium intake is restricted.

A low fat diet is essential for all people with high blood pressure, whether controlled well or badly, because all of them are at increased risk of premature hardening of the arteries. There is also good evidence that a low fat diet reduces blood pressure.

Low sodium diets tend to be tasteless, particularly for the first month or two; after this your taste for salt will gradually lessen, so that what you once enjoyed now tastes too salty. If you are on a low sodium diet, unless you make a conscious effort to reduce fat you may that find you are eating more fat in an effort to make food more tasty.

Targets

Average sodium intake in the UK is about 180 mmol a day for men and 150 mmol a day for women. Your blood pressure is unlikely to fall unless you can get your sodium intake well below 100 mmol a day for men, or 80 mmol for women; that is, between one-half and two-thirds of what you have been used to.

In most diets, salt (sodium chloride) is the main source of sodium, but other sources of sodium may be equally important, notably sodium bicarbonate used to preserve green colour in cooked vegetables, and monosodium glutamate in Chinese food. One portion of a Chinese take-away meal may contain 200 mmol of sodium, more than 2 days' total ration on a low sodium diet! Most convenience foods, fast foods, and tinned foods contain much more sodium than home cooking. One average sized potato contains 0.2 mmol of sodium, compared with 21 mmol in one cupful of instant mashed potato. One portion of Kentucky Fried Chicken contains 75 mmol, and one portion of branded hamburger and chips contains 97 mmol. Lots of foods we generally think of as unsalted actually contain a lot of sodium, for example cheese and bread, particularly bread baked in the French style. On average, about one-third of sodium comes from bread. Low sodium bread can be found by shopping around, but reduction below 50% of the usual level makes it impossible to bake.

The keys to success are to proceed slowly, and to include the whole family, at least for cooked meals. If you gradually reduce sodium intake over about 3 months, your taste sense will have time to adapt. If you try to adopt a strict low sodium diet quickly your food may taste like cardboard or cotton wool, and you may find the diet difficult to maintain. A slow but steady reduction in salty foods may allow the rest of your family to join in, which will make cooking and shopping much easier, as well as being better for their health. The tendency to high blood pressure runs in families, and reduced salt in childhood and adolescence may prevent high blood pressure later on.

Obviously the first step is to stop adding salt to your food at the table, and then gradually reduce the amount used in cooking. Eating at work will be a problem unless you can make some arrangement with the cook. Sandwiches made with ordinary bread will contain a lot of sodium.

High, Low and Middling Sodium Foods

Foods can be divided into three groups: high sodium foods which must be avoided altogether, low sodium foods of which you can eat as much as you like, and 'middling' sodium foods which you can eat sparingly.

Low sodium foods of which you can eat as much as you like include:

- all fresh fruit
- all fresh or home cooked vegetables (but not cooked in sodium bicarbonate)
- rice, spaghetti, macaroni, and pasta of all kinds
- fresh meat, fish and poultry.

Many of these can be made more interesting with the addition of herbs and spices of all kinds, including vinegar, mint, mustard, pepper, paprika, garlic, onion, and lemon juice.

'Middling' sodium foods should be eaten sparingly; they include:

- some breakfast foods: unsalted porridge, Ready Brek, muesli, Alpen, prunes
- milk: not more than half a pint of semi-skimmed a day, yoghurt, ice cream, and cottage cheese
- curries
- low salt bread, preferably wholemeal

- eggs: not too high in sodium, but high in cholesterol; allow yourself two a week
- unsalted butter or polyunsaturated margarine
- unsalted nuts.

High sodium foods must be avoided completely; they include:

- sauces and condiments: bottled sauces, chutneys, Bovril, Marmite, Oxo and laverbread
- smoked and tinned fish: kippers, bucklings, smoked haddock, cockles, mussels, prawns, shrimps, scampi, tinned salmon, anchovies, pilchards and sardines
- most breakfast cereals: Weetabix, Allbran, Rice Krispies, cornflakes, special K, Frosties (Shredded Wheat, sugar puffs, puffed rice, wheat and oats are acceptable.)
- snacks: salted nuts, pork scratchings, Bombay mix and chana chur, pork pies, pasties, pizzas, bahjees and somosas, and peanut butter
- most milk products and cheeses: evaporated and condensed milk, tinned cream, salted butter and margarine, and all cheeses other than cottage cheese; unsalted butter and margarine is acceptable
- most soups: all canned or packet soups have a lot of salt, and home recipes must be modified
- savoury biscuits and pastry: crispbreads, cheese biscuits, cocktail biscuits, self-raising flour (because of sodium bicarbonate), cornflour, baking powder, frozen and packet pastry
- preserved meats: sausages, fried or boiled bacon, fried, cooked or smoked ham, tongue, jellied veal, luncheon meat and pâté
- canned vegetables, baked beans and tomatoes
- dried fruits
- golden syrup, chocolate and toffee
- ordinary bread, whether white, brown or wholemeal.

Measuring your Sodium Intake

Sodium intake is measured in millimoles (mmol). The standard way to measure this is not to measure what goes in, but what comes out (in urine), as in Britain's cool climate these two figures are roughly the same. Only in very hot weather do you lose much sodium as sweat.

In most people, sodium intake, and therefore output, varies a lot from hour to hour and day to day. People who guess their sodium intake, including doctors, are usually wrong. Even analysis of 24-hour urine output is only a rough guide to average intake. A low sodium diet requires a lot of effort for most people, so it is worth knowing accurately how much sodium you normally eat before starting your diet, and what you have achieved, say 3 months later.

The best way to do this is to collect all the urine you pass over 7 days, measuring the total volume of urine each day in a large graduated bottle you can get from your doctor. This will contain a little disinfectant to stop smells. To avoid burning your skin with this, pass urine into another smaller container, and then empty it into the large one with the disinfectant. Empty your bladder into the toilet at the beginning of the trial, and from then on make sure all urine, day or night and at home, work, or wherever, gets into that bottle. You may need several discreet containers to use outside your home, with tight-fitting screw caps. Stick a notice on your toilet to remind you not to use it. For men, a safety pin over their zip may be a useful reminder. At the end of each day (at the same time as the trial began), measure the total volume of urine in the container against the graduations on the side, and write this figure down. Then shake up the bottle to mix all the urine, and pour out 10 ml into a universal container (from your doctor). Take the seven 10 ml containers, together with your record of the seven daily urine volumes, to your doctor's surgery for laboratory analysis.

Appendix 4
Use and Care of
Sphygmomanometers

Blood pressure varies greatly from time to time, depending on patients' physical and emotional state. The aim is to measure average resting pressure.

Common causes of false high readings are:

■ Anger, fear, pain and embarrassment.

The atmosphere should be friendly and unhurried. With new patients you should explain what you are doing while you do it. If you think it may have affected the reading, record your impression of the patient's emotional state: frightened, angry, etc. Pulse rate is an indicator of stress and anxiety, so record this routinely at the same time.

■ A full bladder.

Ask about this discreetly, if you get an unexpected high reading.

■ Cuffs that do not fit or are badly applied to the arm.

The rubber bag inside the cuff should encircle the arm. If it does not, you may get false high readings. You need at least two sizes of cuff: one for normal arms and one for fat arms. If you are to do your work properly, you must insist that you have these.

Common causes of false low readings are:

■ Tightly rolled clothing above the cuff.

Many women must take their arm right out of their dress to get a reliable reading.

■ Dropping the mercury column too fast.

This is a result of bad habits learned in antenatal clinics, to try to save time, or because the control valve on the inflator bulb is leaking and will not hold the pressure.

■ Pressing too hard with the stethoscope over the artery.

The patient should sit comfortably with the arm supported on a table. Use either the left or the right arm on all patients, but not both indiscriminately. Make your readings as accurately as possible; all clinical decisions are based upon them. Lower the mercury slowly, about 2 mm/s (roughly one division on the scale) for each pulse beat at a normal heart rate. Either write down, or (better) speak the pressures as you hear them, or you may find you have forgotten the systolic pressure by the time you reach the diastolic sounds. If you speak the pressures, you will interest your patients and help to involve them more intelligently in their own care; in my experience they usually remember the pressure if they hear it. Make all your readings to the nearest 2 mm down, and try to avoid reading only to the nearest 0 up or down.

Systolic pressure is the first regular sound you hear. Record it accurately, because it is easier and therefore more accurate than diastolic pressure.

Diastolic pressure is defined either as:

- the point where the regular, clear, tapping sound is replaced by a muffled, whooshing sound (phase 4), or
- the point where regular sounds disappear (phase 5).

Your team must make up its mind which of these definitions it will use, and stick to it. Phase 5 is easier and is now generally accepted everywhere as standard procedure.

Patients with an irregular pulse (atrial fibrillation or very frequent extra, ie ectopic, beats) may spin off lots of odd sounds above systolic and below diastolic pressure, so accurate blood pressure may be unmeasurable. If you notice this, write it down; do not invent a blood pressure that is not there. In some patients phase 4 can not be heard, only phase 5. In others the sounds are still audible down to 0. In most of these you can get a diastolic pressure by removing all clothing from the arm, and if that does not work, you can try the other arm. When this fails, if you get the patient back the next day, phase 5 may be clearly audible. An easier alternative is to record phase 4, but if you do this you must write down what you have done; there is an average difference of 8 mmHg between phase 4 and phase 5. Whatever you do, never be afraid to record what you actually hear.

It is very important to check and maintain your sphygmomanometer. Errors arise from mercury manometers in three ways: dirty glass tubes, blocked or leaking valves, and leaking tubing and connections.

Once every 6 months it should be somebody's job to lift out the glass tube and clean it with the long pipe cleaner originally supplied with the instrument. This will remove dirty mercury from the lining of the glass tube, so that the mercury level can be read accurately rather than guessed. Next, the valve at the base of the rubber bulb should be tested by inflating the cuff and then closing the valve right down. Pressure should hold for 1 minute without much loss; if there is a leak, pressure will fall fairly quickly, and the valve should be opened up and the rubber washer replaced. If the valve seems all right, the leak is probably from a crack in perished rubber tubing, or from one of the male-female joints. The tubing can usually be shortened, and joints can be replaced. When the valve is blocked, usually with fluff over the mesh filter, it becomes difficult to squeeze the bulb. The bulb should be removed and the mesh filter cleaned.

Appendix 5
Protocol for Nurse-Run High Blood Pressure Clinics

This protocol was used in Glyncorrwg for many years, before the 1990 Contract; modify it to suit your requirements.

Blood pressure clinics are held once a fortnight, from 16.15 to 18.00 hrs. The clinic is run by a practice nurse, who sees all the patients. A doctor works concurrently, seeing patients with ordinary appointments, but bookings are kept light, so that the roughly one-third of blood pressure patients who want or need to see the doctor as well as the nurse can be fitted in.

Detection, initial diagnostic workup, and the beginnings of patient education are all done in ordinary consulting sessions. The blood pressure clinic is not a screening and detection clinic, but a follow-up clinic. Patients are not referred to it until this initial work has already been done. Most of the patients are on stable medication and are well controlled.

The aims of the clinic are:

■ to keep blood pressures at a safe level, generally below 160/90 mmHg, or below 150/80 mmHg in diabetics
■ to keep patients coming to the clinic, so that they have some supervision at intervals not longer than 3 months
■ to ensure that patients steadily gain understanding of the nature of their problem so that they can either share in management decisions, or take them themselves.

The means of achieving these aims are:

■ to check blood pressure, medication, body weight and current smoking in all treated hypertensive patients at least once every 3 months
■ to get and keep pressures below 160/90 mmHg whenever possible (good control), or at most below 175/100 mmHg (poor control)
■ to verify that patients are taking and understand their medication, explain what they do not understand, and detect side effects
■ to get and keep the BMI below 30
■ in ex-smokers, to verify that they have not resumed; in smokers, to enquire

about chest and throat symptoms, and to discuss selectively the possibilities of stopping, cutting down, or shifting to low tar brands.

Procedures

Whenever a new hypertensive patient is detected in this practice, the doctor or nurse who takes this decision should label the patient's A4 record with blue tape across the spine. He or she should also notify you of the patient's name, address and phone number. These should then be written on a new card for a boxed blood pressure card index,* containing all diagnosed hypertensive patients known to the practice. These should be grouped in 2-weekly clinic date order. At each clinic the receptionist will date stamp the cards of all patients listed for that date, including defaulters. No other information should be written on this card, except personal details which may help to maintain contact, such as details of shift work, or notes about patients who are temporarily or permanently housebound and need a home visit.

One week before the clinic, look through the group listed for it and ask the receptionist to extract all these records. In each, look at the entries for the past 3 months. Where patients have already had a blood pressure check at an ordinary general session, and it was well controlled, note the date this was done on the index card, move the card 3 months ahead from that date, and tell the receptionist, who will notify the patients. If patients are expected to come to the clinic again soon after a patient initiated consultation where blood pressure was checked, your default rate will rise. For patients who seem from the record to be housebound, ask the receptionist to arrange for a doctor or nurse to visit. For all other patients, give your list to the receptionist for her to send out reminder notes with appointment times. For patients who default repeatedly, telephone a reminder the day before the clinic. Although all these reminders are a lot of bother, they cause much less trouble than the consequences of untreated high blood pressure, for the primary health care team as well as the patients.

At the clinic start seeing patients as soon as they begin to arrive. Enter the date on the A4 record. Ask all patients how they have been since the last clinic, and write down any important events, not necessarily medical; for example, losing a job or getting married should be recorded; better too much than too little. Look at the last entry to see if they have consulted with a new medical problem. Ask all patients to show you all the medication they are currently taking, not

---

* This protocol was developed before our records became partially computer held, on the VAMP system. Like most systems, this has facilities for listing patients with high blood pressure, entering, storing, and displaying data on blood pressure, BMI, smoking and blood cholesterol, and for tracking blood pressures (but no other variables) graphically. This obviously supersedes the card index system. For a computer system to work effectively, it is essential that all medical and nursing staff agree on diagnostic criteria and terminology, so that all data entries use the same language.

only blood pressure tablets. Prescriptions for chronic disease normally cover 3 months in this practice, so as a rule there should be few tablets left over. Do not count them, but if there are obviously a lot more than expected, ask if your patient is having difficulty remembering to take them, or thinks they are causing side effects.

Then measure and record the following:

- blood pressure: use phase 5 (disappearance of sound) for diastolic pressure, and record to the nearest 2 mmHg down; let the mercury down slowly about 2 mm per pulse beat; tell the patient the figures, as you hear them
- pulse rate: count pulse over 15 seconds and multiply by four
- current smoking in cigarettes a day, and any attempts or plans to stop smoking
- weight in kilograms: remove upper clothing but not shoes
- peak expiratory flow rate if this was recorded at the last clinic visit.

Ask all patients if, for any reason, they want to see the doctor. The doctor will be seeing other patients, but time should be allowed for about one third of your booked patients to be seen by the doctor, who will therefore be less pressurized than you are.

Refer patients to the doctor for the following reasons:

- if systolic pressure is over 160 or diastolic pressure is over 90 mmHg; before referring the patient, try to find out yourself why blood pressure is poorly controlled; for example, note if the patient seems frightened or upset, ask about today's medication, worries at home or work, or drinking in the past two days.
- if pulse rate is less than 60/min; many antihypertensive drugs slow the heart
- if you think, and the patient agrees, that the time is right for a new attempt to stop smoking
- if you think, and the patient agrees, that the time is right for a new attempt to tackle obesity
- if the patient has not seen a doctor for a year or more
- if you are worried for any reason about the patient.

At the end of the clinic either you or the receptionist should telephone defaulters to find out why they have not come, arrange new appointments, and shift their cards forward to appropriate dates. Give the doctor a list of the defaulters and discuss possible reasons briefly. All treated cases should be seen at least once every 3 months, and if your card index is well maintained you will always know how closely you are approaching this target.

Once every three months check:

- that every record with a blue tape on the spine has a card in the boxed index
- every card in the boxed index to see that all patients have either been seen, or arrangements have been made to see them.

If any of these tasks take more time than you are paid for, raise this matter at the next practice staff meeting.

Appendix 6
Flow Diagram of Ascertainment
in a Practice Population of 2000

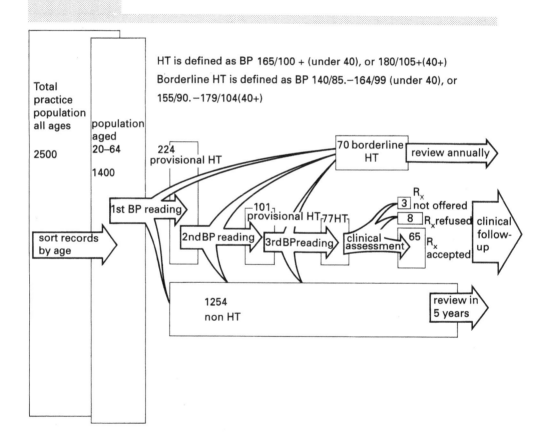

HT is defined as BP 165/100 + (under 40), or 180/105+(40+)

Borderline HT is defined as BP 140/85.−164/99 (under 40), or
155/90.−179/104(40+)

Total practice population all ages

2500

population aged 20–64

1400

224 provisional HT

70 borderline HT — review annually

1st BP reading

sort records by age

101 provisional HT 77HT

2nd BP reading   3rd BP reading   clinical assessment

R_x 3 not offered

8 $R_x$refused

65 R_x accepted

clinical follow-up

1254 non HT — review in 5 years

Appendix 7
Brand and Generic Names and UK Costs of Antihypertensive Drugs

Costs are derived from the *British National Formulary* number 22, September 1991, based on one month's treatment at average maintenance doses as given in the BNF; actual doses and therefore costs may differ considerably from these. Fixed combination antihypertensive drugs including diuretics are included, but diuretics combined with potassium supplements, and slow release beta-blockers are not recommended or included in this list.

Group and Generic name	Brand name	Daily dose (mg)	Monthly cost (£)
Thiazide diuretics			
Bendrofluazide	Generic		
	Berkozide		
	Aprinox, Neo-Naclex		
	Centyl-K	2.5	00.20
Chlorothiazide	Saluric	500	00.53
Chlorthalidone	Hygroton	25	00.57
Cyclopenthiazide	Navidrex	0.25	00.24
Hydrochlorothiazide	Esidrex	25	00.80
	Hydrosaluric	25	00.41
Hydroflumethiazide	Hydrenox	25	00.27
Indapamide	Natrilix	2.5	05.56
Mefruside	Baycaron	25	01.97
Methyclothiazide	Enduron	2.5	00.57
Metolazone	Metenix	2.5	01.22
	Xuret	0.5	03.03
Polythiazide	Nephril	0.5	00.39
Xipamide	Diurexan	20	03.66
Beta-blockers			
Acebutolol	Sectral	400	08.88
+hydrochlorothiazide	Secadrex	200/12.5	08.39
Atenolol	Generic	100	06.74
	Tenormin	100	06.98
+chlorthalidone	Co-tenidone 50/12.5	50/12.5	05.27

	Tenoret 50	50/ 12.5	05.28
	Co-tenidone 100/25	100/ 25	07.50
	Tenoretic	100/ 25	08.33
Betaxolol	Kerlone	40	15.40
Bisoprolol	Emcor	10	08.96
	Monocor	10	08.96
Labetalol	Generic	400	06.35
	Trandate	400	09.02
Metoprolol	Generic	200	04.90
	Betaloc	200	04.80
	Lopresor	200	06.05
+chlorthalidone	Lopresoretic	100/ 12.5	03.73
+hydrochlorothiazide	Co-Betaloc	100/ 12.5	06.65
Nadolol	Corgard	160	15.10
+bendrofluazide	Corgaretic 40	40/ 5	06.07
	Corgaretic 80	80/ 5	08.69
Oxprenolol	Generic	160	01.99
	Trasicor	160	04.09
+cyclopenthiazide	Trasidrex	160/ 0.25	06.73
Pindolol	Visken	30	12.52
+clopamide	Viskaldix	10/ 5	05.72
Propranolol	Generic	240	00.63
	Inderal	240	03.40
+bendrofluazide	Inderetic	80/ 2.5	02.83
	Inderex	160/ 5	07.73
Sotalol	Beta-cardone	200	04.91
	Sotacor	200	06.15
+hydrochlorothiazide	Sotazide	160/ 25	07.12
	Tolerzide	80/ 12.5	04.05
Timolol	Betim	20	04.90
	Blocadren	20	05.94
+bendrofluazide	Prestim	10/ 2.5	03.91
	Prestim Forte	20/ 5	08.23

Vasodilators

Hydralazine	Generic	100	01.54
	Apresoline	100	01.96
Minoxidil	Loniten	20	23.86
Centrally acting			
Clonidine	Catapres Perlongets (slow release)	1	25.48
Methyldopa	Generic	500	01.93
	Aldomet	500	03.28
	Dopamet	500	02.04
+hydrochlorothiazide	Hydromet	250/15	04.26
Reserpine	Serpasil	0.125	00.27
+hydrochlorothiazide	Serpasil-Esidrex	0.15/10	00.53
Alpha-blockers			
Doxazosin	Cardura	4	16.00
Indoramin	Baratol	100	10.64
Prazosin	Hypovase	10	09.07
Terazosin	Hytrin	5	18.54
ACE inhibitors			
Captropril	Capoten	50	12.03
+hydrochlorothiazide	Capozide	50/25	16.07
Enalapril	Innovace	10	11.03
Fosinopril	Staril	20	21.00
Lisinopril	Carace	10	12.13
	Zestril	10	12.13
Perindopril	Coversyl	4	12.13
Quinapril	Accupro	20	13.10
Ramipril	Tritace	2.5	07.70
Calcium–channel blockers			
Amlodipine	Istin	10	17.50
Diltiazem	Generic	180	04.20
	Adizem 60	180	04.41
	Tildiem	180	04.20
Isradipine	Prescal	5	11.39
Nicardipine	Cardene	90	14.83
Nifedipine	Adalat retard (slow release)	40	10.81
	Coracten (slow release)	40	09.74
Verapamil	Generic	240	07.48
	Berkatens	240	07.56
	Cordilox	240	07.48
	Securon	240	07.88

Appendix 8
Procedure for Creatinine Clearance Test

Creatinine is a metabolite of muscle. Daily output and blood levels are fairly constant and largely independent of diet, although huge meat intakes can raise blood levels significantly.

Creatinine is excreted almost completely by glomerular filtration, hardly at all by tubular secretion, so creatinine clearance closely approximates glomerular filtration. Serum creatinine levels begin to rise above the normal upper limit (110 mmol/1) when glomerular filtration is reduced by about 50%.

Your laboratory can calculate creatinine clearance from two values:

■ serum creatinine, estimated from 5 or 10 ml clotted blood, taken at any time

■ urine creatinine, estimated from a complete 24-hour collection of urine. Urine can be collected conveniently at a weekend. Provide a 2 litre glass bottle containing a few crystals of thymol to keep the urine sterile, and a funnel. Warn male patients that these crystals are caustic, so they should avoid any skin contact with the lip of the bottle. Patients should empty their bladders into the toilet before going to bed, noting the time, and from then on all urine must be collected in this bottle. For both sexes, a notice on the toilet reminding them of the collection, and for men, a safety pin across their trouser flies, help to improve compliance. Warn patients to urinate separately before defaecation. At exactly the same time the following day, they should empty the bladder into the bottle. The collection is now complete.

Both the blood and the urine sample should be sent to the laboratory as soon as possible the next day. Patients will usually take it if asked.

Normal clearance in an average adult is 100–140 ml/min. For children, and adults who are either extremely fat or extremely thin, give heights and weights on the request form.

Appendix 9
Determination of Acetylator Status[1]

Give any systemically absorbed sulphonamide in a single dose of about 10 mg/kg body weight. Between 5 and 6 hours later, collect urine for 1 hour, and send this to your laboratory.

The only problem is getting the sulphonamide, as few wholesalers now stock any except sulphasalazine.

Reference

1.   Schroder H (1972) Determination of acetylator status. *Br Med J* 3: 506.

Appendix 10
Dr Chandra Patel's Treatment Plan for Relaxation Training

The treatment involves training in breathing exercise, deep muscle relaxation and meditation using a biofeedback instrument as a teaching aid, plus educational programmes to motivate patients to practice relaxation-meditation regularly and to integrate this behaviour in their everyday lives. Instructions for training are on a cassette audiotape. Training can be done by a nurse, and audiotapes are loaned to patients for practice at home.

The educational programme is carried out by the doctor. Patients attend in groups of 8–10 once a week for 8 weeks of 1-hour sessions. The first 15–20 minutes are used for education. The next 30 minutes are used for practising relaxation-meditation. The last 10–15 minutes are used by the nurse to measure blood pressure, and results are fed back to the patient by the doctor to reinforce active participation.

The educational sequence is as follows.

First Session: explain treatment plan, the ideas of biofeedback and stress response, and possible subjective, behavioural, and physiological signals which can be measured.

Second session: a film by Walt Disney 'Understanding stresses and strains'. Questions answered. Physiological effects of relaxation explained.

Third session: how and why of meditation explained. Questions answered. Positive effects used to reinforce regular practice.

Fourth session: slides shown demonstrating beneficial effects of relaxation-meditation from other studies. Questions answered.

Fifth session: how to integrate into everyday life. Patients are asked to practise breathing relaxation when stopped at red traffic lights, before answering the telephone, in the dentist's waiting room, or in other familiar stressful situations. A coloured spot is stuck to their wrist watch to remind them to relax whenever they are under time pressure.

Sixth session: protective effects of social support. Cultural and community traditions and communication skills discussed.

Seventh session: type A behaviour discussed. Ciba film 'Stress, personality and cardiovascular disease' shown.

Eighth session: general discussion. Anything patients want to bring up. Regular practice and integration of new behaviours into everyday life re-emphasized.

Appendix 11
Historical Note: How High Blood Pressure Became a Disease

Here are the notes of a medical student, John Spicer[1], taken at the London Hospital Medical College, Whitechapel, in 1904. They concern a builder's painter, Thomas Stewart, aged 51.

History
3 weeks ago R eye began to get dim
8 days ago R eye went quite blind
 Never quite himself since April 15 1903 when he suddenly had a kind of fit while at work. Affected whole R side. Paresis of R side gradually passed off in course of week.

Examination
Decidedly pale, pasty and puffy
 Slight oedema both legs
 Pupils large, R>L
 R fundus shows gross optic neuritis. Very pale retina. Papilla swollen, indistinct outline. Arteries tiny. Veins + + and very tortuous. Neuro-retinitis ++. Much fluffy swelling (oedema). White patches especially to outer side of disc. Many small haemorrhages (L fundus similar).
 Urine: slight amount of albumen
 No intracranial symptoms, headache or vomiting
 Pulse 72, regular. Tension raised, arterial wall thick.

October 17
Seen by Dr Percy Kidd who agreed that patient was suffering from granular kidney

October 26
Patient noted to have blood in R anterior chamber
 Large vitreous haemorrhage with secondary glaucoma
 Pain relieved by eserine

November 2

R eye removed. Very large haemorrhage immediately into orbit.

November 14
No further trouble. Patient discharged.

This case shows the evolution of thought on hypertension. Eight years before these notes were made, Riva-Rocci published the details of the first practical sphygmomanometer. In this teaching hospital everything about malignant hypertension was clearly described except its immediate cause; the pressure itself was not a measured quantity, but a perceived quality of pulse and arterial wall at the wrist. The consequences of hypertension were fairly well understood. They were the disease to which the label 'hypertension' was later appended.

The pioneer in Britain of the idea of hypertension was Sir Clifford Allbutt of Leeds. In his Hunterian Society lecture of 1895 he described, under the now obsolete title 'hyperpiesis', a condition defined by a hard pulse in the absence of renal disease, citing five patients as examples.[2] He had detached the precursor from the outcome, and in the climate of opinion and practice of his day, it inevitably became a disease in its own right. A chapter in the 1909 edition of his own textbook of medicine described:

'Irregular and indefinite perturbations of health occurring in persons on the farther side of middle life, the nature of which is indicated by persistent elevations of arterial pressure. This . . . may persist for years, especially if untreated . . . Sir Clifford Allbutt has watched many individual cases of this kind over many years, years of more or less persistent ailment, insomnia, cerebral confusion, despondency and nervousness, but not necessarily of danger to life. Most of these cases . . . are remediable by deobstruent means. And, although in all the condition tends to recurrence, yet in the less inveterate each recurrence is less obstinate to treatment, and recovery may be anticipated.'[3]

During the first four decades of the 20th century, the sphygmomanometer gradually replaced the finger on the pulse. Sphygmomanometers were still not standard issue to general duty medical officers in the British Army in 1940, on the grounds that although customary in specialist practice, they were unnecessary for GPs; my father's request for one was refused, on those grounds. They were, and to a large extent still are, used not to quantify a graded risk, but to consign consulting patients to one of two groups, those with normal pressures appropriate to their age, and those with a disease, hypertension.

The 'Symptoms' of Hypertension

By the 1930s hypertension was firmly entrenched as a disease, sometimes symptomless and discovered on routine examination, but often presenting as:

'. . . dyspnoea on exertion, palpitations, a sense of precordial oppression, inability to sleep on the left side, headaches, giddiness, tinnitus aurium, lack of concentration, irritability, anginal pains, epistaxis, numbness or tingling in the legs, cramp or coldness in the legs . . . '[4]

This passage is taken from the textbook of medicine which was still used by my predecessor in the Glyncorrwg practice, before I took over in 1961. Hypertension was a handy explanation for symptoms otherwise lacking any negotiable label. The experience of the life insurance companies, and the association with occasional end-stage illness such as that of Thomas Stewart, reinforced the credibility of a diagnosis otherwise as unconvincing as floating kidneys, autointoxication from the constipated bowel, visceroptosis, chronic appendicitis, and the rest of the bread and butter mythology of interwar private practice.

Medical Trade and Medical Science

How did it come about that this continuously distributed quantity came to be regarded as a discontinuous quality, a condition that people either had or did not have? How did it come about that a condition that rarely gave rise to symptoms until it had caused disease, became linked in the minds of the public and its doctors with a long list of ill defined feelings traditionally thought to be characteristic of menopausal women, the elderly, and the frightened or depressed of all ages and both sexes?

The reasons lie in the origins of medical trade, and the education built upon it in the late 19th century. The teaching consultants spent their mornings in the great hospitals, giving their services free. In exchange for take-it-or-leave-it treatment of the highest technical quality then available, interesting cases of advanced, end-stage disease, with gross physical signs and every kind of radiological and biochemical disruption, were collected in these museums of living pathology. Here the central features of each disease were defined and taught in their classical form. They were taught as distinct entities, units separate and recognizable in the nosology of disease, as were tigers or cockroaches in the animal kingdom. It was this bestiary of gross end-stage disease that was taught to the students, and which even now forms the core of our beliefs. The 'good' cases were those showing the most florid signs of host destruction, in whom there was least doubt of the presence of an invader. The 'bad' cases (US nomenclature =

'turkeys', UK nomenclature = 'rubbish') were those at the periphery of these central end-stage definitions, at the ambiguous boundary between integrity and invasion, cases that defied simple categorization. Teaching hospitals were for the poor, who earned their right to be there by their possession of obvious, classifiable, and for the most part incurable disease.

That was in the morning. In the afternoons the leaders of medical thought went to Harley Street to meet their private patients, there to apply to a population with fees in their wallets but less advanced and more ambiguous disease, the simple classification elaborated in the death-house in the morning. These consultants were GPs to the rich. They were involved in a care transaction with a powerful customer in a buyer's market. At a time when doctors could do little to alter the outcomes of illness, a doctor's reputation depended mainly on successful prophecy, and a capacity to both mould and meet the patient's expectations. Central to these skills was application of a label, elastic enough to accommodate a wide range of outcomes, but precise enough to give customers 'scientific' names for their problems, if not solutions to them. The labels used for this generally less advanced, less defined, more ambiguous illness were derived from the end-stage classification of the hospitals. The malignant hypertension of Thomas Stewart, seen in the morning, was the firm anchorage for the unverifiable guess-work of the afternoon. Hypertension was found where it was sought. Doctors believed in what they did; and they transmitted their beliefs to their patients, so that now even we who do not believe conform to the expectations of patients who do. As late as 1973, 36% of a random sample of British GPs still thought that hypertension normally causes symptoms, so that patient demand could therefore be depended upon to initiate diagnosis. There was no significant difference between those who had qualified before 1925, and after 1964.[5]

If symptoms do not identify those whose pressures justify treatment, the only rational alternative is that all pressures, in the relevant age-groups, be known. Even this, however, does not of itself evade the consequences of marketed care, as opposed to good husbandry. It is no disadvantage to trade that everyone has a blood pressure; the health-check industry is burgeoning in the United States, without proven net advantage and at the expense of care validated by evidence. Without a fundamental revision of our conceptions of arterial pressure and its control, whole-population screening serves in practice chiefly to lower the threshold of diagnosis and increase the population dependent on doctors. By overloading the medical market with cases of low priority, or who on present evidence do not need drug treatment at all, the number of serious but untreated cases shows little change.

Apparently in all countries (though some more than others) doctors still find it difficult to make quantified responses to quantified risks for disease, rather than the yes or no division appropriate to gross injury. As Sir George Pickering has said, doctors still don't want to count to more than two. If we are to develop the customs needed for effective preventive and anticipatory care, rather than our present ineffective mixture of episodic meddling and heroic salvage, we must discard habits of thought developed to serve an entirely different purpose.

The source of data for natural history is nature, not museums. The enormous debt we owe to our hospitals for the clear definition of disease should not blind us to their shortcomings as a source for ideas about health conservation and maintenance, as opposed to terminal salvage. The complex and usually unknown basis of selection of their cases, their often incomplete follow-up, above all their artificial discontinuity with the population outside, have led to working definitions that cannot be extended to whole populations without modification.

The classical if somewhat vague conception of hypertension as a disease, particularly in Europe, includes progression from a first stage of labile hypertension to a second stage of fixed hypertension. Follow-up of a cohort of 5209 men and women in the Framingham study,[6] with measurements made twice a year for 20 years, showed that variability of pressure was not a consistent characteristic from one examination to the next (r = 0.07). Variability increased with age, and with height of pressure. To be sure, if we defined 'hypertension' as diastolic ≥110 mmHg (or any other arbitrary line), those whose mean pressures are slowly rising will initially fluctuate above and below this line, and later remain above it. In any other sense, the progression from labile to fixed hypertension is a myth, unsupported by evidence.

Slowly at first, but now at gathering speed, the definition of the 'disease' hypertension is becoming an operational one; that is, simply the level of sustained pressure above which we have controlled evidence that reduction is effective in improving net outcome, that health gains exceed iatrogenic losses. The disciplines demanded of treated hypertensives require understanding of the nature of hypertension as a graded risk without symptoms, not a disease. The decision to treat should be the result of measured and matched probabilities of outcome either for treatment, or observation without treatment. Titration of treatment against response should then include the patient's own experience of iatrogenic impairment. Both the decision to treat, and to maintain treatment, should be negotiated contracts in which we are able to give the patient a truthful, albeit simplified, account of probable gains and losses. Science is not about arithmetic certainties, but mathematical probabilities. The latter can be approximated to the former not by strength of belief, but by gathering more and better information from observation and experiment.

Uncomplicated hypertension is not a disease, but its reversible precursor. It is a graded risk factor requiring graded response. How many other 'diseases' will prove to follow this model? And how many other areas in which primary health workers might usefully intervene, have remained at the edge of our attention, because they lacked a disease label?

The figures will compel us.

References

1. Bound casenotes of John Spicer (1904) In the author's possession.

2. Allbutt TC (1896) Senile plethora. Abstract of the Hunterian Society: 77th session, p 38. In: Ruskin A (ed) (1956) *Classics in arterial hypertension.* Thomas, Springfield, Illinois.

3. Allbutt TC and Rolleston HD (1909) *A system of medicine, vol 6.* Macmillan, London.

4. Beaumont GE (1935) *Medicine: essentials for practitioners and students.* J & A Churchill, London.

5. Hodes C, Rogers PA and Everitt MG (1975) High blood pressure: detection and treatment by general practitioners. *Br Med J* 2: 674.

6. Kannel WB, Sorlie, P and Gordon T (1978) Labile hypertension: a logical fallacy. Abstracts of the 18th annual conference on cardiovascular disease epidemiology 1978. *CVD Epidemiology Newsletter 25.* American Heart Association, Dallas, Texas.

Index